DASH Diet

W9-ADC-110

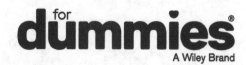

for dummies®
A Wiley Brand

DASH Diet

2nd Edition

by Sarah Samaan, MD, FACC, FACP, FASE; Rosanne Rust, MS, RDN, LDN; and Cindy Kleckner, RDN, LD, FAND

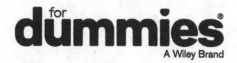

A Wiley Brand

DASH Diet For Dummies®, 2nd Edition

Published by: **John Wiley & Sons, Inc.**, 111 River Street, Hoboken, NJ 07030-5774, www.wiley.com

Copyright © 2021 by John Wiley & Sons, Inc., Hoboken, New Jersey

Published simultaneously in Canada

No part of this publication may be reproduced, stored in a retrieval system or transmitted in any form or by any means, electronic, mechanical, photocopying, recording, scanning or otherwise, except as permitted under Sections 107 or 108 of the 1976 United States Copyright Act, without the prior written permission of the Publisher. Requests to the Publisher for permission should be addressed to the Permissions Department, John Wiley & Sons, Inc., 111 River Street, Hoboken, NJ 07030, (201) 748-6011, fax (201) 748-6008, or online at http://www.wiley.com/go/permissions.

Trademarks: Wiley, For Dummies, the Dummies Man logo, Dummies.com, Making Everything Easier, and related trade dress are trademarks or registered trademarks of John Wiley & Sons, Inc., and may not be used without written permission. All other trademarks are the property of their respective owners. John Wiley & Sons, Inc., is not associated with any product or vendor mentioned in this book.

LIMIT OF LIABILITY/DISCLAIMER OF WARRANTY: THE CONTENTS OF THIS WORK ARE INTENDED TO FURTHER GENERAL SCIENTIFIC RESEARCH, UNDERSTANDING, AND DISCUSSION ONLY AND ARE NOT INTENDED AND SHOULD NOT BE RELIED UPON AS RECOMMENDING OR PROMOTING A SPECIFIC METHOD, DIAGNOSIS, OR TREATMENT BY PHYSICIANS FOR ANY PARTICULAR PATIENT. THE PUBLISHER AND THE AUTHOR MAKE NO REPRESENTATIONS OR WARRANTIES WITH RESPECT TO THE ACCURACY OR COMPLETENESS OF THE CONTENTS OF THIS WORK AND SPECIFICALLY DISCLAIM ALL WARRANTIES, INCLUDING WITHOUT LIMITATION ANY IMPLIED WARRANTIES OF FITNESS FOR A PARTICULAR PURPOSE. IN VIEW OF ONGOING RESEARCH, EQUIPMENT MODIFICATIONS, CHANGES IN GOVERNMENTAL REGULATIONS, AND THE CONSTANT FLOW OF INFORMATION, THE READER IS URGED TO REVIEW AND EVALUATE THE INFORMATION PROVIDED IN THE PACKAGE INSERT OR INSTRUCTIONS FOR EACH MEDICINE, EQUIPMENT, OR DEVICE FOR, AMONG OTHER THINGS, ANY CHANGES IN THE INSTRUCTIONS OR INDICATION OF USAGE AND FOR ADDED WARNINGS AND PRECAUTIONS. READERS SHOULD CONSULT WITH A SPECIALIST WHERE APPROPRIATE. NEITHER THE PUBLISHER NOR THE AUTHOR SHALL BE LIABLE FOR ANY DAMAGES ARISING HEREFROM.

For general information on our other products and services, please contact our Customer Care Department within the U.S. at 877-762-2974, outside the U.S. at 317-572-3993, or fax 317-572-4002. For technical support, please visit https://hub.wiley.com/community/support/dummies.

Wiley publishes in a variety of print and electronic formats and by print-on-demand. Some material included with standard print versions of this book may not be included in e-books or in print-on-demand. If this book refers to media such as a CD or DVD that is not included in the version you purchased, you may download this material at http://booksupport.wiley.com. For more information about Wiley products, visit www.wiley.com.

Library of Congress Control Number: 2020947088

ISBN 978-1-119-74079-7 (pbk); ISBN 978-1-119-74080-3 (ebk); ISBN 978-1-119-74081-0 (ebk)

Manufactured in the United States of America

SKY10024459_012621

Contents at a Glance

Recipes at a Glance

Table of Contents

Introduction

Hypertension, or high blood pressure, is a serious health concern affecting about 45 percent of the world population. According to the Million Hearts Initiative, nearly one out of every two adults in the United States has hypertension. More concerning, only one in four have their blood pressure under control. Because hypertension often has no symptoms, it may go undetected for years, damaging the heart, blood vessels, and kidneys.

Fortunately, in the 1990s, researchers discovered two amazing things: that diet can lower blood pressure without medication and that certain foods seem to play an important role in this. And thus, the Dietary Approaches to Stop Hypertension (DASH) diet was born. Of course, it's not a diet in the traditional sense, because it neither deprives nor restricts you. Instead, it enlightens you to find new ways to add healthful foods to your plate and helps you plan and cook flavorful meals. Experts around the world agree: DASH really works. It's no wonder that in 2013, the American Heart Association and the American College of Cardiology issued a joint statement urging a DASH-style diet to help achieve a healthy blood pressure and improve heart health.

This book fills you in on the DASH diet, how your heart works, and the lifestyle changes that support lowering blood pressure and better health. We begin by filling you in on how DASH was created (so you can understand the science behind why it works), how it can help with numerous health conditions, and how to apply DASH eating principles in your everyday life. To that end, we provide a variety of recipes to get you started. We also include valuable information about making lifestyle changes, such as becoming more physically active and managing stress. Making these sorts of healthy lifestyle changes is easier than you may think, and we're here to show you how. By following the DASH diet and setting simple goals that will improve your life and long-term health, you *will* lower your blood pressure and become healthier to boot. Have no fear — living a healthier life feels good, and the food tastes delicious!

About This Book

This book is your personal reference guide to the DASH diet and heart health. Don't read it from cover to cover (unless that's your style), and don't feel like you have to read the sidebars (they're interesting but not essential). Do, however, flip to the topics or recipes that interest you.

Speaking of recipes, all of our recipes adhere to DASH guidelines and provide a foundation for a heart-healthy, blood-pressure-lowering diet. Some of them may seem slightly higher in sodium and/or saturated fat; when you make them, simply try to balance them out with lower-sodium meals and more fruits and vegetables the rest of the day. It's all good food. And yes, fruits, vegetables, and low-fat dairy are just as important in the DASH diet as reducing sodium — if not more so — and we show you plenty of ways to incorporate more of them into your day-to-day living.

Here are a few ground rules relating to the recipes:

>> All oven and cooking temperatures are measured in degrees Fahrenheit; flip to the appendix for information on converting temperatures to Celsius.

>> All eggs are large.

>> All onions are yellow (unless otherwise noted), but feel free to use Vidalia or white.

>> For measuring purposes, dry ingredients are lightly spooned into a standard U.S. measuring cup or spoon and then leveled with a knife. Liquids are measured in glass, standard U.S. measuring cups. Check out the appendix if you need help converting to metric measurements.

>> All sugar is granulated.

>> All flour is all-purpose.

>> The term *lightly browned* indicates when the food just begins to change color.

>> All herbs are dried unless specified as fresh.

>> Lemon and lime juice are freshly squeezed.

>> All ground pepper is freshly ground black pepper.

>> Some higher-sodium ingredients (kalamata olives, capers, and Parmesan cheese, for example) are used in very small quantities to enhance the flavor of a recipe. Measure these ingredients carefully to avoid increasing sodium levels significantly.

>> References to *percent daily values* or limits on nutrients are based on a daily intake of 2,000 calories.

>> Recipes marked with the tomato icon (🍅) are vegetarian.

One final word: This book isn't intended to be a substitute for medical care. If you have a family history of high blood pressure or have it yourself, you may still need medication. We recommend you see your doctor to determine your personal medical needs and have your blood pressure monitored regularly.

Foolish Assumptions

We wrote this book assuming that you, our dear reader, already have hypertension or are at risk for developing it. We also took for granted that you want to improve your lifestyle and health, meaning you're willing to make a few informed changes in your habits. You're ready to get a deeper understanding of how diet and lifestyle affect blood pressure, and you're willing to spend a little time in the kitchen whipping up tasty, healthy foods. We're not assuming you're a master chef, which is why we share helpful cooking preparation and technique tips in as simple a way as possible.

Icons Used in This Book

Like any *For Dummies* book, *DASH Diet For Dummies* features some helpful icons, which are like little guideposts that point out useful information as you read:

REMEMBER

Keep your eyes peeled for paragraphs marked with this icon, which highlights the most important actions you can take and facts to keep in mind to beat hypertension.

TECHNICAL STUFF

This icon indicates information that's interesting but not essential to your basic understanding of reducing high blood pressure with the DASH diet.

TIP

Want a tip? Read information with this icon to get helpful hints on how to easily make the DASH lifestyle fit within your life.

WARNING

Halt! Stop! Whoa, Nelly! When we place this icon next to a paragraph, it means we want you to pay attention so you don't make a mistake that could impact your health or your recipe.

Beyond the Book

We could only include so much information in the book, which is why we've put up some additional goodies online:

» Check out www.dummies.com/cheatsheet/dashdiet for an at-a-glance breakdown of DASH nutrition guidelines and advice for making positive lifestyle changes.

» Visit www.dummies.com/extras/dashdiet to discover how the low-fat dairy promoted in DASH helps out your bones, which items are the most DASH-friendly at the grocery store, no-cook meal ideas, and more.

Where to Go from Here

You're welcome to head straight to Chapter 1 for an overview of what you'll find in this book, but you certainly aren't required to. If you want to get cooking, start browsing the recipes in Part 4. Wondering what the blood pressure numbers are all about and how your heart works? Head to Chapter 6. Want some help convincing a family member of all the ways eating the DASH way can benefit your health and blood pressure? Head to the chapters in Part 2. You get the idea. Where you go next — both in this book and in your heart-health journey — is up to you!

1
Getting Started with the DASH Diet

Get your feet wet with an overview of the DASH diet —
including its basic dietary guidelines and the lifestyle
changes that help promote normal blood pressure and
support a healthy heart — before diving into DASH
completely to improve your chances of making DASH a
way of life.

Discover the core science behind the diet. That's right:
DASH isn't one of the numerous fad diets out there; it's a
well-researched approach to eating that has been
benefiting people with high blood pressure for more
than 20 years.

Recognize all the ways DASH can have a positive effect
on your health, from the obvious (lowering blood
pressure and reducing the risk of stroke and heart
attack) to the not-so-obvious (fighting diabetes and
decreasing cancer risk).

Understand that adopting DASH is a lifestyle change and
figure out how to ease into the DASH way of eating.
Trust us, setting realistic goals really helps!

Know which foods you can eat on the DASH diet — there
are loads of them, particularly fruits and vegetables,
nuts, whole grains, lean protein, and low-fat dairy served
up in delicious ways.

Chapter 1

What Is DASH?

ypertension, or high blood pressure, affects one in three of the world's adult citizens, including nearly half of all U.S. adults, and contributes to millions of deaths from heart disease, stroke, and kidney failure every year. Although medication is usually very effective, in many cases hypertension can be prevented or lessened simply by choosing a diet and lifestyle that promote good health. The Dietary Approaches to Stop Hypertension (DASH) diet was developed as a holistic, yet medically sound, method to lower blood pressure safely while also promoting wellness and vitality of the whole body. In short: The DASH diet uses food as part of the medical treatment.

This chapter shines a spotlight on what makes DASH so powerful for heart health — and good health in general — and what makes it different from all the other diets out there. It also explains how to find true success with DASH: by making a commitment to changing your current lifestyle for a healthier one that incorporates DASH dietary guidelines and increased activity. Change may seem intimidating, but DASH makes it easy and accessible, incorporating foods you already know and love to help you achieve your goals and live your life to the fullest. There's no time like the present to throw on some sneakers, grab a healthy snack, and jump right in!

Understanding the DASH Difference

Twenty-five years ago, if you were diagnosed with hypertension, your doctor may have simply sent you on your way with a prescription and advice to cut back on salt. However, over the past two decades, the medical community's understanding of the effects that diet, body weight, and lifestyle have on blood pressure has expanded tremendously. Studies by physicians, scientists, dietitians, and others have concluded that controlling blood pressure is about far more than just the salt. The following sections trace the history of DASH and explain why DASH is more than just another trendy diet.

Exploring the origins of DASH

The acronym *DASH* comes from a landmark 1997 *clinical trial* (a well-controlled human research study) that tested the effects of specific types of food on blood pressure. Instead of just telling people with hypertension what to avoid, the study sought to gauge the effects on blood pressure of a variety of readily available, inexpensive whole foods known to support good health.

REMEMBER

Study participants following the DASH diet experienced impressive results: By eating a diet rich in fruits, vegetables, whole grains, and low-fat dairy foods and low in saturated fat, they reduced their blood pressure just as much as if they had taken a single prescription drug. The drop in blood pressure was evident within two weeks, even though the participants were on the DASH diet plan for eight weeks. DASH researchers estimated that the improvement in blood pressure could mean a 15 percent drop in heart attack risk and as much as a 27 percent reduction in stroke risk.

TECHNICAL STUFF

It's worth noting that study participants who followed the DASH diet minus the dairy also reduced their blood pressure, but the decrease was less. That's why including low-fat dairy is recommended for maximum effectiveness.

Having confirmed that healthy and delicious food could lower blood pressure just as effectively as a pharmaceutical drug, the DASH researchers next turned their attention to salt. The study, known as DASH-Sodium, found that by cutting salt to about 1,500 milligrams daily, blood pressure improved even more than with DASH alone. In fact, even a little reduction in salt made an important difference in blood pressure. The effect was seen in people with borderline high blood pressure, as well as in those with true hypertension.

For a deeper dive into the science behind the DASH study, see Chapter 2. Less interested in the science than in finding advice on how to create a healthy diet plan that works for you? We help you out in Chapter 4.

CONVINCING REASONS TO TRY THE DASH DIET

Hypertension, or high blood pressure, is an incredibly widespread problem, affecting people of all ages, shapes, sizes, colors, and nationalities. If you don't have hypertension, chances are your parents, siblings, or friends do. And you may too one day because the prevalence of hypertension increases with age. If you live long enough, you have a 90 percent probability of hypertension.

Although some cases of hypertension are due purely to genetics (as we explain in Chapter 6), many times the problem can be prevented or lessened by simple lifestyle changes. That means you may have more control than you realize. Around the world, access to fast food, processed food, and convenience food, along with an increasingly sedentary way of life, means that more people are becoming hypertensive every year. In fact, it's estimated that if things keep going along the way they are, a jaw-dropping 60 percent of adults around the world will be hypertensive.

Many medications exist that are effective at treating hypertension, and the average person with hypertension requires at least two to three of these medications to really get the problem under control. But due to costs, side effects, and complications, many people never achieve normal blood pressure numbers. Why not save yourself some hassle and prevent hypertension in the first place by following the DASH diet?

Recognizing why DASH isn't just another trendy diet

It seems like every year a new diet book comes out, full of promises and complete with enthusiastic endorsements from the celebrity-du-jour. Is the DASH diet really any different? Absolutely, 100 percent. No doubt about it.

DASH is science-based. It was developed based on reams of scientific research that identified certain foods as being especially beneficial for blood pressure. The DASH team put their highly educated heads together and came up with a diet that incorporated those foods into an easy-to-follow, inexpensive program that they believed would really make a difference. And make a difference it does. Not only can DASH help lower blood pressure, but it can also help with weight loss (thanks to eating more fiber-rich whole grains, fruits, and vegetables), reduce diabetes risk (thanks to complex carbohydrates), and more. Head to Part 2 for an in-depth look at all the benefits DASH provides for your health.

A HEALTHY EATING PLAN FOR THE WHOLE FAMILY

DASH isn't just for adults who have or are at risk for hypertension. It's an approach to eating that's healthy for most children as well. Why talk about DASH and kids? Consider the fact that since the 1970s, American children between the ages of 6 and 11 are now consuming

- Triple the amount of salty snacks
- Nearly double the amount of candy
- More than 40 percent fewer vegetables
- Half the amount of milk
- Twice the amount of soda

It's no wonder that more than one-third of U.S. kids are overweight or obese and are at risk for developing a condition known as the *metabolic syndrome* (the result of a cluster of risk factors including obesity, high blood pressure, abnormal blood lipid levels, and elevated blood sugar), which substantially raises the risk of heart disease, stroke, and diabetes. The good news is that the DASH diet has the potential to help kids who are heading down this road. For instance, a British study of girls with metabolic syndrome found that after spending just six weeks on DASH, blood pressure and insulin levels were improved compared to those who weren't assigned to DASH. Another study that simply tracked the diets of young girls over the course of ten years reported that those whose diets simply included two or more servings of dairy and at least three servings of fruits and vegetables daily were one-third less likely to have high blood pressure by the time they hit their late teens.

When it comes to kids, it's up to parents to provide healthy food options and keep unhealthy snacks to a minimum. DASH keeps it simple by giving you a structure that you can follow to put together nutritious meals for your family. And of course, in Part 4 of this book, we share loads of great recipes that can help you get started. As always, get your pediatrician's or family doctor's approval before jumping right in.

TECHNICAL STUFF

Scientists know that sometimes an idea can make perfect sense on paper and fail miserably when put to the test. Without a scientific study that randomly assigns individuals to one diet or another, with as many variables as possible controlled by the research team (what scientists call a *randomized, controlled trial*), you're just going on an assumption. You also need to set your goals ahead of time and then conduct the study in such a way that it's as unbiased as possible. Next, when it's all said and done, you need to do a detailed statistical analysis and then tidy up the whole mess into a neat and obsessively thorough report. Finally, you submit your work for review by other well-respected and uninvolved scientists (what's known as *peer review*). This meticulous attention to detail and strict scientific method are what set DASH apart from so many other diet plans.

DASH: A Dietary Prescription for a Healthier Lifestyle

Unlike some medical prescriptions, DASH works for just about anyone. It includes enough variety and room for modification so that most people, even those with dietary restrictions, can make it their own. You just have to follow some simple dietary guidelines and commit to making positive lifestyle changes, as we explain in the next sections.

The basic dietary guidelines

Every type of food included in DASH has a purpose, as you can see from the following list:

TIP

>> **Whole grains give you plenty of fiber, potassium, magnesium, and antioxidants, all of which help support the health of your cardiovascular system and lower your blood pressure.** A world of difference exists between refined flour and whole-grain flour because after the rough part of the grain is stripped away, most of the nutrients are gone as well.

If you need to steer clear of gluten (a protein abundant in wheat, barley, and rye products), you have a variety of interesting whole-grain options to choose from, including quinoa, millet, rice, and oats.

>> **Fruits and vegetables offer blood pressure–friendly nutrients galore, including a wide range of vitamins and antioxidants, plus potassium and fiber.** Although whole grains also provide a similar list of healthy elements, the variety supplied by fruits and vegetables is very different. Your body is an incredibly complex system, so you can't rely on just one category of food to give you everything you need.

>> **Low-fat dairy foods have been strongly linked to a lower risk for hyper-tension because they're rich in vitamin D, calcium, magnesium, and potassium; high in protein; and low in saturated fat and calories.** There's also good evidence that dairy foods may reduce the likelihood of stroke, a common complication of high blood pressure.

TIP

If you're lactose intolerant, check with your doctor and see whether a lactase supplement may help you enjoy these healthy foods. We provide more pointers on how dairy can fit into your DASH diet in Chapter 11.

» **Lean meats, fish, and poultry provide plenty of protein to build a healthy and strong body, while limiting your exposure to saturated fats and calories.** Although DASH hasn't been specifically tested in vegetarians, it's easily adaptable, especially because animal protein is a proportionately smaller part of the plan than it is in a typical Western diet. If you're a vegetarian, try substituting soy products or other high-protein, vegetable-based options. Of course, nuts and seeds (see the next bullet) also supply some protein. In Chapter 21, we whip up some terrific meat-free recipes to help get you started.

» **Nuts, seeds, and legumes provide heart-friendly, plant-based protein, along with healthy fats, fiber, and magnesium.** Peanuts and soy nuts are, technically speaking, members of the legume family, which also includes beans, chickpeas (found in hummus), and lentils. Although the calories can add up quickly, especially if you're a nut lover, they come from healthy fats and are a much better choice than typical snack-food fare.

DASH is important not only for the foods it includes but also for those it limits:

» **Fats and oils are limited but not out of bounds in the DASH diet.** Since the time that DASH was developed in the 1990s, more recent research has confirmed the benefit of foods rich in omega-3 fats, such as oily fish, as well as monounsaturated fats like olive oil. A second set of studies known as *Omni-Heart* confirmed that switching out a small portion (about 10 percent) of carb-based calories and replacing them with healthy monounsaturated fats can make DASH even more effective, as long as the calories remain the same.

» **Sugary and high-fat treats aren't forbidden on DASH, but they're kept to a minimum.** If you're like us, you probably need a little indulgence from time to time. Severely restrictive diets aren't always realistic and may even cause you to jump ship, giving up on a healthy eating plan altogether. DASH allows you a little leeway to enjoy the foods you love, but don't be surprised if you find that, after a few days on DASH, you feel so good that snack foods no longer hold the same appeal.

Table 1-1 shows the quantities you should eat of different food groups when following DASH and examples from each group. If what you see here looks a bit basic or maybe kind of daunting, don't despair. We share more than 40 great-tasting recipes in Part 4 that really make the DASH diet come alive. (*Note:* The servings listed in Table 1-1 are based on a 2,000-calorie diet. Some people need more calories than that; others need fewer calories.)

TABLE 1-1   **The DASH Diet (Based on 2,000 Calories/Day)**

Type of Food	Number of Servings for a 2,000-Calorie Diet	Example Serving Sizes
Grains and grain products	6–8 per day	1 slice bread, 1 cup dry cereal, ½ cup cooked cereal, rice, or pasta
Fruits	4–5 per day	10 grapes, ½ grapefruit, 1 small banana, 2 tablespoons raisins, 1 medium apple
Vegetables	4–5 per day	1 cup raw, ½ cup cooked
Low-fat or nonfat dairy products	2–3 per day	1 cup milk or yogurt, 1 ounce cheese
Lean meats, fish, poultry	2 or fewer per day	3–4 ounces cooked per day
Nuts, seeds, legumes	4–5 per week	1/3 cup nuts, 2 tablespoons nut butter, 2 tablespoons seeds
Fats and oils	3–4 per day	1 teaspoon margarine, butter, or oil; 2 tablespoons salad dressing
High-fat/high-sugar extras	5 or fewer per week	½ cup sorbet or frozen yogurt, 1 "fun-size" candy bar, 8 pieces of gummy-type candy, 1 tablespoon jam; 1 ounce dark chocolate (70 percent to 85 percent cocoa)

That's the DASH diet in a nutshell; for a deeper look at DASH nutrition, see Chapter 5.

REMEMBER

By choosing DASH, you'll achieve better blood pressure deliciously. And with such a wide range of foods to choose from, it's easy to see how you can tailor DASH to your personal taste.

The most powerful lifestyle changes

Just as you need a balanced blend of healthy foods to achieve good health and better blood pressure, your body also requires balance in other areas. Throughout this book, we help you cultivate healthy habits to support the vitality, energy, and overall well-being that you're craving. Although making changes to your daily routine may seem intimidating at first, it's surprisingly simple. You just have to take it one step at a time.

We tell you much more about the way lifestyle impacts your health in Chapter 16, but to get started, check out the following sections to get a feel for the simple things you can do or change that may help reduce your risk for hypertension, heart disease, stroke, and a wide array of other conditions.

Moving more

Being active daily is essential for a healthy lifestyle. Before you start calculating the cost of a gym membership and fancy workout clothes, it's important to understand that getting more daily activity can be as simple as putting on your sneakers and walking out the door. Combat the modern sedentary lifestyle by looking for simple ways to add daily activity: taking a ten-minute walk break, choosing to use the stairs, walking where you may normally drive, sweeping the porch more often, or committing to housework or yard maintenance.

While you're busy getting more active, why not add in some exercise? It's nearly impossible to be healthy without regular exercise. By exercising two and a half hours each week, you'll lower your blood pressure, reduce your stress level, burn some calories, and cut your risk of heart disease, stroke, and dementia a well-worth-it 30 percent. If hitting the gym's your thing, go for it! If you're a weight lifter, just make sure you get a good balance of aerobic exercise along with the resistance training. Yoga and Pilates are also terrific ways to take care of your body and encourage serenity of mind, but adding in some walking, running, biking, or swimming to your weekly routine helps keep your heart even stronger.

REMEMBER

Exercise isn't just for the young and fit. Just about anyone can do it, and you can usually find something that works with any limitations you may have. Remember, though, that anytime you're beginning a new exercise regimen or bumping up the intensity of a current routine, you need to check in with your doctor to be sure your plan makes good health sense for you.

TIP

Because exercise can lower blood pressure, blood sugar, and cholesterol, you want to keep track of your numbers when you get started. If you have hypertension, high cholesterol, or diabetes, don't be surprised if, eventually, you don't require as much medication to keep the problem under control.

Cutting back on caffeine, alcohol, and smoking

DASH doesn't put caffeine off-limits, and for many people, a cup or two of tea or coffee is a great way to take a break and recharge. It turns out that these plant-based drinks actually offer a boost of healthy antioxidants along with the caffeine, but don't go overboard. (Caffeinated sodas and energy drinks may give you a similar jolt, but they don't have the same health benefits.) Doctors used to shake their fingers at people with a coffee habit, but the research on coffee and tea strongly suggests that they have health benefits when consumed in moderation — generally considered 3 cups or fewer per day.

REMEMBER

Although coffee can cause a temporary bump in blood pressure, it doesn't appear to cause hypertension. Of course, some people can't take a sip of tea or coffee without experiencing heart flutters or heartburn, and if that's you we're talking about, then it's best to avoid a cup of brew or switch to decaf.

Whether or not to drink alcohol is a personal decision. Any form of alcohol enjoyed in moderation appears to offer health benefits for the heart and brain, although red wine is especially beneficial. "Moderation" means one drink for women and one to two for men. More than that and you're more likely to develop high blood pressure, especially if you binge drink. Additional downsides of overindulging in alcohol include alcoholism, a higher risk of cancer, poor decisions made under the influence (perhaps including extra calories from junk food), and of course weight gain from the extra calories.

WARNING

We'd be remiss if we didn't touch on smoking. If you don't already know that smoking is bad for your health, we have to assume that you've been in hibernation for the past 50 years. Not only does it raise your risk for numerous particularly nasty forms of cancer, but it also drastically raises your chances of developing heart attacks, aneurysms, blocked leg arteries, and strokes. It may not affect your blood pressure much, but it can hurt you in just about every other way. Quitting isn't easy, but it's well worth the effort.

Reducing stress

Not all stress is created equal. There's good stress, which you have control over, and then there's the bad kind, which leaves you feeling overwhelmed and powerless. Guess which form of stress is harmful? Of course, it's the second type. Sometimes you can get away from this sort of stress, but sometimes it's just a part of your work or family life.

TIP

Stress can seem like so much a part of everyday life that it becomes hard to recognize, but the truth is that it can affect your health. Perhaps you don't realize it, but when you're stressed you may be more apt to reach for a cookie or a soda rather than an apple or a handful of nuts. Sometimes these cravings mean that you're searching for an instant energy boost, but processed foods only serve to cause a vicious cycle of craving and hunger. Keep these foods out of reach and you may find that you're better able to manage the stress that comes your way.

Not surprisingly, stress can also have a direct influence on your blood pressure. By leaving an unhappy job or a difficult relationship, you may suddenly find that your blood pressure is much easier to manage. Of course, sometimes you can't, or don't want to, get away from the situation that's causing the problem, but many times there's something about it that you can change for the better. Don't give up on yourself just because it seems difficult. Your health depends on you taking good care of yourself.

Stress can also cause poor sleep, which itself may lead to high blood pressure and cravings for unhealthy food. Getting to the root of the problem may help you sleep better.

When dealing with stress above and beyond the daily annoyances, it often helps to enlist the services of a well-qualified counselor. By doing so, you'll find it much easier to get your life back on track, and the healthier choices may begin to come more naturally.

TIP

Preparing for Success with DASH

By choosing DASH, you're affirming a commitment to good health and vitality. Unlike many other diet plans, DASH doesn't explicitly tell you what to do; there are no gimmicks, supplements, or products that you need to make it work. Instead, DASH offers a range of options that you can use to build a diet that works specifically for you. Though this framework may seem a little intimidating at first, you'll find that such flexibility is exactly what makes DASH so useful and so doable. Choices abound in the real world, and DASH gives you a structure that helps you make healthy sense of the options.

Choosing foods that support your health

Does the word *diet* make you think of dreary, boring meals; deprivation with nothing to look forward to; and miserable nights spent alone avoiding social situations where food may appear? We promise that's not the life you'll be living when you adopt DASH. Although the word *diet* is often used in conjunction with DASH, we're here to show you how DASH is different and how it can be part of a healthy, vibrant, and delicious way of eating and living.

One of the really wonderful things about DASH is that it gives you such broad leeway to make your own personal choices about the foods that you eat. Studies of DASH have incorporated the plan into menus all over the world, including the United States, Asia, Europe, South America, and the Middle East. The thing really works!

For many people, the number of servings of fruits and vegetables is an eye-opener. If you follow DASH, you'll naturally start to peruse the produce aisles with more curiosity, and you'll probably begin to take some chances, bringing home unfamiliar produce to try at home. You can think of it as a great adventure!

The DASH diet is lower in sodium than a typical Western diet, which may take some adjustment for you. Be patient with your taste buds as you cut back on the salt because it may take them several weeks to adapt. If you cut back slowly, it won't seem like you're giving something up, and you'll probably find that you're enjoying the natural flavors of foods so much more than ever before.

REMEMBER

TIP

Sweets and other simple carbs may be a bit harder to renounce, but, just like salt, you'll eventually realize that, first of all, many packaged sweets usually don't taste as good as advertised, and second, you'll actually feel better if you limit portions to just a small taste of something homemade and really good. Plus, as you cut back on sweets, you'll crave them less often.

We share additional guidance on adopting a DASH way of life in Chapter 11, as well as a 14-day meal plan you can follow. For help setting up your kitchen for your new cooking adventures, see Chapter 13. Or for advice on following DASH when dining out or traveling, see Chapter 15.

PUTTING FOOD BEFORE SUPPLEMENTS

It's tempting to think that rather than having to bother with healthy eating, you may be able to get your nutrition from a pill or a powder. It often seems all *Willy Wonka and the Chocolate Factory,* but like those hapless kiddos who fell victim to the magical "three-course meal in a stick of gum," it just doesn't work out the way you'd think it should. You may be surprised to know that the world of supplements is largely unregulated, so manufacturers face little accountability.

Over the years, trends have come and gone for a wide variety of supplements, including vitamin E, high dose folic acid, selenium, L-arginine, and others. When put to the scientific test, these supplements and their counter-mates have often had unintended consequences, including a greater risk for certain cancers, diabetes, and heart disease. Other supplements used for weight loss and energy may put you at risk for heart rhythm disturbances, heart attacks, and strokes. And while a multivitamin probably won't hurt you, there's little evidence that it will do you much good, either.

Whole foods are very different from supplements. Their natural goodness is balanced in a neat package created by Mother Nature, with literally dozens of nutrients in a single bite. Your body was designed to use foods in their natural form. By overwhelming your system with massive doses of a single substance, you may be setting yourself up for unintended consequences.

Of course, there are exceptions. For instance, many people are deficient in vitamin D, and in these cases, a supplement can be helpful. The same may apply to iron and certain B-vitamins. Your doctor can test you to see whether your levels are low. Other supplements, like fiber, can help with constipation and even lower cholesterol. And sometimes a protein shake can be a reasonable replacement for a single meal. But before you take a product's claim on faith, check in with your doctor or a registered dietitian.

Creating lifestyle changes that stick

Hypertension, diabetes, heart disease, obesity. All these conditions, and more, can be impacted by your lifestyle, and they can weigh you down if you allow them to. Fortunately, you don't have to. Making positive changes in the way you eat and the way you choose to spend your time can have a lasting impact on your health and the overall quality of your life. No matter what challenges you may have in your life, never give up or give in. Life is too precious.

TIP

Don't think of DASH as "going on a diet." That implies a temporary situation. What you're after here is making a lifestyle change that you can live with — one that doesn't make you feel deprived or drained, but rather, one that you can celebrate! Our recipes and tips throughout this book will help you accomplish this, and you'll find lots of tips in Chapters 4, 11, and 16.

By following the DASH diet, you'll be able to create a plan that will support your health and empower you with more energy. Consequently, exercise will seem less daunting, and you'll find it easier to change other habits that have been keeping you back.

REMEMBER

Track your successes and forgive your slip-ups. Reach out for support from professionals or a friend when you need encouragement or focus. Making healthy changes may seem difficult at first, but by taking it one step at a time, you'll find that you can accomplish a great deal.

A DASH of Caution

Although DASH is a fabulous plan that promotes better health and well-being for most people, it's not for everyone.

One advantage of DASH is the fact that it's high in potassium. For most people, that helps their kidneys regulate blood pressure more efficiently. However, people with advanced kidney disease may need to limit the potassium in their diet.

WARNING

If you have a chronic medical condition or take prescription potassium, it's important to discuss any major changes in the foods you choose with your doctor. In some cases, you may need more careful monitoring of blood work, and in other situations, it may be possible to cut back on the potassium pills when you switch to DASH.

Of course, if you have high blood pressure, DASH may lower it enough that your medications will need to be adjusted. That's a really good side effect, but not one that you want to overlook. When you commit to DASH, it's important to monitor your blood pressure closely, especially in the first one to two months and whenever you find yourself losing weight. Let your doctor know of any changes. Doctors love it when patients can ditch a pill or two.

It goes without saying that if you're gluten intolerant, you need to modify a bit, but there are plenty of tantalizing, gluten-free, healthy grains, including buckwheat, quinoa, millet, and wild rice.

If you're lactose intolerant, yogurt and other dairy products may not be right for you (although kefir, a cultured milk product low in lactose and high in healthy probiotics, may be an option). Consider calcium-fortified soy milk, almond milk, and other such products.

WARNING

If you have a disease or disorder that requires medical nutrition therapy (MNT), you need to consult with a registered dietitian/nutritionist (RDN) for individual nutrition counseling prior to starting the DASH diet. Talk to your doctor about a referral or find an RDN near you by checking out "Find a Registered Dietitian" at www.eatright.org.

Finally, despite the fact that some people eat way too much salt, others need more salt, and not everyone needs to cut back. Competitive athletes and people working outdoors in the heat are the obvious examples. A small minority of people suffer from low blood pressure, and in those cases, extra salt is often the treatment of choice.

The great thing about DASH is that it can be easily adapted for a wide variety of tastes and conditions. Because everybody is different, check with your doctor before jumping in with both feet, and let her be a partner in your path to wellness.

IN THIS CHAPTER

» Tracing the origins of DASH to its
original study

» Examining the relationship between
DASH and sodium intake

» Looking at other diets similar
to DASH

» Seeing some of the positive potential
effects of DASH

Chapter **2**

The DASH Diet and Wellness: What Scientists Know

espite its catchy name, the DASH diet is based on hard science. It was created to help fight and reverse high blood pressure. It also has some remarkable benefits for the body as a whole. Incorporating decades of medical and nutritional research, the DASH diet is a delicious way to boost your health and keep your taste buds happy all at the same time. By choosing to eat the DASH way, you're making a commitment to a healthier, happier, and more vibrant you. In this chapter, we fill you in on the science behind the DASH diet to help you better understand why it was created and how it works.

You may want to skip ahead so you can get started on the DASH diet and dig in to all the great recipes right away, and there's nothing wrong with that. But knowing the hows and whys can help keep that motivation going.

Exploring the Science behind the Diet

Hypertension (or high blood pressure) is more common than the common cold — and a lot more deadly. All told, in the U.S., hypertension affects upwards of 1 out of every 13 people in the under-40 set and more than 30 percent of folks in their 40s and 50s. By age 60, nearly two-thirds of individuals have full-on hypertension. And if you make it to 90, you're nearly guaranteed full membership in the hypertension club. That adds up to more than 100 million Americans and over one billion people worldwide potentially popping a lot of pills every single day, and though that may make the drug companies happy, it's not so good for everyone else.

More than just a number, high blood pressure affects the health of your heart, brain, and kidneys. Most research suggests that an ideal natural blood pressure is around 115/75. Those numbers may vary depending on your age and other health conditions, a topic we delve into in Part 2 of the book. For a typical adult age 40 through 70, it's been estimated that for every 20-point elevation in systolic blood pressure (the top number) or 10-point rise in diastolic pressure (the bottom number) above these ideal numbers, your risk for heart attack or stroke doubles.

Although the link between diet and blood pressure had long been suspected, for years, no one had scientifically put a healthier diet to the test in average Americans with borderline to high blood pressure. In the 1990s, a group of physicians, nutritionists, nurses, and other medical researchers from five medical centers across the United States, along with scientists from the National Heart, Lung, and Blood Institute, set out on a mission to find out whether straightforward changes in diet could have an important impact in blood pressure. They wanted to create a plan that was easy to follow, accessible, and would work well for a variety of individual tastes. Auspiciously, the researchers called themselves the DASH group, for *Dietary Approaches to Stop Hypertension.* Who says scientists don't know how to have fun?

Setting up the study

The scientists set up their research as a randomized, controlled trial, which means they followed strict scientific principles to limit any deviation from the study, provided all the meals, and monitored the research subjects very closely.

For their first experiment, the DASHers recruited 459 brave men and women, all of whom had borderline to high blood pressure. To be included, the participants' baseline systolic pressure couldn't be higher than 160, and the diastolic readings could range from 80 to 95. No one was on blood pressure medication.

Women have often been under-represented in medical studies, but the DASH researchers were smart enough to avoid that mistake. About half of those enrolled were female. The researchers also made sure to enroll a large number of African-American participants, about 60 percent of the total group, because they knew that high blood pressure is especially prevalent in African Americans (currently about 46 percent, compared to around a third of whites, Hispanics, and Asians).

REMEMBER

DASH hasn't been studied on a large scale in Hispanics, Asians, or other ethnic groups, but small studies have found similar benefits in Hispanic Americans and in Chinese men and women, and it is easily adaptable for a wide variety of dietary preferences. No matter who you are or where you're from, if you have high blood pressure or are at risk for it, you owe it to yourself to check out the DASH diet.

The people studied were also diverse in other ways. Some were low-income; others middle-to-upper-middle class. Their average age was 44, but the range of ages was wide. Most were overweight, but some were obese.

Conducting the research

After all the subjects were recruited and screened, the fun began. In what was termed the *run-in* phase, everyone was given a standardized control diet for the first three weeks, which included all their meals and snacks. Next, each person was randomly assigned to spend eight weeks on one of the three experimental diets: control, fruits and vegetables, or DASH. All the food was prepared for them to keep everything as strictly regimented as possible.

Throughout the study, researchers measured the participants' blood pressures at strict intervals, administered a questionnaire about symptoms and activity, and did urine tests to objectively assess potassium, magnesium, calcium, and protein intake (and to be sure everyone was onboard with the assigned diets).

REMEMBER

In DASH, researchers kept the subjects' calories constant throughout the study to keep body weight stable so they could evaluate the effect of the diet itself. Because they knew that weight loss lowers blood pressure, they had no reason to reinvent the wheel. (In reality, it's easy to cut calories and lose weight on DASH, but that wasn't the point of this particular study.)

The initial DASH study also kept sodium intake constant at about 3,000 milligrams per day. Although 3,000 milligrams is a pretty high daily dose of sodium, it's still somewhat lower than the typical 3,400 milligrams found in a standard Western diet. To keep it simple, the DASH group wanted to first determine whether certain foods people eat may have an impact on blood pressure, regardless of salt.

» **The control diet:** Because the control diet was designed to mimic a typical American diet, it included a hefty quantity of fat, plenty of meat, paltry amounts of fiber, and meager servings of fruits and vegetables. It was fairly low in potassium, magnesium, and calcium. In short, it was the type of diet that keeps cardiologists in business.

» **The fruits-and-vegetables diet:** The fruits-and-vegetables diet group included on average more than 5 servings of fruit and more than 3 servings of vegetables each day, or nearly 2½ times the amount of plant-based food as the control diet. As a result, this diet supplied more than three times the amount of fiber as the control diet, and much more potassium and magnesium as well. This particular diet wasn't designed to test a vegetarian diet, so it included about the same amount of fat and the same amount of meat, poultry, and fish as the control diet. However, it included one-third the number of snacks and sweets.

» **The DASH diet:** In addition to incorporating the added fruits and vegetables, the DASH diet group included 2 servings of low-fat dairy per day, something neither of the other diets did. DASH dieters received about one-third the amount of meat as the other groups but similar quantities of poultry and a little more fish. Added fats, such as oils and salad dressing, were reduced by more than half, and sweets and snacks were severely curtailed.

Analyzing the results

The results of the DASH study were conclusive: A reduced-fat diet rich in low-fat dairy, along with plenty of fruits and vegetables, can lower blood pressure substantially. Compared with the control diet, the fruits-and-vegetables diet dropped systolic pressure 2.8 points and diastolic 1.1 points. That doesn't sound very impressive, but it's meaningful in terms of stroke and heart disease risk reduction. The DASH diet was more powerful, lowering systolic pressure by 5.5 points and diastolic by 3 points.

More important, in those people diagnosed with hypertension at the beginning of the study, blood pressure fell by an average of 11.4 points systolic and 5.5 points diastolic, which is on par with the results you would expect from medical therapy. The improvement happened quickly, with results seen within two weeks on the diet, and improvement was seen across race and gender. Speaking of gender, DASH was actually somewhat more effective in women over the age of 45 compared to men. (Other studies focusing on salt restriction have also found that women do at least as well as their male counterparts over the long term, substantially reducing their risk for stroke and heart disease.)

TECHNICAL STUFF

Some people may worry that a plant-heavy diet could cause intestinal upset, but the DASH researchers found the opposite. In fact, constipation was reported in 10 percent of those on the typical Western-style control diet but in only 4 percent of those on DASH.

REMEMBER

Overall, the researchers estimated that the drop in blood pressure seen by simply following the DASH diet had the power to reduce heart disease by 15 percent and cut the incidence of stroke by 27 percent. That's a lot of lives saved and misery prevented.

Responding to America's Salt Obsession and Addressing Controversies

Sodium consumption in the United States and around the world has skyrocketed over the past few decades. This growth can be traced directly to a growing reliance on fast foods, restaurant meals, and processed foods. In the United States, the average diet includes about 3,400 milligrams of sodium every day, yet the human body requires a mere 500 milligrams for normal function.

REMEMBER

Overload your system with salt, and your blood pressure is likely to rise. Why? Because sodium causes the body to retain water, which in turn affects the kidneys' ability to properly regulate blood pressure. High sodium may also have directly harmful effects on the arteries that feed the heart, kidneys, and other vital organs. What's worse, a low potassium diet tends to cause the body to retain salt, aggravating the problem. Potassium comes chiefly from fruits, vegetables, and milk. The fact that DASH is relatively high in these natural sources of potassium is probably one reason that it works so well.

Though a number of studies over the years have convincingly implicated salt as a bad guy when it comes to hypertension, the DASH researchers took on the challenge of directly comparing the impact of three different levels of sodium intake when added to a healthy, blood pressure–friendly DASH diet versus a less healthy, more typical control diet. Enter the DASH sodium study.

Participants included 412 adults with blood pressures higher than 120/80. More than half were women, more than half were black, and 40 percent had hypertension. Most were overweight.

The study included both the higher-fat, control, Western diet and the healthier DASH diet, and it tested three different levels of sodium intake: 3,450 milligrams, 2,300 milligrams, and 1,150 milligrams. Everyone started out on the high-sodium control diet for the first two weeks, and each was then randomly assigned to one of the two diets at one of the three sodium levels. After 30 days, researchers changed the sodium dose such that each individual was tested at the low, intermediate, and high levels of sodium. As in the original DASH study, the researchers prepared all the participants' food and kept their calories constant.

Not surprisingly, the lower the salt intake, the better the blood pressure. The impact of sodium was greater with the less-healthy control diet than it was in the DASH diet, but the DASH group had lower blood pressure overall. Cutting sodium was especially effective in people who had hypertension to begin with, indicating they were more sensitive to salt's effects.

THE CASE FOR SALT REDUCTION

Although it's true that a few studies haven't confirmed a link between sodium and high blood pressure, the overwhelming majority of research conducted over the past 50 years (analyzing more than 250,000 individuals, we might add) has established a strong, stepwise connection between salt intake and high blood pressure.

If stodgy scientific research is hard to make heads or tails of, consider this: In those dwindling societies that exist outside of the grasp of modern life, free of modern grocery stores and fast food, hypertension rarely happens, even in old age. This phenomenon has many reasons, of course, but one important contributor appears to be the low-salt, high-potassium diet of these literally down-to-earth cultures.

An analysis by the World Health Organization estimates that by simply cutting average salt consumption around the globe by 15 percent, more than 8.5 million lives would be saved over the next 10 years. That's a hard statistic to argue with.

Although this is a goal that shouldn't be difficult to achieve, the average American diet includes about 3,400 milligrams of salt daily. Cutting this amount by 15 percent would get down to about 2,900 milligrams daily, which is still substantially higher than the recommendations by the Centers for Disease Control and Prevention (CDC). For optimum health, the CDC recommends a maximum daily sodium intake of 2,300 milligrams for most people age 50 and under. For those over 50, African Americans of any age, and people with hypertension, diabetes, or congestive heart failure, the recommended limit is 1,500 milligrams. The CDC also advises obese individuals to adopt a lower-salt diet because obesity tends to increase salt sensitivity and fluid retention. Overall, though, far fewer than 10 percent of Americans stay within these guidelines.

Remember: If your blood pressure tends to run low, or if it drops when you stand up, then a low-sodium diet may not be right for you. For some people, this may be a sign of dehydration or anemia. If you have low blood pressure or symptoms of dizziness, be sure to check with your doctor before making a change.

When pitted against the high-sodium control diet, the low-sodium DASH diet dropped systolic blood pressure by 11.5 points in people with hypertension. The effect was even greater (12.6 points) for black people. Women benefited more than men. Even those without hypertension saw their blood pressures fall by about 7 points. Diastolic blood pressure dropped as well, but the effect wasn't as dramatic, averaging about a 4.5-point difference between the high-sodium control diet and the low-sodium DASH group.

TECHNICAL STUFF

Because most people consistently eat too much salt, you may worry that a sudden change in sodium intake could cause side effects, even if, in the long run, it's better for you. To the contrary: There were fewer headaches and no differences in any other symptoms reported.

Omni-Heart: A Variation on the DASH Theme

In 2003, a group of researchers from Johns Hopkins University and Harvard University decided to test the theory that by increasing high-quality protein, and slightly decreasing carbohydrates, the DASH diet could be made even better. Funded by the National Institutes of Health, the Optimal Macronutrient Intake Trial to Prevent Heart Disease — also known as Omni-Heart — included 164 individuals similar to those enrolled in DASH. The average age was 54, 45 percent were women, and 55 percent were black. Most were overweight or obese. Everyone's blood pressure was at least 120/80 at baseline.

Three different diets were tested:

>> **The carbohydrate diet** was very similar to DASH, except that it was a little heavier in carbs and a bit lighter in protein. (Carbohydrates made up more than 55 percent of the calories in the original DASH diet; protein made up 18 percent.)

>> **The protein diet** had 25 percent of calories coming from protein, about half of which were of plant origin (think soy, beans, and nuts). Carbs were cut to 48 percent, as compared to 58 percent in the DASH-like carb diet.

>> **The unsaturated fat diet** provided 37 percent of its calories from fat (compared with 27 percent in the other two options), more than half of which was monounsaturated (typical sources include olive oil, canola oil, peanut oil, avocado oil, avocados, and almonds). Protein content was the same as in the DASH-type diet, while carbs were kept to 48 percent.

To put it more simply, the Omni-Heart researchers played with just 10 percent of the DASH diet calories, boosting protein in the protein diet and bumping up monounsaturated fat in the unsaturated fat diet, both at the expense of carbohydrates. Omni-Heart wasn't a low-sodium study. Everyone received the same amounts of sodium (a middle-of-the-road 2,300 milligrams) and similar amounts of blood pressure–friendly potassium, magnesium, and calcium. Omni-Heart wasn't a weight loss diet, so calories were kept constant to maintain a stable body weight.

Much like in the original DASH study, Omni-Heart researchers prepared all the food for participants. Each person spent about six weeks on each of the three diets, with the sequence of the diets (carb versus protein versus mono-fat) randomly assigned.

Compared with baseline blood pressure readings, blood pressures improved on each of the three diets. However, both the diet higher in protein and the one with more monounsaturated fat had a significantly greater impact on blood pressure control for those people who already had high blood pressure. To be more precise, on the DASH-style diet, systolic blood pressure plunged by an impressive 13 points in people with hypertension. Nice! But both the higher protein and the higher monounsaturated fat diets surged ahead with a 16-point drop over baseline. Likewise, diastolic pressure fell by a respectable 6 points in the DASH-like diet but tumbled more than 8 points with the other two options. Lipid numbers (HDL, or "good" cholesterol; LDL, or "bad" cholesterol; and triglycerides) were also somewhat better on both of the alternative diets, although all three options improved LDL cholesterol readings compared to baseline.

REMEMBER

The results of Omni-Heart show that by cutting carbs just a bit and adding a small dollop of good fat or high-quality protein, the DASH diet can be enhanced and enriched. More important, these results reveal that you shouldn't be afraid to reduce grain servings (to 5 to 6 servings) in DASH just a little, as long as you substitute high-quality protein and healthy monounsaturated fats. Healthy food should never be boring. Whether simply made or worthy of a master chef, a good meal is not only sustenance but also one of life's true and pure pleasures.

DASH: Wellness through Optimal Nutrition

People have known for more than a century that high blood pressure is harmful, yet effective treatments didn't hit the market until the 1950s. Thanks to the hard work of medical researchers around the world, a wide variety of medications are now available. This is great, but medications can be costly, and even the very best options have potential side effects. Take a look at these stats:

- » More than two-thirds of people with hypertension need at least two drugs to keep their numbers under control.

- » Blood pressure medications can be lifesaving, but, depending on the pill, side effects can occur in up to 15 percent of people.

- » A typical blood pressure pill lowers blood pressure about 10 points — about the same reduction you see when following DASH.

- » By cutting sodium to 1,500 milligrams, à la low-sodium DASH, the effect could be equal to two different drugs (take a look at Table 2-1 to see just how effective reducing your daily sodium intake to 1,500 milligrams can be).

TABLE 2-1 **Effects of a 1,500-Milligram Sodium DASH Diet on Reducing Both Systolic and Diastolic Blood Pressure**

Characteristics	Systolic Blood Pressure (in Millimeters of Mercury)	Diastolic Blood Pressure (in Millimeters of Mercury)
Hypertensive	–12 mm Hg	–6 mm Hg
Pre-hypertensive	–7 mm Hg	–4 mm Hg
Age over 45	–12 mm Hg	–6 mm Hg
Age under 45	–6 mm Hg	–3 mm Hg
African American (all)	–10 mm Hg	–5 mm Hg
White and others (all)	–8 mm Hg	–4 mm Hg
Male	–7 mm Hg	–4 mm Hg
Female	–11 mm Hg	–5 mm Hg

Source: Study from the New England Journal of Medicine, 2001.

REMEMBER

Ironically, health experts know more about how to lower blood pressure with diet and lifestyle than ever before, but rates of hypertension continue to rise. That's because people are eating more of the wrong stuff and less of the good stuff, exercising less, and carrying more weight. You don't have to be a genius to see that you can save a lot of dough and feel better if you get in sync with DASH.

An analysis from researchers at the University of California, San Francisco reported that if Americans simply shaved off a third of their average daily sodium intake, the following would occur:

- » New heart disease cases could be cut by up to 120,000 per year.

- » Strokes would be reduced by as many as 66,000.

PRESENTING THE "BEST OVERALL DIET"

In January 2013, *U.S. News and World Report* reviewed 29 different diets designed to improve health and well-being and awarded DASH "Best Overall Diet." The publication based this designation on several criteria, including the following:

- Nutritional value
- Heart health
- Diabetes
- Safety
- Ease of use
- Effectiveness for short- and long-term weight loss

When the results were tallied, DASH came out ahead of the pack, which included the Mediterranean Diet, the Mayo Clinic Diet, and the Therapeutic Lifestyle Changes Diet (from NIH). DASH has remained at or near the top of the rankings ever since. When heart doctors and jaded journalists can agree on something this important, it's worth taking note.

>> As many as 99,000 heart attacks could be averted.

>> 92,000 lives could be spared.

If those numbers don't impress you (and we're not sure why they wouldn't), consider this: If everyone trimmed their salt habit, healthcare cost savings in the U.S. alone could amount to as much as $10 billion to $24 billion annually. And this doesn't even get into the benefits that may surface if everyone chose to put a little more DASH into their lives. That's powerful medicine indeed.

IN THIS CHAPTER

» **Seeing how DASH fights high blood pressure**

» **Understanding the DASH diet's effects on cholesterol**

» **Losing weight with DASH**

» **Tackling diabetes with DASH**

» **Considering how DASH can lessen your risk for cancer**

Chapter **3**

Improving Your Overall Health

ASH is a dietary multi-tasker. If you follow a DASH-worthy diet, you'll reduce your risk of numerous life-changing and potentially deadly cardio-vascular conditions. You may also drop your cholesterol, maintain a healthier weight, cut your risk for diabetes, and even reduce your likelihood of developing certain types of cancer. We explain how in this chapter. (For an in-depth look at the conditions we cover in this chapter, head to Part 2.)

Fighting the Silent Killer: Hypertension

Hypertension can lead to a number of cardiovascular ailments, including heart attacks, congestive heart failure, heart rhythm disorders, and stroke. (We tell you more about these surprisingly common conditions in Chapter 6.) Hypertension is also a leading cause of kidney failure and can contribute to dementia and eye disease.

WARNING

Because it usually causes no symptoms until one of these serious conditions develop, hypertension is often known as the "silent killer." The tragedy is that high blood pressure is easily diagnosed and can usually be effectively treated. Even better, it can often be prevented.

The DASH diet was created specifically to test the effects of a dietary pattern that includes a variety of foods known to help lower blood pressure. In fact, it was one of the first mainstream attempts to test the potential of what is now known as *functional medicine*. Although DASH has other very beneficial effects on your health and well-being, it was born to prevent or reduce hypertension. The following sections break down exactly why blood pressure concerns are relevant for everyone and how adopting a DASH lifestyle can help alleviate those concerns.

Why blood pressure matters

High blood pressure causes serious wear and tear on your heart, brain, and kidneys, so it's critical that you take it seriously. Although a brief rise in blood pressure isn't likely to cause permanent harm, your body isn't designed to handle continuously high pressure. Just think of a garden hose gushing at full blast and imagine what that might do to your tender blood vessels.

The human body is built to be resilient, but over time, the nonstop strain of high blood pressure can cause the following:

>> Abnormal thickening and stiffness of the heart muscle, which can lead to heart failure

>> Microscopic tears, stiffening, and scarring in the arteries of the heart and brain, raising the risk for heart attack, stroke, and dementia

>> Irregularity of the heart rhythm, which may also raise the risk for stroke

>> Damage to the blood vessels that feed the kidneys, leading to kidney failure and, in severe cases, dialysis

>> Weaknesses in the walls of the blood vessels of the eyes, causing blurry vision or even blindness

REMEMBER

Some of these problems can be stabilized or even reversed if they're caught early. But why put yourself in harm's way? Don't ignore your high blood pressure. Follow the treatments prescribed by your doctor. High blood pressure can almost always be treated safely and effectively. Even better, it can often be prevented.

How DASH can help

High blood pressure usually develops over time, starting with a condition known as *pre-hypertension*, an important health issue we tell you more about in Chapter 6. Note that these numbers are lower than they used to be. The High Blood Pressure Guidelines were modified in 2017. Picture-perfect blood pressure is pegged at around 115/75. Doctors don't classify blood pressure as hypertensive until the systolic blood pressure (the top number) gets to 130 to 139 or the diastolic blood pressure (the bottom number) hits 80 or above (see Chapter 6). In between, you have *elevated* blood pressure when your blood pressure is running at about 121 to 129 over 80. As many as 50 percent of Americans, fit this profile. More concerning is that about 20 percent don't even realize they have hypertension, so it's important to get your blood pressure checked regularly.

When you're living in the pre-hypertensive zone, you carry a higher risk for heart disease and stroke than someone whose pressure is normal. To be more precise, every 20-point rise in systolic blood pressure or 10-point rise in diastolic blood pressure doubles the risk of heart disease and stroke. In this range, medications aren't recommended. Instead, pre-hypertension is a wake-up call to get working on a healthy way of life. Say hello to DASH.

REMEMBER

DASH is often thought of as a high blood pressure diet, but it was designed to help people with pre-hypertension as well. In order to get into the study, a blood pressure higher than 120/80 was required. If you're pre-hypertensive, you can expect to drop your systolic blood pressure by a very respectable 7 points. For many people with pre-hypertension, that's enough to move back into the normal range.

How does DASH work its magic on blood pressure? For starters, it's abundant in fruits and vegetables. Plants provide a wealth of health-boosting vitamins, antioxidants, and phytochemicals (see Chapter 5 for more about these disease-fighting substances), and they're loaded with blood pressure–friendly potassium. Potassium works in opposition to sodium, lessening its effect on blood pressure. It may also have beneficial effects on the tone and health of your blood vessels. A potassium bonanza, DASH provides twice the amount of potassium found in a typical Western diet. Of course, it's also low in sodium.

DASH also promotes consumption of low-fat dairy, and research has found that a diet rich in low-fat dairy products such as yogurt and low-fat milk and cheese has consistently been linked to lower blood pressure. In the National Heart, Lung, and Blood Institute's Family Heart Study, those with the greatest intake of dairy products were about one-third less likely to have hypertension. Not only do these foods provide a great source of calcium, which helps keep your arteries strong and flexible, but with DASH, they also replace less-healthy saturated fats and processed foods.

WARNING

Wondering whether you can pop some potassium and calcium supplements and get the same effect as if you were eating foods rich in these nutrients? Forget it! Your body is an expert at extracting nutrients from food, but unless you have a medical deficiency, supplements won't do the same job. In addition, DASH promotes modest weight loss, which also leads to lower blood pressure. You can't expect to eat a burger and fries followed by a potassium chaser and get the same effect.

DASH and Cholesterol

Your doctor, your family, and even your TV set are always nagging you about cholesterol. Why do they care, and what exactly is the stuff, anyway? *Cholesterol* is a waxy substance that comes from your diet but is also made by your body. Although it's often lumped in with fats, it's technically a *lipid*, a broader category that also includes fats. There's a lot of confusion between dietary cholesterol and the cholesterol made by your body, so we want to clear things up.

REMEMBER

Everyone's body creates some cholesterol. Some people are genetically super-producers; others naturally manufacture pretty meager amounts of the stuff. That's why cholesterol in the diet doesn't have a huge influence on the cholesterol level in the blood. It's the type of *fat* in the diet that you want to focus on. Metabolic studies have long determined that a high level of *saturated* fat in the diet leads to higher cholesterol levels in the blood. Always check out the amount of saturated fat on the food label. Fiber also helps reduce blood cholesterol levels, especially the soluble fiber found in plant foods. Total recommended fiber intake (insoluble and soluble) is 25 to 35 grams per day. Eating 5 to 10 grams of soluble fiber (barley, oats, quinoa, beans, legumes, vegetables, fruits) a day has been shown to reduce cholesterol by 5 to 10 points or more. Learn more about fiber in Chapter 12.

Why cholesterol matters

The two types of cholesterol circulating around in your blood that you need to concern yourself with are *low-density lipoprotein* (LDL) and *high-density lipoprotein* (HDL).

>> LDL is the "bad" cholesterol because it's the one that clogs up arteries. You need a little bit of it to keep your cell membranes healthy, your brain working smoothly, and your hormones at healthy levels, but most people's bodies make far more than they need.

REMEMBER

Most of the LDL swimming through your bloodstream is generated in your liver, a highly creative organ that can make cholesterol out of just about any sort of food. Dump in a load of *saturated fat* (coconut oil, animal fats) and it goes to town. *Trans fat* (found in partially hydrogenated oils, especially hard margarine and shortening, and many processed baked goods) revs up the liver's cholesterol-creation system even more. Carrying around some extra body fat, especially the type that collects around your tummy, also boosts LDL production. Smoking does too.

» HDL is the good stuff that works to protect your blood vessels. It works in opposition to LDL, pulling bad cholesterol out of the arteries and taking it back to the liver to be processed and eliminated. In general, the higher the HDL the better. Monounsaturated fats (from olive oil, avocados, and nuts), exercise, and alcohol in moderation raise HDL.

TIP

Think "*H* is for happy; *L* is for lousy" if you have trouble remembering which cholesterol is which.

If your LDL level is high, then you may be more likely to suffer a heart attack or stroke, whereas high levels of HDL may help protect you. The optimal levels vary, depending on your other risk factors. These include hypertension, diabetes, smoking, and whether you've already started to develop cholesterol plaque in your arteries. For more about cholesterol and how to figure out your ideal numbers, check out Chapter 7.

TAKING A CLOSER LOOK AT YOUR LIPID PROFILE

Sometimes doctors refer to *non-HDL cholesterol*. Basically, this includes LDL and all the other forms of not-so-good cholesterol, including VLDL (very low-density lipoprotein) and IDL (intermediate density lipoprotein). These two bad actors are closely connected to triglycerides, another undesirable.

Triglycerides aren't technically in the cholesterol family, but they're part of the standard lipid profile blood test. These "blood fats" go up with foods that are high on the glycemic index (that is, foods with simple carbohydrates that quickly raise blood sugar and insulin response). Total carbohydrate intake isn't as important as the intake of those simple carbs. Processed sugary foods are triglycerides' best friends. It's no surprise that a high triglyceride level is often considered a marker for an unhealthy lifestyle. High levels of triglycerides in the blood have been linked to higher risk of heart attack.

How DASH can help

The effect of a strict DASH diet on cholesterol is modest yet still meaningful. In a study comparing DASH to a standard Western control diet, with no weight loss allowed, LDL dropped nearly 11 points. The diet, if followed to the letter, will actually drop HDL a little and have no effect on triglycerides.

REMEMBER

If those results sound underwhelming, remember that the great thing about DASH is that you can modify it to suit your needs. For example:

>> If your LDL needs some work, back off the red meat, baked goods, and coconut oil, and add in more fiber (oats, beans, apples) and some soy-based foods (such as soy nuts, edamame, and tofu).

>> If your HDL is running low, try working in a few more monounsaturated fats and omega-3 fatty acids, found in foods such as olive oil, nuts, and fatty fish.

We show you more ways to make the DASH diet work for you in the recipes in Part 4.

Battling the Bulge

If you're struggling with your weight, you have plenty of company. More than two-thirds of Americans are overweight, and more than 40 percent are medically obese. A DASH meal plan can help reduce risk factors for heart disease, diabetes, and cancer. According to the Centers for Disease Control and Prevention (CDC), heart disease, stroke, type 2 diabetes and certain types of cancer that are some of the leading causes of preventable, premature death.

Globally, the numbers continue to grow. As of 2017, 39 percent of adults were overweight with 13 percent classified as obese. Though genetics may play a role, there are three times as many people struggling with obesity as there were in the 1960s. These statistics result in 4.7 million premature deaths annually.

Why weight matters

Stepping on the scale may feel like an act of courage, and sometimes it's just easier to convince yourself that maybe your body weight is only skin-deep. In truth, it's much more than a cosmetic issue. People come in all sizes and shapes, and there's a wide range of healthy body weights, but after you cross the threshold into obesity, you open yourself up to a host of medical problems.

WARNING

High blood pressure is a serious but easily overlooked consequence of being overweight or obese. If you are overweight, consider a 10 percent body weight loss for improved blood pressure and improved health. Losing just 10 pounds, however, can lower blood pressure as much as 10 points. We've also personally seen clients and patients reduce the amount of — and even eliminate — blood pressure medications they take after they commit to losing weight.

Obesity doesn't just help blood pressure rise. It also aggravates other issues related to high blood pressure. For instance, heavier people tend to retain more fluid, which can lead to swelling in the legs, hands, and face, and in severe cases, congestive heart failure. Additionally, the more weight you carry, the more sensitive you may become to salt, which in turn raises blood pressure.

It's estimated that obesity shortens the average life span by 10 to 20 years. That's because that extra weight also raises your risk for

>> Arthritis

>> Cancer

>> Dementia

>> Diabetes

>> Heart disease

>> Intestinal disease

>> Lung disease

>> Stroke

We tell you more about these serious consequences of body weight in Chapter 8.

How DASH can help

DASH wasn't designed as a weight-loss program, but it's perfect for the job. Why, you ask? Because a DASH diet is not overly restrictive, is chock-full of green leafy vegetables and fruit, is high in fiber (so it fills you up), and includes health-promoting foods that are lower in calories.

By choosing to eat the DASH way, you'll add plenty of low-fat dairy products such as Greek yogurt. (Greek yogurt is higher in hunger-squashing protein than regular yogurt, and it's a great source of calcium to boot.) Be sure to check flavored yogurt labels for *added* sugar (some of the sugars in yogurt are from its natural lactose). We like to use plain yogurt and add our own fruit or crunchy toppings like granola, nuts, or seeds. Plain yogurt is great for cooking and baking as well. Nuts are another DASH-friendly treat that calm the hunger beast with heart-healthy fats (just be sure to measure your portions, because nuts are calorie-dense).

Need more evidence? Consider the results of a 2010 study from Duke University, which evaluated the effects of a calorie-cutting DASH diet plus exercise for overweight and obese men and women. The four-month program, designed with a weight-loss goal of one half to a full pound per week, was tested against the DASH diet without weight loss and against a typical American diet. At the end of the four months, those on the weight-loss plan were down more than 20 pounds on average. Compared to their baseline numbers, systolic blood pressure had dropped by about 16 points, and diastolic by 10. DASH dieters without weight loss, on the other hand, lowered systolic blood pressure a respectable but not as impressive 11 points, and diastolic 7.5 points. On top of all that, those who lost weight with DASH were at lower risk for diabetes, had better lipid profiles, and could exercise for longer.

Fighting Diabetes

Diabetes is an illness that affects how the body processes glucose. When you eat, the body converts food into the most common form of energy: glucose. Glucose circulates in your bloodstream to be used as fuel for many parts of the body. In response to this, insulin is secreted to metabolize the glucose (in other words, deliver it to cells). *Insulin* is the hormone responsible for ensuring that the glucose in your bloodstream is put to work. All people with diabetes have problems with either producing or using insulin.

Since the 1970s, the prevalence of diabetes has more than doubled, and the number continues to rise. At the time of this writing, 34.2 million people in the U.S. have diabetes and more than 425 million people worldwide are living with diabetes. Many more are at high risk for developing the disease. It's estimated that 1.5 million people are diagnosed in the U.S. alone each year. The vast majority of diabetes cases are the type 2 variety and in most cases are a direct consequence of diet, lifestyle choices, and obesity. Once known as *adult-onset diabetes*, this term is now a misnomer because more and more young children are being diagnosed with type 2 diabetes.

Why diabetes matters

When the body's various systems become overloaded with glucose, the situation is anything but sweet. High blood sugar and high insulin levels are directly damaging to the lining of your blood vessels. This accounts for many of the tragic consequences of diabetes, including the following:

>> Blindness

>> Heart disease, including heart attacks and heart failure

>> Intestinal disease

>> Kidney failure

>> Liver disease

>> Nerve damage

>> Poor healing, which may lead to dangerous skin and bone infections, sometimes requiring amputation

>> Stroke

WARNING

Complications from diabetes can usually be managed with medication and surgery, but they can't be undone. It doesn't take a medical degree to recognize that an ounce of prevention is worth a pound of cure.

How DASH can help

Rest assured that diabetes will change your life, but it's usually preventable, and DASH can be part of the solution. With its emphasis on healthy whole foods and limits on sugary foods and snacks, DASH is a great fit for people with diabetes. Critics of DASH cite its relatively high carb count, but it's important to remember that not all carbs are the same, and the fiber content of DASH is quite beneficial to anyone with diabetes. In addition, the carbohydrate balance is reasonable and can be adjusted (anywhere from 45 percent to 50 percent of your total calories). DASH includes plenty of nutritionally rich complex carbohydrates, including fruits, vegetables, and whole grains, but it eliminates sugary beverages, candy, chips, pretzels, salty processed crackers, high-sugar snack bars, and other highly processed foods.

TIP

The DASH creators weren't dummies. They realized that everyone needs to sneak in a little treat from time to time, so the diet allows for up to five not-so-healthy snacks per week. It's up to you to make those goodies count. If you have diabetes, you'll need to account for all carbohydrates and calories.

You don't have to take our word that DASH works. Several important studies have evaluated the effect of DASH on type 2 diabetes showing that adherence to DASH can help reduce the incidence of type 2 diabetes. In the Insulin Resistance Atherosclerosis Study (a mouthful if there ever were one), more than 850 non-diabetic individuals ages 40 to 69 filled out a detailed food questionnaire. After five years, those whose diets were most like DASH were 70 percent less likely to become diabetic compared to those whose eating habits strayed the farthest from the diet.

OMNI-HEART TACKLES DIABETES

Due to physicians' and dietitians' nagging concerns about potential negatives of a high-carb, lower-fat diet, the Omni-Heart researchers tested their higher protein and higher monounsaturated fat diets against DASH. In diabetes, the body becomes less sensitive to insulin, so the Omni-Heart researchers' goal was to find out whether DASH or a higher protein or high mono-fat version of the diet (substituting for some of the carb content) would improve sensitivity to insulin, potentially cutting the chances of developing diabetes.

Although the higher protein diet didn't seem to make a difference, the mono-fat version of the DASH diet, which included more olive oil, canola oil, nuts, and seeds, improved participants' insulin sensitivity. Not only do they taste good, these healthy-fat foods are also known to be heart-smart, brain-protecting, and hunger-busting. It makes sense to make them part of your healthy eating plan.

In a study published in 2011, a cooperative endeavor between American and Iranian researchers, people with diabetes who spent eight weeks on DASH

>> Dropped blood sugar levels nearly 30 points

>> Lowered LDL cholesterol 17 points

>> Increased HDL cholesterol more than 4 points

>> Lowered systolic pressure nearly 14 points

>> Dropped diastolic pressure nearly 10 points

Tackling Cancer

Cancer is a term fraught with dread. It makes people miserable, often requires horribly draining chemotherapy and radiation treatments, and may even be disfiguring. But what exactly is it? *Cancer* is really a catch-all term for a wide variety of diseases that happen when cells stray from their normal function, mutate, and begin to divide and grow out of control. Eventually, these growths can interfere with the body's ability to carry out its day-to-day, life-sustaining processes.

There are more than 100 different types of cancers. Some you can live with for decades and never know they're there. Others can be deadly within months or less. Often, doctors have no idea why a particular cancer strikes a particular individual.

It's possible to live an entirely pure way of life and still be struck down by the disease. Others engage in every possible vice and yet live well into their 90s. Be that as it may, some triggers are guaranteed to drastically raise your risk for one or many forms of cancer. Smoking is the obvious offender. So is long-term unprotected exposure to sunlight. But body weight and lifestyle can play a factor too, both positive and negative.

Why cancer matters

Many cancers, including breast cancer, colon cancer, and pancreatic cancer, are strongly linked to diet and lifestyle. It's estimated that as many as 40 percent of cancers can be prevented with simple lifestyle changes. None of these changes are radical, but all require some effort on your part. For example, if you're a smoker, dropping the habit can significantly reduce your risk for lung cancer, cancers of the mouth and throat, and more.

Body weight and the food you eat are two very important and modifiable risk factors for cancer. When you commit to a heart-healthy diet like DASH, you cut your risk for cancer and boost your chances of staying healthy for the long term.

How DASH can help

With its emphasis on fruits, vegetables, and whole grains, combined with limited amounts of sodium, sugar, red meat, and processed foods, DASH is spot-on for reducing the risk of some cancers.

TIP

Fruits and vegetables not only are great sources of powerful antioxidants and other cancer-fighting nutrients but also provide loads of colon-friendly fiber. Whole grains likewise deliver another wide spectrum of equally important nutrients and fiber. Diets rich in these healthy foods have long been associated with a lower likelihood of cancer.

WARNING

Red meats, especially processed meats such as bacon and lunch meats, have been clearly linked to a higher risk for colon cancer. DASH keeps these high-sodium foods to a minimum, with the option of avoiding them altogether. And because a high-salt diet may raise the likelihood of esophageal and stomach cancers, choosing DASH can make all the difference.

Finally, obesity itself contributes to a spectrum of cancers, including cancers of the breast, esophagus, pancreas, colon, uterus, and prostate. Combining DASH with calorie-cutting and exercise can get you back on the right track.

IN THIS CHAPTER

» **Establishing new lifestyle routines**

» **Increasing the good stuff in your diet and decreasing the bad**

» **Setting specific dietary goals and tracking them**

» **Anticipating obstacles so that you stay on track**

Chapter **4**

Gearing Up for a DASH Lifestyle

The great thing about Dietary Approaches to Stop Hypertension (DASH) is that it's an eating plan for life. Unless you have specific food sensitivities or other medical issues that require medical nutrition therapy (see Chapter 1), DASH is a great eating plan for the whole family, not just those with (or at risk for) high blood pressure. You do have to be willing to make a few adjustments to your eating schedule and food choices, though.

Specifically, you need to eat on a fairly regular schedule and include more fruits, vegetables, and dairy foods in your diet. (If you have an intolerance to dairy or lactose, you can still adopt the plan; see Chapter 5 for more on dairy.) No super-exotic foods are required with DASH, but you may encounter vegetables you don't eat too often or whole grains you haven't tried. Dare yourself to become a more adventurous eater as part of your journey to a healthier diet. (We share numerous tantalizing recipes in Part 4 that make moving ahead in your food adventures easy and tasty.)

In this chapter, you find out how to get ready to modify your current diet. You also discover how to set goals, track your progress toward those goals, and overcome pitfalls that could otherwise hinder your progress.

Setting Yourself Up for a DASHing Success

Creating and practicing a new routine is part of establishing a new habit. If your diet is low in fruits and vegetables and high in salt and fat right now, you can't expect to do a complete turnaround overnight. You have to establish a few small goals at a time and work on those goals until they become new habits. After you adopt a few new habits, you can move on to the next few goals.

You can successfully follow a DASH diet plan by keeping these tips in mind:

» Make a commitment to change your *habits* for the long haul, not just your food and beverage intake.

» Be open to learning more about how your body works and why diet truly has an impact on health.

» Replace overeating behaviors with other strategies for coping with stress, boredom, and other situations where emotions rule eating.

» Stay open-minded about trying new foods.

» Understand that modifying your diet to include DASH diet principles isn't a quick fix, nor are the overall lifestyle changes you'll make.

» Realize that you'll have setbacks — and that you can forgive yourself and move on.

» Seek a support system to help you meet your eating and exercise goals.

Of course, before you make any changes in your diet or lifestyle, you have to be in the "action phase" of readiness, which is the fourth stage of the classic five-stage model for successful behavioral change:

» **Precontemplation:** In this stage, you're not even thinking about changing your diet or lifestyle, and you may not even realize that you have a problem (for instance, if you're overweight or your doctor has told you that your diet is affecting your health).

» **Contemplation:** During this stage, you're willing to consider making some changes, but you may be on the fence.

» **Determination:** The fact that you're holding this book in your hands probably means you're at least in the determination stage. You've thought about it, you're making a plan, and you're ready to commit to some action.

» **Action:** In this stage, you may also be sharing your goals with others, making you more accountable. During this stage, you continue to work on your plan by setting goals and tracking progress. Success breeds success! The success you have (whether it's lower blood pressure, weight loss, lower blood cholesterol, or just feeling better) is a huge motivator to keep on track. You may be in the action stage for at least three to six months, and this leads to maintenance.

>> **Maintenance:** This stage is a lifelong endeavor where you address the ups and downs and get through situations that are challenging (vacations, holidays, and other special occasions).

Generally, most people go through each stage and often have setbacks along the way. Provided you recover from them, those setbacks are A-OK because the DASH lifestyle isn't a quick-fix fad diet; it's an eating plan to adopt for a lifetime of healthy living.

REMEMBER

Your long-term goal is to develop a healthy eating and exercise plan that you can live with for the rest of your life. You can do this by making gradual changes, following the dietary guidelines at least 80 percent of the time, and recovering quickly when you do get off track. (For the specifics on DASH dietary guidelines, see Chapter 5.)

TIP

Setting up an appointment with a registered dietitian/nutritionist (RDN) can help you get started with a plan that's just right for you. An RDN will review your personal medical history and provide a nutrition assessment and personalized plan. Give your local medical center or your primary physician a call about referral to a local RDN. You can also look online at www.eatright.org and click "Find a Registered Dietitian" to find one near you using your ZIP code.

More of This, Less of That

As outlined in Chapter 1, the DASH diet includes lots of fruits and vegetables and some nuts and whole grains but limits saturated fat, desserts, and salt. For many people the "lots of fruits and vegetables" aspect is tricky, but those foods are essential for the full benefits of the DASH diet plan.

No worries! We have you covered with easy suggestions to help you meet your goals of adding more fruits and vegetables to every meal. Even if some vegetables are on your don't-like list or eating spinach at breakfast seems completely weird to you, open your mind to some of our sneaky healthy-eating suggestions in this section and give fruits and vegetables another chance. Before you know it, you'll find them much tastier and more convenient than all those processed foods you may be used to.

Increasing the quantity of fruits, vegetables, nuts, seeds, and beans

The first strategy for adding more plant foods to your diet is making sure you have them available. Face it — you won't eat right if all you have in the fridge is a jar of mustard and some pickles. Adding fruits and vegetables to your weekly shopping list is a must. These foods contain a good amount of potassium, an important mineral for healthy hearts.

Having easy, ready-to-eat access to these foods in the refrigerator is helpful. When you purchase vegetables, store them in the crisper bin in the refrigerator; they'll last longer. Keep some washed, cut, and ready to eat in airtight containers so grabbing them is easy. The same goes for fruit: Keep it stored in a fruit bin, and keep fruits that perish more quickly (bananas, berries, and so on) on your running grocery list so you always have them on hand.

Try these time-saving strategies to help get you eating more fruits and vegetables:

>> When you bring home melon, take a few minutes to cut it, remove the rind, and cube it for snacking. Keep it in an airtight container in the refrigerator. If fruit is clean and ready to grab when you want to eat it, you'll eat more of it and throw less away.

>> Keep a vegetable snack box in the fridge too. Put sliced celery sticks, sweet bell pepper slices, and mini carrots into a zippered bag and keep it in sight when you open the refrigerator. Use these as snacks before dinner or pack them in your lunch. Dip them into a yummy Greek yogurt dip and enjoy.

>> Keep bananas on the counter where you can see them and easily grab one on the go. Eat one each day, before they go brown (although those make great DASH muffins). Add them to oatmeal or yogurt or just eat them as is for a quick snack.

>> Wash and freeze stemmed grapes for a refreshing snack in warmer months, or try cutting a banana into 1-inch chunks, dipping one end in melted dark chocolate, and freezing — a delicious, potassium-filled frozen treat!

>> Swap the salt-ridden taquitos that may have once inhabited your freezer for frozen fruits and vegetables — a quick and economical choice.

>> Spread peanut butter lightly onto whole-wheat toast or an oat bran English muffin and top with sliced strawberries or bananas and a sprinkling of flax seed for a midday snack.

>> Make a yogurt parfait with nonfat plain Greek yogurt, 2 tablespoons granola, and fresh fruit.

TIP

>> Cook spinach the night you bring it home, even if you don't eat it then. Cooked spinach lasts a few more days in the refrigerator and is easy to reheat in a microwave or saucepan and add to eggs or a pasta or rice dish. You can also cook half of it and use the rest as sandwich toppers for your lunches.

Spinach only takes about 5 minutes to cook. Bring a large pot of water to a boil, add the spinach, cover, let simmer for 2 to 3 minutes, and drain. You can also sauté it with onion and garlic in a smidge of healthy olive oil.

>> Keep dried fruits such as apricots, raisins, and cranberries on a prime pantry shelf for a quick snack or to add to salads and other recipes.

>> Mix up a fruit smoothie for breakfast or for an after-work snack while you're getting dinner together. Place 1 cup of frozen or fresh berries or a frozen banana into a high-speed blender with ½ cup of Greek yogurt (if you're using fresh fruit, pop in two to three ice cubes). Blend until smooth.

>> Keep canned beans and canned tomato products on hand. Some of these items are higher in sodium, but they're loaded with important antioxidants. And you can remove some of the sodium by rinsing and draining beans before using.

>> Keep frozen peas or other no-salt vegetable blends on hand for a quick side dish or to add to pasta or rice dishes.

When you first glanced at the DASH diet, you may have said out loud: "What? Eat 4 to 5 servings of vegetables every day? And eat 4 to 5 servings of fruit too?!" But alas, friends, there is comfort in the answer to the question "What is a serving?" Table 4-1 gives you the lowdown.

TABLE 4-1   **Serving Sizes of Fruits and Vegetables**

Food	1 Serving
Apple, orange, peach, pear	1 medium
Kiwifruit	1
Banana, medium-large	½
Raisins, dried cranberries, dried cherries	¼ cup (or 4 tablespoons)
Frozen, canned, or fresh mixed fruit	½ cup
Fruit juice	6 ounces
Raw vegetables	1 cup
Cooked vegetables	½ cup
Low-sodium vegetable juice	6 ounces

So with the information in Table 4-1, you know that if you slice up a large apple or a large banana for your midday snack, you can count that as 2 servings. Most dinner salads at restaurants are also 2 servings. Add 4 tablespoons of dried fruit to that salad and you've got another serving of fruit. Throw 1 cup of frozen strawberries into the blender with some low-fat yogurt and you just included another serving of fruit! See how easy this 4-to-5 servings rule is?

REMEMBER

In addition to the fruit and vegetable groups, you want to add nuts, seeds, and dried beans to your diet. These high-protein foods are considered to be part of the meat/protein food group. In addition to protein, they provide nutrients and fiber. Serving sizes are important here too. Just ⅓ cup of nuts equals 1 serving. A serving of seeds is just 2 tablespoons, and a serving of beans is ½ cup.

Decreasing the amount of saturated fat, cholesterol, and sodium

In general, you should choose less packaged, processed food. The DASH diet is low in saturated fat, so keep an eye out for the amounts you see on food labels. Look for foods that have less than 1.5 grams of saturated fat per serving. DASH is also low in cholesterol and total fat and limits sugary foods and beverages.

The DASH diet is lower in sodium, recommending no more than 2,300 milligrams per day. The 2010 dietary guidelines for Americans advise people who already have high blood pressure, or have diabetes or kidney disease, to consume no more than 1,500 milligrams of sodium per day. This guideline also applies to middle-aged or older adults. Younger, healthy folks can handle a bit more sodium, but staying under 2,300 milligrams per day is a good bet. However, even with sodium levels at around 3,000 milligrams a day, when all other DASH guidelines were employed, blood pressure was still reduced. Still, the DASH research shows that eating plans that are lower in sodium lower blood pressure even more. Table 4-2 shows the breakdown of various nutrients used in the DASH studies.

Of course, because one of the goals of the DASH diet is also to maintain a healthy body weight, you must figure out how many calories you need. To lose weight, you must create a calorie deficit. See the sidebar "How many calories do you need?" for help calculating the amount of calories needed to maintain your weight.

TABLE 4-2 **Daily Nutrient Goals Used in DASH Diet Studies**

Macronutrient	Percentage of Daily Calories
Total fat	27%
Saturated fat	6%
Protein	18%
Carbohydrate	55%

Nutrient	Amount
Cholesterol	150 milligrams (mg)
Sodium	2,300 mg
Potassium	4,700 mg
Calcium	1,250 mg
Magnesium	500 mg
Fiber	30 grams

Source: National Heart, Lung, Blood Institute

Creating Goals for Dietary Change

Imagine a stronger, healthier you. Visualizing yourself accomplishing your new diet and exercise goals is one way to begin the goal-setting process. Consider writing down some of the aspects of your vision. For example: I will feel better, I will be more fit, I will look great in new clothes, I will have more energy, I will learn more about myself as I keep a daily journal, and so on.

After you've visualized yourself living a healthier lifestyle, you can start setting the goals that will ultimately help you get there. For the best chance at success, keep your goals specific and realistic. You also need to track your progress toward your goals to hold yourself accountable. We help you do both in the next sections.

Being SMART

SMART goals are Specific, Measurable, Attainable, Realistic, and Timely. What does all that mean, exactly? Well, the specific aspect is pretty self-explanatory. Instead of setting a bunch of general goals, give yourself specific ones that you can better hold yourself accountable to. We list some examples in Table 4-3.

TABLE 4-3   **Setting Specific Goals**

General Goal	Specific Goal
I will eat more fruit.	I will pack an apple or orange every day for work.
I will lose weight.	I will record my daily food intake and follow my meal plan, working toward a 10- to 20-pound weight loss over the year.
I will eat more vegetables.	I will have a variety of fresh, frozen, and low-sodium canned vegetables on my weekly grocery list and try a new recipe each week that includes them.
I will exercise more.	I will schedule a workout for an hour every Tuesday and Thursday right after work.
I will eat out less often.	I will cook dinner at home at least four days a week using simple recipes from this book.

Specific goals are more measureable. Measureable goals are easier to track and help you visualize your progress. Work on one or two measurable goals at a time. To measure some of the goals from Table 4-3, simply keep a journal for the week. Let's say your initial goal is to eat 3 servings of fruit daily. You can easily measure that by recording your intake daily and comparing it to the goal.

You can do the same for exercise, but you can also measure the activity itself (not just completing it, but the intensity or duration of it). If you begin a walking routine and it takes you 60 minutes to walk 3 miles, you may consider setting a goal to improve your speed. Measure this goal by using a watch and timing your walks, and then you can easily see your progress.

You can also take some baseline measurements right before you make changes in diet and lifestyle and then come back and measure them in three months (fruit/vegetable servings, weight when starting DASH, waist measurement, and so on).

TIP

The scale is an objective measurement tool, but don't get overly obsessed with it, especially if it isn't budging or your weight loss is slow going. Body weight is one aspect of health, but there are others. Meeting your weekly exercise goals and goals to improve the quality of your daily diet is wonderful progress in the right direction. Sometimes getting overly concerned with the number on the scale can be negative feedback that sends you off track.

Consider using your smartphone or a fitness tracker (like a Fitbit) to track your sitting and standing goals. Let's face it, we sit too much. Simply working toward more movement and standing in your day-to-day life helps keep your metabolism revving. You can set goals into your program and continue to track and improve.

Also consider how attainable your goal is. Losing 30 pounds by next month isn't attainable, but breaking that goal into smaller, doable goals — such as "I will lose 2 pounds over the next week" — feels a lot more attainable. Setting attainable goals is all about being realistic and *not* setting yourself up to fail.

Setting realistic goals helps you move forward and stay on track. Realistic goals aren't self-defeating; they're doable. Try to be honest with yourself. If you've never eaten fruits and vegetables on a daily basis, then don't set yourself up for failure by setting the unrealistic goal that starting tomorrow, you're going to eat 8 servings of fruits and vegetables a day. It probably won't happen. Start small, and then build on that. A small step forward is still a step in the right direction.

Goals should be timely too. While you want them to be realistic, it's still helpful to look down the road a bit and set the bigger goals you want to achieve. For instance, maybe you started jogging a mile a day. You may set a goal to add a quarter mile to that every week, to be able to run 3 miles in 8 weeks, and to enter a 5K race in 12 weeks. Placing goals on an incremental timeline helps you achieve them more successfully.

TIP

Recording an end date can keep goals timely and help make sure they happen. Whether you set goals for behaviors that need to occur daily, weekly, or over a period of months, putting the timeline in place helps you stay on track:

>> I will plan my meals and snacks.

>> I will weigh myself every Tuesday to track my weight-loss progress.

>> I will begin eating two extra servings of fruit per day.

>> I will cook two new vegetables this week.

Having a visual goal sheet in writing can help you stick to your plan and be accountable. Figure 4-1 provides an example of how you may record your goals.

Goal: _____

Specific:
Measurable:
Achievable:
Realistic:
Timely:

Obstacles: Solutions:

FIGURE 4-1: Sample goal worksheet.

© John Wiley & Sons, Inc.

REMEMBER

Setting too many goals all at once can be overwhelming and unproductive. Try to work on two to three goals at a time. After a goal becomes an everyday habit, check it off and move on to a new goal.

HOW MANY CALORIES DO YOU NEED?

Several clinical formulas can determine how many calories a person needs, but you can use a phone app or this general rule of thumb to give you a good estimate: Multiplying your body weight in pounds by 10 or 15 (use 10 if you're older or more sedentary and 15 if you're regularly active) gives you the approximate number of calories you burn daily. If you're overweight or obese, you need to reduce this amount to lose weight. The following table breaks down the daily calorie needs for women:

Age (Years)	Calories (Sedentary)	Calories (Moderately Active)	Calories (Active)
19–30	2,000	2,000–2,200	2,400
31–50	1,800	2,000	2,200
51+	1,600	1,800	2,000–2,200

Here are the daily calorie needs for men:

Age (Years)	Calories (Sedentary)	Calories (Moderately Active)	Calories (Active)
19–30	2,400	2,600–2,800	3,000
31–50	2,200	2,400–2,600	2,800–3,000
51+	2,000	2,200–2,400	2,400–2,800

Remember: If you need to lose weight, you have to create a calorie deficit by either reducing your intake of calories or burning more calories through exercise — or, ideally, both. And it's not just about calories. The balance of nutrients is important, too. Including enough healthy fat and protein, as well as plenty of fiber, in your diet helps with nutrition and satiety, so make smart choices.

Tracking your progress

Keeping a record of your food intake and exercise routine can help you measure your success. Writing these things down helps you organize your goals, stay on track, and ultimately lower your blood pressure.

For instance, say you set a goal to add more low-fat dairy foods to your diet. Ask yourself: "How many more servings of dairy am I consuming every day now?" Perhaps you've also set some goals to increase physical activity: "Have I accomplished my goal to exercise for an hour three days a week?" Keep in mind that your goals are specific to you and they change over time.

TIP

It's a good idea to keep a food and exercise record every day for the first week or two after you begin the DASH lifestyle. After the first couple of weeks, you can just check in with yourself two or three days a week and record those days. The purpose of tracking your progress is to help you see what's missing in your diet and help you focus on specific goals. You'll be surprised how much it helps you focus and stay on track.

After a goal becomes habit, you can move on to the next goal. Some people find setting up a reward system motivating. Perhaps one of your dietary goals is to replace the candy bar you eat every afternoon with a piece of fruit or a yogurt parfait. You can set up a reward system related to the goal, like treating yourself to a manicure or a movie on Saturday if you skip the candy bar every day that week.

Of course, everyone has setbacks, and you may occasionally blow off your diet and exercise plans. If this happens after you stop recording your progress, resume writing down what you eat and when and how much you exercise. It's also helpful to create a simple to-do list for the following day after you've overindulged. This can be something as simple as, "Tomorrow, I'll have yogurt, a banana, and one slice of whole-grain toast for breakfast; I'll go for a walk at lunchtime and order a salad; and I'll cook dinner at home." You can also consider writing out a meal plan for the next few days as well. That way, when it's time to eat, you don't even have to think about it.

TIP

If you're looking for a tool to help you learn how to write goals and track them, check out coauthor Rosanne's book *Calorie Counter Journal For Dummies* (Wiley). You can also check out the many phone apps that are available and record your progress there.

Planning around Obstacles

Consider any barriers that may be present as you set and track your goals. First and foremost, think of the eating habits of the people you live with. Do you have children in the house who enjoy cookies or ice cream regularly? Does having these foods around tempt you to go overboard? Speak openly with your housemates about why it's important to you to make lifestyle changes toward better heart health. Although children may have a bit more leeway when it comes to raiding the cookie jar, they still require several servings of fruit, vegetables, and dairy each day too, so setting a heart-healthy example actually benefits the whole family.

Vacations, holidays, and special events (like your coworker's wedding or the upcoming family reunion) can also hinder your progress toward a healthier lifestyle — if you let them. It's totally fine to enjoy yourself, but regroup the week after a big event. We know we sound like a broken record, but a good plan will help you avoid getting completely off track and losing all the progress you've made. Although we want you to enjoy these special occasions, we also know you'll feel better if you take care of yourself by eating well and exercising during these special times. Modify your goals during busy times (instead of a 45-minute walk, schedule a 20-minute walk) and use the tips in Chapter 15 to get you through vacations and special times.

Perhaps your fatal flaw when it comes to changing your lifestyle is your schedule — or lack thereof. A routine can keep you on track, meaning less snacking and skipping of meals. Although no two people's schedules are the same, establishing your own daily routine helps you achieve your daily and weekly goals. Consider this:

>> Plan to eat three meals a day, and include two snacks.

>> Space meals and snacks out throughout the day to keep hunger in check and also to give you opportunities to fit in all the food groups.

>> Schedule your exercise into your week on specific days at specific times. Consider morning exercise, as people who exercise first thing in the morning tend to be more consistent.

One of the best things you can do to improve your odds of achieving your goals is to plan ahead for pitfalls so you can more easily address problems as they surface. Following is our handy list of recommendations for avoiding troublesome situations:

>> **Have a snack plan in place.** Because one of the goals of DASH is to increase fruits and vegetables, aren't they a great snack option at least once daily? Keep those vegetables clean, sliced, and ready to eat in your fridge. Have fruit available on the counter so that you're cued to grab a piece, and pack two pieces of fruit to bring with you to work each day. Because you'll also want to include healthy fats like nuts and olives each week, these are other snack options to have a few times a week.

>> **Remove temptation.** If you keep snack crackers or candy at your desk, remove them. Instead, replace those unhealthy snacks with small portions of dried fruit and nuts, small cans of low-sodium vegetable juice, or a bowl of clementines.

>> **Make healthy swaps.** Swap healthier snacks for not-so-healthy ones. Enjoy a banana spread with a tablespoon of nut butter or have a fruit-yogurt parfait. You can also make exercise a healthy swap for midday stress eating by getting up for a ten-minute walk instead. If you find yourself getting antsy at work midafternoon and start heading to the vending machine, change it up. Take a walk up two flights of stairs, get a drink of water, and walk back to your desk refreshed. Or step outside and walk around the block and back. A five-minute change of scenery can do wonders midday to relieve tension that sometimes results in emotional eating.

>> **Plan ahead to avoid overeating.** If you sometimes eat past the point of being full or eat out of boredom or simply pleasure, consider ways to plan ahead. Be mindful of portions and set an intention to serve yourself half your usual portion and slow down at the table.

>> **Take a break.** Sometimes your body just may need a reset. There's evidence that intermittent fasting or time-restricted eating may help with appetite control. Consider only eating during a 10- to 12-hour period (say, from 7:30 a.m. to 7:30 p.m.) and having fewer calories one day a week (eat three healthy meals, but skip the in-between snack).

>> **Seek out support.** Find a friend to help keep you on track, whether it's an exercise partner or someone that you can simply talk to about your dietary goals. A cheery support system can do wonders when your attitude needs adjusting!

Chapter **5**

Presenting Your DASH Nutrition Primer

re you ready and raring to start eating your way to a healthy heart, lower blood pressure, and improved overall health? Great! Just promise us you'll read this chapter first so you can get a truly solid understanding of the principles of the DASH diet. First, we help you recognize where salt — long considered an enemy in the battle against hypertension — is lurking in your life. Then we help you figure out just how much sodium you need in your diet and how to start reducing your intake to get to that level. Finally, we get you excited about all the delicious foods you'll be *adding* to your diet when you start following the DASH diet framework.

Revealing Where Sodium Hides

Many factors influence the development of high blood pressure, as we explain in Chapter 6, but sodium is one of the components of the DASH diet that requires your attention, and for good reason. In scientific tests analyzing sodium's effect on blood pressure, about half of participants with high blood pressure were labeled *salt-sensitive* (salt sensitivity also increases with age). This label means that their blood pressure decreased with a very low sodium diet, then increased when a sodium solution was offered. Why the increase? Too much sodium in the diet promotes water retention in the body, which can affect the kidney's ability to regulate blood pressure.

REMEMBER

These two electrolytes are important to normal body function. A diet low in potassium causes the body to retain sodium too. When potassium levels are low, the body hoards it and consequently holds on to sodium, too. This causes the fluid retention. DASH provides you with plenty of potassium when you meet your fruit, vegetable, and dairy goals. Adding certain fish (salmon, snapper, mahi-mahi, and tuna) to the diet helps add potassium, too.

So, how can you reduce your sodium intake? First, you need to understand where the sodium is coming from in your current diet. The following sections help you do just that.

Processed foods

According to the U.S. Centers for Disease Control and Prevention, most of the sodium Americans consume comes from processed and restaurant foods. Only a small amount comes from salting food or adding salt during cooking (which is why it's okay to add a pinch in your cooking here and there). Generally speaking, the more processed the food, the more likely it is to have a higher sodium content. Table 5-1 gives you an idea of what we mean. Even with a quick glance, you can see that the farther a food gets from its natural state, the more sodium it has.

TABLE 5-1   **Comparing Sodium in Foods**

Food	No or Low Sodium	Moderate Sodium	High Sodium
Condiments and spices	Herbs, spices, low-sodium mustard, and red pepper sauce	Salted herb/spice blends, barbecue sauce, ketchup, steak sauce, salad dressing, tomato sauce/puree, and Worcestershire sauce	Seasoning salts, soy sauce, teriyaki sauce, dried soup mixes, and bouillon cubes
Grains	Low-sodium breads and crackers, oatmeal (not instant), rice, and pasta	Regular breads and rolls, dry cereals, muffins, instant hot cereals (like oatmeal), pancakes, waffles, pastries, cakes, and cookies	Canned spaghetti, refrigerator biscuit and cookie dough, boxed mixes for pancakes and macaroni and cheese, boxed potatoes, stuffing mixes, and salted crackers, chips, popcorn, and pretzels

Food	No or Low Sodium	Moderate Sodium	High Sodium
Fruits and vegetables	Fresh fruit, fruit juices, fresh or frozen unsalted vegetables, no-salt-added canned vegetables	Canned vegetables	Pickles, olives, pickled vegetables, canned vegetable juice, and frozen vegetables with sauces
Meats, eggs, beans, and nuts	Fresh beef, pork, poultry, eggs, low-sodium canned tuna, and unsalted nuts	Canned beans (rinsed), frozen "healthy" entrees (with less than 500 mg of sodium), fresh fish, deli meats, peanut butter, and low-sodium canned soups	Hot dogs, sausage, bacon, smoked meats, canned soups, frozen dinners, packaged lunchmeats, raw poultry or pork products that are injected with sodium solution, and canned tuna, clams, crab, and salmon
Dairy	Milk, sherbet, ice cream, and ricotta	Buttermilk, yogurt, aged hard cheeses, feta cheese, Parmesan cheese, cottage cheese, and pudding	Processed cheese (like American) and blue cheese

REMEMBER

Some high–sodium foods (like olives) are still healthy. You just have to balance that sodium out during the day with all the foods you choose. On the other hand, choosing fresh meats over processed ones and skipping boxed mixes of foods like rice or potatoes is always a good idea.

You can also find sodium tucked away in a variety of common foods:

>> **Bottled salad dressings and tomato sauces:** Making your own salad dressings and tomato sauces can help you cut back on your sodium intake.

>> **Breads and cereals:** Some varieties are higher than others in the sodium department, so compare labels before you buy. Note the sodium listed on the Nutrition Facts label and choose the varieties with the lesser amounts.

>> **Canned foods:** Canned goods, including beans and vegetables, are convenient because they have a long shelf life and because all you have to do is heat them up. Unfortunately, sodium is the reason their shelf life is so long. Look for no-salt-added canned foods and rinse all canned beans and vegetables before you eat them to help reduce their sodium content.

>> **Cheesy foods, pizza, sausage, hot dogs, bacon, deli meats, ready-to-eat foods, canned soups, canned pasta, boxed dinner mixes, pouch recipe kits, and frozen meals:** Yes, all these foods add convenience to dinnertime chaos, but they also have lots of sodium. Making more homemade foods can help you reduce your intake of these high-sodium culprits. Find tips about stocking your pantry and freezer in Chapter 13.

- » **Condiments and sauces:** Although they add zing to dishes, condiments and sauces can be surprisingly high in sodium. For instance, 1 tablespoon of soy sauce contains 1,800 milligrams of sodium. Use smaller amounts of condiments and sauces or look for low-sodium varieties to reduce the amount of salt you eat.

- » **Flavoring packets that come with foods, such as quick-cooking rice dishes and other packaged "all-in-one" pasta dishes:** If the packet is separate from the rice or pasta, use just half of it to flavor the dish and reduce the sodium. Better yet, go for plain rice and pasta and add your own fresh seasonings.

- » **Frozen, processed chicken breasts:** Salt is added as a preservative to many frozen chicken breasts. Check the label and buy fresh chicken breasts instead (to save money and time, you can always buy them in bulk and freeze the unused breasts for later use).

- » **Rotisserie chicken:** Store-bought rotisserie chicken is higher in sodium than fresh chicken. If you're in a real pinch and don't have time to roast your own chicken, go ahead and use the store-bought one, but try to choose lower-sodium sides to balance out the meal (think a tossed green salad or steamed frozen green beans tossed with olive oil and herbs). Removing the skin also cuts sodium, and if you're going to use the chicken for shredding (as in soft tacos or a salad), you can also rinse it and pat dry.

- » **Spice or herb blends:** Spice blends often aren't labeled with the word *salt* but have salt added anyway. Look for *salt-free* on the front of the package or read the ingredients list in search of *salt*.

REMEMBER

When you're trying to figure out whether something you're about to eat is too sodium-heavy, keep in mind this general rule of thumb: The fresher the food, the lower the sodium content. Similarly, the more processed the food, the higher the sodium.

A SURPRISING SODIUM SOURCE

You probably never guessed you'd have to worry about getting salt from medicine. Well, think again. Sodium hides in many over-the-counter (OTC) meds. We recommend checking the labels before you buy and talking to your doctor if one of your regular OTC meds is pretty high in sodium. He may be able to suggest a lower-sodium alternative.

Table salt alternatives

Today's grocery store shelves are lined with coarse salt, grinding salt, kosher salt, Italian sea salt, Hawaiian sea salt, regular sea salt, and so on. Having a different name or flavor doesn't mean they're healthy. In fact, the sea salt, gourmet salt, and potassium chloride alternatives to traditional table salt *aren't* healthier, they're just different.

The broad term *sea salt* describes salt derived from the ocean or sea. It's harvested by channeling ocean water into clay trays and allowing the sun and wind to evaporate the water, leaving behind salt crystals. As a result, sea salt is generally less processed than table salt. You may notice a subtle difference in flavor, but its nutritional profile is essentially the same as traditional table salt.

TIP

The one benefit to using sea salt may involve table use. If you grind sea salt instead of using refined table salt from a shaker, you may find that you use less because grinding takes more time. Also, table salt pours so easily that you may accidently add too much, so grinding keeps you from overdoing it by accident. Still, the sodium content of each is about the same by weight, so don't add double the salt just because it's sea salt. Also, keep in mind that table salt is fortified with iodine, an essential nutrient, so do use some regular table salt in your cooking. All added salt should be used in small amounts, however.

Figuring Out How Much Sodium You Really Need

Sodium is a mineral that's important to good health, but many people consume way more sodium each day than they actually need. The tricky thing is that the recommendation for sodium intake varies. According to the 2010 Dietary Guidelines for Americans (DGA), it's 1,500 milligrams (mg) daily. The American Heart Association (AHA) recommends no more than 2,300 milligrams a day (but ideally only 1,500 milligrams), and the World Health Organization (WHO) recommends consuming less than 2,000 milligrams daily (and adds that you should also consume 3,510 milligrams of potassium). The bottom line? Reducing your sodium intake helps reduce high blood pressure.

TECHNICAL STUFF

Although there are no guidelines in place for a minimum requirement for sodium, there are Adequate Intake (AI) and Upper Limit (UL) guidelines. According to the U.S. Department of Agriculture, AI is defined as "the recommended average daily intake level based on observed or experimentally determined approximations or estimates of nutrient intake by a group (or groups) of apparently healthy people that are assumed to be adequate — used when an RDA cannot be determined."

The AI for sodium is 1,500 milligrams per day. The UL — the highest average daily nutrient intake level that is likely to pose no risks of adverse health effects — set for sodium is 2,300 milligrams daily for adults.

Although the organizations that issue nutrition guidelines can't seem to agree on sodium, you can be confident in one thing: Reducing sodium intake to 1,500 to 3,000 milligrams daily is good for the heart (and conveniently part of the DASH diet). The DASH-Sodium study checked out three sodium levels — 3,000, 2,400, and 1,500 milligrams — and showed that along with the DASH diet principles, blood pressure was reduced at each sodium level but was reduced twice as much with the 1,500-milligram sodium level.

Reducing Your Salt Intake by Retraining Your Taste Buds

Human taste buds recognize several types of flavors: sweet, sour, bitter, salty, and umami (savory). Some people are more naturally drawn to sweeter flavors, and others are drawn to saltier ones. Habit plays a role, no matter what the food preference may be.

So why does it seem that salt makes some foods taste better? Salt can reduce the bitterness in vegetables and therefore make them more appealing to some people. There also seems to be a link between the increasing amounts of sodium in the food supply and people's desire for salty foods. In other words, the more high sodium your intake, the more used to that salty flavor you get.

REMEMBER

If you're accustomed to using a lot of salt, reducing your salt intake is a must if you have high blood pressure, but doing so often means training your taste buds to prefer less-salty foods. It'll take some effort, but it's doable. Your palate will adjust, although it may take a few months. In addition, aging can bring changes in smell and taste. Your taste buds become less sensitive to sweet, salty, sour, and bitter. We share our advice for reducing sodium intake in the next sections. In Chapter 13 and the recipe chapters, you find out how to boost flavor and set up a DASH-friendly kitchen.

Stepping away from the salt shaker

While processed foods make up the majority of a high-sodium intake, not all the sodium in your diet is secretly tucked away in a loaf of bread or a can of tomato sauce. In fact, a lot of the salt that makes its way into your diet may be right out in the open — in the form of the salt shaker. Table salt itself adds a lot of sodium to the diet. Just one level teaspoon of salt provides 2,300 milligrams of sodium.

Here are some tips to help you start cutting back on how often you use the salt shaker:

>> Taste food before salting it. If you're in the habit of shaking salt onto your burgers, fries, or other foods before you even taste them, try having a few bites first to make sure additional flavor is really necessary. If you need a little more kick, add some ground black pepper or a dash of red pepper flakes rather than salt.

>> Don't shake salt inside the skillet or pan when cooking. Instead, stock your spice rack with new spices. Using sodium-free spices and herbs, such as basil, curry, garlic, ginger, mint, oregano, pepper, paprika, rosemary, and thyme really will kick up the flavor of your food. Look for salt-free spice blends, too.

>> Instead of salting meats or vegetables when sautéing, add balsamic vinegar or wine to the pan.

>> Enjoying some high-fiber popcorn? Hold the shaker! Another way to use less is to load your pepper shaker with salt (it has fewer holes). Try shaking the salt into your hand first to see it; you'll use less this way. You can also find salt-free seasoning powders to add zing to your corn.

>> When cooking eggs, add flavor with vegetables and other ingredients rather than pouring on the salt.

>> Going out for happy hour with friends? Skip the salted rim on that margarita!

REMEMBER

If you're a true-blue salt lover, don't lose heart. When you're on the DASH diet, keep in mind that low-sodium doesn't mean no-sodium. In fact, most of the recipes in this book contain some sodium and even a pinch of salt. Although some recipes may be higher in sodium than others, they represent only one item or meal in your diet. You can balance out a saltier meal with less-salty meals the rest of the day.

Employing table salt substitutes

Sometimes physicians prescribe *potassium chloride*, a salt composed of potassium and chlorine, to treat low blood potassium levels. Potassium chloride is a salt, like sodium chloride. Although people often think of sodium chloride when they use the term *salt*, chemically there are many types of salts (another example is the calcium chloride used to salt roadways in the winter).

You can also find "light" salt mixtures or *salt substitutes* at the supermarket in the salt or spice section. These salt substitutes contain less sodium and often include potassium chloride. Potassium salts taste similar to sodium chloride, but they have a slightly bitter or metallic aftertaste on the tongue. Some salt substitutes may contain potassium and *lysine* (an amino acid that has a salty taste). A "light" salt may be a mixture of sodium chloride and potassium chloride (thereby cutting the sodium by half).

WARNING

Don't use a salt substitute without first checking with your physician. Depending on your complete medical history (and especially if you have kidney disease), using a potassium chloride product may be harmful. For this reason, we encourage you to use natural alternatives, such as herbs and spices, rather than salt substitutes.

Examining the DASH Diet Framework

The DASH diet involves eating less of certain types of foods and more of others. The focus is on lowering sodium and increasing potassium. The fruit and vegetable group supplies lots of potassium, as does the dairy group. In general, eating the DASH way means reducing the portion sizes of all meats (chicken, beef, pork, lamb, and fish) and increasing the portion sizes of plant foods. (For a bonus, you can add some nuts and seeds to your meals.) We offer up numerous recipes in Part 4, but here we focus on breaking down the components of the DASH diet one by one.

REMEMBER

Although there isn't complete proof that eating certain foods or exercising regularly allows you to live to be 100, there's no question in our minds that lifestyle changes add life to your years. Making healthy changes in your diet and lifestyle help you bring down your blood pressure, improve your overall heart health, have more energy, and generally feel better, allowing you to do the things you love. (For help identifying lifestyle changes you can make aside from modifying your eating habits, see Chapter 16.)

2 to 3 servings of low-fat dairy

The clinical trials that led to the DASH diet, which we describe in Chapter 2, showed that the greatest reductions in blood pressure correlated to an intake of low-fat dairy products, which is why DASH calls for eating 2 to 3 servings of low-fat dairy each day. If you're overweight, choosing low-fat dairy products helps keep calories under control. (As an added bonus, studies have shown that drinking low-fat milk helps promote weight loss.)

TECHNICAL STUFF

Dairy isn't just helpful for blood pressure. Several studies have concluded that intake of nonfat or low-fat dairy products is associated with reduced risk for diabetes, hypertension, and cardiovascular events. Other studies have shown that calcium can reduce LDL (bad cholesterol) and increase HDL (good cholesterol). In addition, adequate calcium throughout life is important to bone health, and most milks are fortified with vitamin D, which helps the body absorb more calcium.

Adding calcium to your diet is a DASH-certified strategy for reducing high blood pressure. You can get about 100 to 150 milligrams of calcium per cup from vegetables such as broccoli, kale, beet greens, or bok choy, but an 8-ounce glass of nonfat milk easily provides more than 300 milligrams of calcium.

REMEMBER

Although low-fat dairy was used in the DASH trials and, in general, helps support weight-loss efforts if you're overweight, you can still choose some full-fat dairy if you like. New research has suggested that full-fat dairy products are not associated with heart disease risk. Instead, it seems that the positive benefits of consuming dairy products for heart health outweigh any risk.

TIP

Here are some sample servings of low-fat dairy, with each serving providing about 300 milligrams of calcium:

>> **8 ounces nonfat (skim) or 1% milk:** You can drink it with meals or use it in cooking or baking.

>> **½ cup part-skim ricotta:** Although it's higher in fat, it's also much higher in calcium than cottage cheese.

>> **1 cup pudding made with skim milk:** This is a great calcium-rich dessert that can fit into DASH.

>> **8 ounces nonfat yogurt:** Look for yogurt that's non-sweetened (plain) or lightly sweetened or that uses a non-caloric sweetener.

Choosing a scoop of nonfat frozen yogurt rather than a scoop of ice cream can save you about 8 grams of fat per serving. Additionally, each ½-cup serving provides 100 milligrams of calcium, compared to 60 milligrams in a ½-cup serving of most ice cream brands.

Check out Table 5-2 to see which common foods have the most calcium for the fewest calories. The foods in the table are listed from highest to lowest in terms of their calcium content.

TABLE 5-2

Calcium and Calories in Common Foods

Food	Amount	Calcium (mg)	Calories
Yogurt, plain, low-fat	8 ounces	225	155
Cheddar cheese	1.5 ounces	300	180
Milk, 1%	8 ounces	300	100
Yogurt, fruit, low-fat	8 ounces	200	240
Cottage cheese, 1% fat	1 cup	140	160
Spinach, cooked	½ cup	120	40
Frozen yogurt, soft-serve	½ cup	100	120
Kale	1 cup	95	35
Ice cream, vanilla	½ cup	85	200
Broccoli	½ cup	20	25

Clearly, nonfat and low-fat dairy products are the way to go to meet your daily calcium needs. But just what are those needs? Adults ages 19 to 50 need about 1,000 milligrams of calcium daily. After age 51, the National Institutes of Health recommends females up their intake to 1,200 milligrams daily, whereas most sources say men can maintain 1,000 milligrams.

So if your calcium intake should be 1,000 milligrams per day, perhaps you can try consuming a glass of 1% milk with breakfast, a half-cup of yogurt mid-morning, a scoop of cottage cheese on your salad at lunch, a side of spinach with dinner, and a scoop of frozen yogurt for dessert. Not so bad, huh?

REMEMBER

Dairy foods also add some potassium to the diet, about 360 milligrams per 8-ounce cup. (For comparison's sake, a banana has about 420 milligrams of potassium.) Potassium is an important mineral for blood pressure and heart health.

TIP

What can you do if dairy's not for you? If you don't enjoy plain milk, it's okay to add some flavoring. Adding 1 to 2 teaspoons of chocolate syrup only adds about 35 calories and still delivers all the calcium in the milk. You can also make a smoothie or smoothie bowl, an iced mocha, or a tea drink. To make a smoothie bowl, check out the Breakfast Smoothie Bowl recipe in Chapter 17. To make an iced mocha or latte just add 4 ounces of nonfat milk to 4 ounces of plain coffee (for mocha, add 1 teaspoon of chocolate syrup, too) or brewed tea. Shake with ice and enjoy. If your body can't tolerate milk because of lactose intolerance or some other issue, you can try soy milk, calcium-fortified almond milk, or calcium-fortified orange juice. You can also try out milk that has had the lactase enzyme added to it.

PLANT-BASED ALTERNATIVES TO COW'S MILK

Cow's milk alternatives — such as almond, cashew, oat, or soy milk — are gaining popularity, but they aren't nutritionally the same. Cow's milk offers calcium, potassium, vitamin D, vitamin B12, and protein. Nutritionally speaking, soy milk is the most equivalent to cow's milk in terms of protein and potassium. Almond milk and cashew milk are fortified with calcium, but they aren't a good source of protein.

Choosing a plant-based milk is fine if you enjoy the flavor, are vegan, or are lactose intolerant. Just keep in mind that the DASH research was based on including cow's milk to further reduce blood pressure.

THE SCOOP ON CALCIUM SUPPLEMENTS

Most experts agree that getting your calcium from your diet is your best bet, but you can check with your doctor to see whether supplements are a good option for you. Calcium supplements fall into two categories: calcium carbonate and calcium citrate. Calcium citrate works well for people with reflux who have reduced stomach acid because of taking acid-blockers, whereas calcium carbonate is readily available, well absorbed, and generally less expensive.

When checking out various supplements, look at the amount of elemental calcium on the Nutrition Facts label. For instance, a 500-milligram calcium carbonate pill may provide only 200 milligrams of elemental calcium (the pill itself isn't pure calcium and only supplies 40 percent calcium by weight; calcium citrate supplies only about 20 percent calcium by weight). In general, look for the USP seal on a supplement (dietary supplements are poorly regulated, so having the United States Pharmacopeia approval assures quality and standards).

It's probably not necessary to take a supplement that promises more than 100 percent of the daily requirements. Research has suggested that issues may be inherent in over-supplementing with calcium. Keep in mind that a calcium pill is a *supplement* to the dietary calcium you ingest. We can't say it enough: Check with your doctor before taking any supplements.

4 to 5 servings of vegetables

The DASH diet calls for 4 to 5 servings of vegetables daily, which is no surprise because vegetables are a valuable source of nutrients that are important for heart health. Vegetables provide a wide variety of important minerals, one of which is potassium. Potassium plays a role in muscle contraction and is crucial to heart function. A diet low in potassium has been associated with an increased risk for hypertension and stroke. Conversely, a diet higher in potassium has been associated with lower blood pressure.

Vegetables are also full of vitamins, several of which are antioxidants. Antioxidants protect against *free radicals,* molecules that damage cells in the body. Vitamins A, C, and E plus beta carotene are all antioxidants. You can also find *phytochemicals* in vegetables; these are substances in plants that may have protective properties. (To find out more about phytochemicals, check out the nearby sidebar.)

TIP

The best — and most fun — way to incorporate vegetables in your diet is to eat the rainbow: red, orange, yellow, green, blue, and violet. Blue food, you say? Yes, sir, and we're not talking cotton candy. Believe it or not, there are naturally occurring foods that can add every spectrum of the rainbow to your diet. So pick up those purple potatoes or that green cauliflower the next time you're at the grocery store.

Adding more vegetables to your day is easier than you may think. Here's an example:

>> Slice a ripe tomato onto your cheese-topped English muffin for breakfast or add some chunky salsa and vegetables to your two-egg omelet.

>> Add shredded cabbage to your wrap and have a cup of low-sodium vegetable soup or a spinach salad with lunch.

>> Nosh on sugar snap peas at your desk midday.

>> Make it a habit to create a mixed green or tomato and cucumber salad as a side with dinner each night. Or add lots of extra chopped vegetables to a homemade pasta salad.

>> You can also add a handful of greens to a smoothie with sliced apples or berries, ½ avocado, and a teaspoon of honey. The fruit masks the greens' bitterness, and your body will appreciate the quick nutrition boost.

>> Grill some asparagus or zucchini to go along with your evening meal.

PHYTOCHEMICALS

Scientists are still figuring out all the benefits of a phytochemical-rich diet, but suffice it to say, eating plant foods with these nutrients promotes heart health, helps you retain healthy vision, likely reduces some cancer risk, and even offers anti-aging perks. Several important phytochemicals are present in plant foods. In addition to serving all the afore-mentioned purposes, many phytochemicals (specifically plant sterols, flavonoids, and sulfur-containing compounds) found in fruits and vegetables also act as antioxidants in the body, potentially protecting your body's cells from disease, including cancer. With all those benefits, why not eat as many phytochemicals as you can? A few of the best phytochemicals include

- **Allicin:** This sulfur-containing compound is found in garlic and onions and may be important to heart health because of its antiplatelet (anti-blood-clotting) properties.

- **Anthocyanins:** Look to blue and purple foods for these flavonoids that have been shown to help with memory and urinary tract health. They also have anti-aging benefits.

- **Carotenoids:** Contained primarily in red and orange foods (but also in some green foods), carotenoids help promote healthy vision and may reduce cancer risk. Lycopene is an example of a carotenoid found in red foods.

- **Flavanols:** Found in red foods such as apples, berries, red grapes, and red wine, and also in yellow and green foods such as yellow onions, kale, and broccoli, flava-nols promote heart health and may help reduce stroke risk. Flavanols are also present in chocolate and teas.

- **Flavanones:** Found in citrus fruits and juices, flavanones can lower your risk of gastrointestinal cancer.

- **Indoles/isothiocyanates:** Found in green and white cruciferous vegetables, such as broccoli, cabbage, cauliflower, and kale. Indoles and isothiocyanates have anti-cancer qualities.

- **Lutein:** Green and orange foods — including egg yolks, mangoes, peaches, sweet potatoes, spinach, romaine lettuce, honeydew, pears, and avocados — contain the antioxidant lutein, which supports eye health.

- **Phytosterols:** Whole grains, legumes, and nuts contain phytosterols, which lower cholesterol.

4 to 5 servings of fruit

The DASH diet also includes a daily intake of 4 to 5 servings of fruit. You know that fruits are healthy because they provide essential vitamins and minerals, especially antioxidants and potassium, that your body needs. But did you know that thanks to their generally sweeter taste they can help satisfy sweet-tooth cravings while providing fiber as well?

TIP

Fruits can even help you reduce your sodium and help boost the flavor of a variety of main dishes, salads, and sides. This may sound a little unorthodox, but it works. For example, you can zest the peels of lemons, oranges, and limes into salad dressings, pasta salads, and potato dishes or onto fish or poultry to add a tasty punch without adding salt. You can also add dried fruits to stuffing to add new flavors to a stuffed turkey or chicken. When you sauté onions, add some chopped fresh peaches or mango to top baked fish.

You can also marinate poultry in the juices of fruits to avoid using salty sauces and store-bought marinades. Soak chicken pieces in ½ cup of orange juice along with your favorite fresh herbs to add flavor and moisture the next time you fire up the grill. After meat has marinated for an hour or more, place on the grill (always discard leftover marinade to avoid foodborne illness). Orange juice works well for baking mild white fish, too. Simply place fish into a glass baking dish, pour about a cup of orange juice over the fish, add fresh chives, and bake for 20 to 30 minutes at 350 degrees.

You can make traditional homemade salsas with tomatoes, but try adding some minced seasonal fruit to them for a sweet-hot flavor. Peaches, nectarines, mango, and pineapple all work well. Or put the fruit right on the grill. Adding any grilled fruit to beef or pork provides added flavor that helps you cut down on salt. Try grilled peach halves or pineapple slices alongside a small steak or grilled pork loin chop.

TIP

Eating the rainbow is a good approach to take with fruits (as well as vegetables, as we note in the preceding section). Having a banana every day is great, but don't stop there. Choose foods from the red, blue, and tan groups to include at other meals too! It's your diet over the week that matters, so don't worry if you come up short on one day. Mix and match by whipping up a healthy smoothie using apple and spinach, blueberries and banana, or strawberries and carrots. Pick out some of your favorite fruits in each color:

- **Green:** Apples, avocados, grapes, honeydew, kiwi, limes

- **Orange and deep yellow:** Apricots, cantaloupe, grapefruit, mangoes, papayas, peaches, pineapples

- **Purple and blue:** Blackberries, blueberries, cranberries, plums, prunes

- **Red:** Cherries, cranberries, pomegranate, red grapes, red/pink grapefruit, tomatoes, watermelon

- **White, tan, and brown:** Bananas, brown pears, dates, white peaches

6 to 8 servings of grains

Foods from the bread/grain/cereal group are an important component of the DASH eating plan because they supply fiber and a variety of vitamins and minerals. Based on a daily 2,000-calorie intake, the DASH plan recommends 6 to 8 servings of grains. The important thing here is portion. Although you should aim to make at least half of your grain choices whole grains, you can incorporate some refined grains (such as white, Italian, or French breads; regular pasta; and rice or corn cereals) into your diet. Better choices include whole-wheat or oatmeal breads, whole-wheat pasta, brown rice, whole-wheat crackers, whole-wheat cereals, bran cereals, oat bran, and oatmeal.

REMEMBER

When choosing whole-grain breads, look for the word *whole*. Don't assume that brown-colored "wheat bread" is a great choice. Check the Nutrition Facts label: Whole-wheat flour or another whole-grain flour should be listed as the first ingredient, and the bread should have 2 or more grams of fiber per serving. By comparison, a slice of white bread provides only 0.6 grams, or less, of fiber. Refined grains have the bran and germ removed, which eliminates the fiber. The vitamins and minerals taken with it are replaced after the milling process (this is what the term *enriched* means).

WARNING

It's easy to go overboard on grains, so make sure you understand what a single grain serving looks like. One serving of grains is one slice of bread, half a small bun, half an English muffin, ¼ of an average bakery bagel, ½ cup pasta or rice, one small waffle or half a Belgian waffle, or one 4-inch pancake. These may seem like smaller servings than what you're used to. Remember that if you eat the whole Belgian waffle (which is considered a treat, not your best day-to-day grain choice), it counts as 2 servings. One large bakery bagel represents 4 servings!

As you work at improving your diet to lower your blood pressure, consider venturing out into some new grain territory:

>> Barley

>> Brown rice and wild rice

>> Buckwheat

>> Bulgur (cracked wheat)

>> Oats

>> Quinoa

>> Whole-wheat couscous

Small servings of better fats

You've probably heard by now that fat isn't a problem; the real issue is whether you choose to eat what we call "better fats." DASH calls for small servings (2 to 3) of "better fats" daily, meaning the unsaturated fat that comes primarily from plant products and fish. These fats may help lower your blood cholesterol levels. Fat also helps with satiety. Adding some healthy fat to your meals will help you stay full longer and could actually help with weight management. You want to work at replacing most of the saturated fat (which comes mostly from animal products and packaged baked goods) in your diet with unsaturated fats.

Sources of good fats include fish, plant oils (but not palm or coconut oils), nuts, and seeds. Salmon, trout, olives, walnuts, avocado, and vegetable oils such as soybean, safflower, sunflower, corn, canola, and olive oils are all good choices. Unsaturated fats include both polyunsaturated and monounsaturated fats, and both of these may help lower cholesterol by lowering LDL.

WARNING

There is some evidence that omega-6 fatty acids (found in corn oil and soybean oil) may cause more inflammation in the body than other fats. Because DASH recommends swapping saturated fat for unsaturated fat, and a low-fat diet overall, this probably isn't a concern. Still, we recommend mostly cooking with olive, canola, or avocado oil, instead of corn oil or soybean oil.

REMEMBER

Palm oil and coconut oil are plant-based oils but are highly saturated. Some research shows that coconut oil may increase HDL, but we're uncertain how it impacts heart disease or cholesterol levels overall, so it's best to use it sparingly.

TIP

One serving of fat is equal to about 5 grams of fat. This represents 1 teaspoon or 1 tablespoon of fat, depending on the type. Check the Nutrition Facts label.

Cooking with healthy vegetable oils, adding nuts to salads and other dishes, and including fish on the menu through the week are some ways to add these good fats in. And we're on your side, too — the recipes we present in this book help you add these healthy fats to your diet. Try the Roasted Broccolini with Toasted Sesame Seeds in Chapter 20 or our Seared Scallops with Pistachio Sauce or Curry-Crusted Roasted Salmon in Chapter 19.

TIP

Look for ways to sneak good fats into your breakfast, lunch, or snack routine. Here are a few ideas to get you started:

>> Add chopped walnuts or pecans to your morning oatmeal.

>> Use canola oil to make homemade pancakes or muffins.

>> Try a small handful of almonds for a midday snack.

>> Enjoy 2 teaspoons of all-natural peanut butter on a banana or apple slices.

>> Make your own simple salad dressings using olive oil and vinegar.

>> Slice avocado for a sandwich topping.

>> Add olives to your tossed salad.

>> Add nuts to your stir-fry, pasta, or rice dish.

2 servings of lean proteins

Your body actually needs less protein than you realize, particularly on the DASH diet, because you'll be getting some protein from vegetables, grains, nuts, and seeds. Consequently, you need just 4 to 6 ounces of lean meat, fish, or poultry daily.

TIP

Choosing a meal with fish — preferably baked, grilled, or broiled — twice a week is a good habit to get into. Most any type of fish is fine, as long as you limit deep-fried fish to no more than once every couple of months. Fish varies in fat content, but fatty fish delivers healthy omega-3 fatty acids and is higher in monounsaturated fat and lower in saturated fat than beef or pork. Most fish is lower in calories as well.

In the case of poultry, you can choose from a variety of white and dark meats — without the skin. Removing the skin trims away more than half the total fat and nearly 70 percent of the saturated fat.

Choosing leaner cuts of beef and pork helps reduce your overall saturated fat intake, which is important for controlling blood cholesterol. In all cases, you can reduce the fat by trimming most of the visible fat from the meat before cooking. Limit your intake of high-fat cuts of beef (such as prime rib and chuck roast) and pork (like bacon, pork ribs, and shoulder) or avoid them altogether. Table 5-3 shows you how to size up lean meat portions. Each trimmed 3-to-4-ounce portion provides only about 3 to 10 grams of fat.

TABLE 5-3 **Making Lean Beef and Pork Choices**

Type	Cut	Portion
Beef	Sirloin	3–4 ounces
	Filet mignon	4–6 ounces
	Eye of round	4–6 ounces
	Loin roast	3–4 ounces
Pork	Tenderloin	4–6 ounces
	Loin chops	3–4 ounces
	Loin roast	3–4 ounces

4 to 5 servings of nuts, seeds, and legumes

DASH recommends you eat 4 to 5 servings per week of nuts, seeds, and legumes (lentils, beans, peas, and peanuts) to add even more protein, folate, and fiber to your diet.

Nuts and seeds are included in the DASH diet because of their healthy fat profile, magnesium, and fiber. Fiber has a multitude of health benefits for your heart and gut. Its heart-healthy benefits include helping your body keep cholesterol and fatty acids in check. Plus, it also helps with hunger and weight control by keeping you full longer. The omega-3 and omega-6 fatty acids provided by nuts and seeds can help keep your heart healthy.

TIP Omega-3 fatty acids are essential fats. Your body needs them to function properly, but it can't generate them, which means you need to consume these types of fats through your diet. Nuts and seeds, especially walnuts and flaxseed, contain ALA (alpha-linolenic acid). ALA is a type of omega-3 fatty acid that helps support heart health, appearing to protect the heart by reducing inflammation in the arteries, stabilizing the cell membranes, reducing the risk for blood clots, and lowering triglycerides. Omega-6 fatty acids, found in soybean, safflower, sunflower, and corn oils, as well as sunflower seeds and nuts, are also essential. There is some research that suggests omega-6 fatty acids are inflammatory, but when eaten in moderation, small amounts are fine. Like just about everything else, omega-3 and omega-6 fatty acids from food appear to be more protective than supplements.

TIP Most nuts are also a good source of potassium too, providing around 150 to 200 milligrams per ounce (an ounce of pistachios provides almost 300 milligrams; an ounce of nuts is less than ¼ cup). Choose unsalted nuts most often to keep sodium in check.

Nuts and seeds deliver quite a bit of fat, so it's a good idea to eat those only a few times a week or in very small amounts daily. (If eaten daily, consider about 10 to 15 peanuts, walnuts, almonds, or cashews to be a small daily portion.) See Chapter 14 for more on serving sizes. Legumes, on the other hand, are very low in fat and high in fiber and nutrients, so incorporating these into at least one meal a week is a super idea. Legumes are also great for controlling weight and preventing heart disease.

New to eating beans and legumes? Try our Black Bean 'n' Slaw Sliders in Chapter 21 to discover just how delicious they can taste.

2
DASHing toward Better Health

Find out what you need to know about pre-hypertension and hypertension, as well as what your blood pressure numbers really mean. Then take control of the situation with DASH.

Reduce your risk for heart disease, stroke, and kidney failure by making simple changes such as bumping up the servings of whole grains, fruits, and vegetables and lessening your intake of animal protein and saturated fat.

Recognize how excess weight can contribute to many serious health conditions, including diabetes, heart disease, and cancer. Although DASH wasn't created as a weight-loss diet, it can help you shed extra pounds thanks to its focus on portions and good nutrition.

Get the scoop on what factors contribute to diabetes, why it's such a serious health problem, and what you can do to prevent or reverse the disease. (Here's a hint: Adopting the DASH diet can help.)

Discover how DASH can protect the kidneys, improve brain function (especially as you grow older), and reduce cancer risk, regardless of your age, gender, or ethnicity.

IN THIS CHAPTER

» **Understanding the mechanics of heart function**

» **Homing in on how blood pressure is measured and classified**

» **Defining primary and secondary hypertension and examining risk factors**

» **Exploring the medical and dietary treatments used to treat high blood pressure**

Chapter **6**

Taking Charge of Hypertension

Hypertension is a fancy way of saying "high blood pressure." More than 100 million Americans (that's nearly half of all American adults) suffer from hypertension, yet close to 20 percent of those individuals are unaware they have a problem. According to the Centers for Disease Control and Prevention, hypertension contributes to more than 472,000 deaths each year in the United States alone. Worldwide, the death toll attributed to high blood pressure exceeds 7 million, or nearly 13 percent of all deaths, according to the World Health Organization (WHO). Many more will suffer life-changing and disabling complications of the disease. The majority of people who experience heart attacks, stroke, heart failure, and kidney failure suffer from hypertension, and in many cases, they could have avoided those devastating complications simply by lowering their blood pressure.

You don't have to be hyper or tense to develop hypertension, and most people with hypertension have no symptoms to tip them off. The silent existence of hypertension means you can be living with this dangerous condition without knowing it. Although genetics and age both play important roles in developing hypertension, lifestyle choices contribute enormously, and that means you have the power to take steps to keep your blood pressure in a safe range. This chapter helps you understand how your heart operates, what those mysterious blood pressure numbers indicate, and what kinds of hypertension exist. It also breaks down hypertension risk factors in simple language and surveys the types of medications you may need to treat hypertension in combination with the DASH diet.

A Crash Course in Cardiology

Your heart is a remarkable organ. In its natural, healthy state, it beats strong and steady, delivering freshly oxygenated blood from your lungs, through your arteries, supplying all your vital organs. After the blood is depleted of its life-sustaining oxygen, it's recycled through the veins, transferred back to the heart, and delivered to the lungs to be resupplied with oxygen. This cycle happens second after second, day after day, year after year.

TIP

To help you get a better mental picture (and understanding) of your heart as the extremely complicated yet compact organ that it is (see Figure 6-1), think of it like the cardiologists do — as consisting of pumps, pipes, and electrical wiring. If you're a kid, your heart is about the same size as your fist, and if you're a healthy adult, your heart is about the same size as two fists put together.

>> **Pumps:** The pumps are made up of your left and right ventricles, as well as the smaller left and right atria. The *left ventricle* is what propels the blood through the *aorta* (a muscular artery resembling a garden hose), through an intricate network of arteries, and then to your entire body. *Veins* (less muscular than arteries) carry the blood back toward the heart, eventually dumping it back into the right atrium by way of the superior and inferior venae cavae. From the right atrium, blood is rhythmically released into the *right ventricle,* which sends it back to the lungs. From the lungs, the blood enters the left atrium on its way back to the left ventricle, and the cycle starts all over again. Weakening or stiffening of the pump can cause congestive heart failure.

>> **Pipes:** The pipes are your *coronary arteries.* These small yet very important blood vessels siphon off some of the blood from the aorta to feed the heart muscle. A blockage in one of these arteries will lead to a heart attack.

>> **Wiring:** The wiring is what keeps your heart ticking in rhythm. Your heart is full of electrical tissue. Although the electricity usually flows in an orderly fashion, sometimes the wiring gets old and frayed, and that deterioration can cause the heart to slow down or beat erratically. Other times, you may have a short circuit or a rogue patch of electrical tissue that fires out of time with the rest of the heart, causing your rhythm to go haywire.

REMEMBER

Problems with one part of the heart can affect its other functions. For instance, a heart attack may damage the wiring as well as the pump. Hypertension can cause the pump to become weak or stiff, which in turn can lead to electrical problems. But even when the heart becomes damaged or overworked, it does its best to keep on ticking.

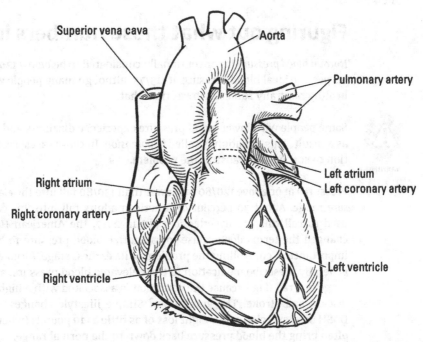

Superior vena cava

Aorta

Pulmonary artery

Right atrium

Left atrium
Left coronary artery

Right coronary artery

Left ventricle

Right ventricle

FIGURE 6-1:
The inner workings of the human heart.

Illustration by Kathryn Born

Zeroing In on Blood Pressure Basics

Blood pressure is a measure of the force that blood pulses through the arteries in the body. It's usually measured with a blood pressure cuff that consists of an inflatable arm cuff and a pressure gauge called a *sphygmomanometer.* The cuff inflates to a point that the *brachial artery* (the main artery in the arm) is briefly closed off. Then air is gradually released until a pulse is either heard with a stethoscope placed in the crease of the elbow or detected by an electronic machine. When medical staff folks take your blood pressure, they're listening for two things:

>> The point at which they hear sound is the *systolic pressure,* and it occurs when the heart contracts and blood is forced through the arteries.

» The point at which the pulse is no longer audible is the pressure when the heart relaxes; it's called the *diastolic pressure.*

TECHNICAL
STUFF

Blood pressure is measured in millimeters of mercury (mm Hg), a term that derives from the time of the original mercury-based blood pressure gauges. To keep things simple and avoid clutter, we just use the numbers by themselves.

Figuring out what those numbers indicate

Normal blood pressure is conventionally considered to be below 120/80. Some studies peg the ideal blood pressure at 115/75, although many people who are perfectly healthy naturally run even lower than that.

WARNING

Some people with lower blood pressure experience dizziness and lightheadedness as a result. This situation is called *hypotension.* In those cases, seek medical attention to sort out the cause of the problem.

Pressures at or above 120/80 but lower than 130/80 fall into the *elevated blood pressure* range. About 30 percent of American adults fall into this category. Doctors used to call this *pre-hypertension,* but in 2017, the American Heart Association changed the terms doctors use to categorize blood pressure to better reflect the importance of controlling the problem at its earliest stage. Although doctors don't generally prescribe medication to treat elevated blood pressure, a pressure in this range is a red flag because the condition is associated with a higher risk for heart disease and stroke. The good news? Simple lifestyle changes — including the DASH diet, exercise, and weight loss of as little as 10 pounds (when needed) — can often bring the blood pressure back down to the normal range.

REMEMBER

Blood pressure varies from individual to individual, but here are the ranges for normal, borderline, and high blood pressure. If the numbers seem lower than what you remember from years past, you're right. The categories were revamped in 2017 after new research found that damage to the heart and other organs begins at blood pressure levels previously thought to be normal:

» **Normal:** A systolic (upper) number less than 120 mm Hg *and* a diastolic (lower) number less than 80 mm Hg

» **Elevated:** A systolic (upper) number of 120–129 mm Hg *and* a diastolic (lower) number less than 80 mm Hg

» **Hypertension, stage 1:** A systolic (upper) number of 130–139 mm Hg *or* a diastolic (lower) number of 80–89 mm Hg

» **Hypertension, stage 2:** A systolic (upper) number of 140 mm Hg or higher *or* a diastolic (lower) number of 90 mm Hg or higher

>> **Hypertensive crisis:** A systolic (upper) number higher than 180 mm Hg *and/or* a diastolic (lower) number higher than 120 mm Hg

Understanding high blood pressure readings

Blood pressure isn't a single set of numbers. On a typical day, your blood pressure is likely to fluctuate up or down by about 20 percent. That's why your doctor will probably want to obtain at least three different readings on three different days before diagnosing you with hypertension. (Of course, if you have dangerously high blood pressure, you usually don't need to wait to start treatment; we cover the medical treatments of hypertension later in this chapter.)

Sometimes high blood pressure isn't really high blood pressure but rather "white coat hypertension" — also known as the spike in blood pressure that occurs when you visit the doctor. In fact, a study from the VA hospital system found an average 10-point difference between home blood pressure readings and office measurements. That's why having your own blood pressure machine at home is so useful. (We explain how to measure your own blood pressure in the nearby sidebar.) Although white coat hypertension is usually just a nuisance, nearly half of all individuals with the condition eventually develop persistently high blood pressure.

On the flip side, some people may experience *lower* readings in a doctor's office and higher readings at home. This situation is referred to as "masked hypertension," and it's yet another reason why keeping tabs on your own blood pressure is a good idea.

Although you can have both systolic and diastolic hypertension, elevations in just one or the other of the two numbers are common. People under the age of 50 are more apt to have high diastolic pressures, whereas those over 50 tend to have higher systolic numbers. That's because the systolic pressure often reflects hardening of the arteries, which is more common as people age. *Remember:* Both numbers are important, so you can't ignore your readings just because only one of the two is high.

TECHNICAL STUFF

Just to make matters a little bit trickier, guidelines published in *The Annals of Internal Medicine* in 2017 recommended that for folks over 60 without a history of stroke or high risk for cardiovascular disease, blood pressure medication shouldn't be started until the systolic pressure is consistently over 150. That doesn't mean that 150 is an ideal systolic blood pressure; it simply recognizes that medications have benefits and risks, and that in many cases, you should hold off on drug treatment a little longer and work even harder on creating and maintaining a healthy lifestyle. The guidelines left room for doctors to make judgement calls based on the particular characteristics and conditions of each individual. That's because, for many seniors, the benefits of a lower blood pressure outweigh the potential risk of side effects of medical therapy.

MEASURING YOUR OWN BLOOD PRESSURE AT HOME

Although your doctor may use a manual device, known as a sphygmomanometer, electronic cuffs are typically used for home blood pressure monitoring, and they're a great investment in your health. When choosing a blood pressure machine, opt for a cuff that fits over your upper arm rather than your wrist because upper arm cuffs are usually more accurate than wrist cuffs, which tend to overestimate blood pressure. Also, make sure the cuff size is appropriate for you. Usually, the cuff has a marking on it that shows you whether it's a good fit. If yours doesn't fit correctly, buy a separate cuff in the correct size. If you don't, your readings aren't likely to be accurate.

Before you start taking blood pressure readings at home on your new machine, we recommend getting your machine checked at your doctor's office or at the local fire station to be sure it's working properly.

Last but not least, a few pointers for measuring your own blood pressure:

- Before you check your blood pressure, sit quietly for five minutes with your feet on the floor.

- Keep your arm relaxed and at heart level while measuring your blood pressure.

- Save a record of your blood pressure readings to take with you when you visit your doctor. A series of readings is much more helpful than a single measurement.

Distinguishing between Primary and Secondary Hypertension

Hypertension is easy to diagnose, is often preventable, and can usually be treated successfully. The first step in beating the problem is developing an understanding of what hypertension actually means and what it means to you. Hypertension comes in two types: primary and secondary.

Primary hypertension accounts for 95 percent of cases and is the product of a mishmash of age, genetics, and the things you do (or don't do) to your body. Although age and genetics are out of your control, in many cases, the simple choices you make every day can both influence your likelihood of developing primary hypertension and affect how well your blood pressure responds to medications. These factors include

- » Being overweight or obese
- » Excessive alcohol use
- » Excessive salt in the diet
- » Inadequate sleep (including sleep apnea)
- » Lack of exercise
- » Not enough fruits and vegetables
- » Smoking
- » Stress
- » Too much fat in the diet, especially animal fats

Several less common but important and correctable causes of hypertension are the result of treatable medical conditions. This type of hypertension is known as *secondary* hypertension. These conditions account for only 5 percent of hypertension, but it's important to keep them in mind because after the underlying cause is treated, the blood pressure problem often goes away. These conditions include

- » **Coarctation of the aorta:** This *congenital* condition (meaning it's something you're born with) means the aorta, the body's main blood vessel, is pinched in the middle, potentially causing high blood pressure in the upper part of the body and low pressure in the blood vessels feeding the legs. It's usually diagnosed in childhood with an *echocardiogram,* which is a special ultrasound of the heart and blood vessels. In adults, a CT scan may be necessary.

- » **Hyperaldosteronism:** This condition causes the adrenal glands (which sit on top of your kidneys) to produce too much of the hormone *aldosterone.* A blood test showing an unexpectedly low potassium level is a red flag, but additional testing is needed to confirm the diagnosis. Recent research suggests that this condition may account for more cases of hypertension than was previously suspected.

- » **Medical therapy:** Steroids, some decongestants, nonsteroidal anti-inflammatories such as ibuprofen, and birth control pills can raise blood pressure. Though not everyone who takes these medications will have high blood pressure, it makes sense to monitor blood pressure if you're taking these drugs for extended periods of time.

- » **Pheochromocytoma:** A rare but important cause of hypertension, this is a tumor that produces adrenaline and other similar chemicals. It can cause severe spikes in blood pressure, headaches, and palpitations. A blood or urine test usually detects this condition.

>> **Renal artery stenosis:** This ailment refers to a blockage of the arteries that feed your kidneys. If these arteries become blocked, the kidney senses a low blood pressure and sends out signals to the body to raise the blood pressure. The blockage may be due to cholesterol buildup, in which case opening up the artery will sometimes help the blood pressure. In younger patients, a rare condition called *fibromuscular dysplasia* (say that fast three times!) can cause a membrane to form inside the artery, restricting flow. Breaking up the membrane with a balloon on the end of a *catheter* (a small flexible tube inserted into the artery) often improves blood pressure. An ultrasound or CT scan is ordered when renal artery stenosis is suspected.

>> **Supplements:** These are well-known blood pressure culprits, especially those marketed for weight loss. Ephedra (also known as ma huang) and bitter orange (also called citrus aurantium) are frequent offenders. Because supplements aren't directly under the oversight of the Food and Drug Administration (FDA), you can't always be sure what's in that little pill. Shady supplement dealers have been known to spike their products with steroids and stimulants. If you're taking a supplement, let your doctor know. Just because it's "natural" doesn't mean it's good for you.

>> **Thyroid conditions:** These are conditions that affect the thyroid gland, which sits in the middle of the neck. An underactive thyroid *(hypothyroidism)* tends to raise diastolic blood pressure, whereas an overactive thyroid *(hyperthyroidism)* raises systolic blood pressure. A simple thyroid blood test usually diagnoses the condition.

TIP

When needed, screening tests for secondary hypertension are readily available. Your doctor can go over these options with you and decide whether you need to be tested.

Examining the Factors That Contribute to Primary Hypertension Risk

A number of factors contribute to boring old primary hypertension (defined in the preceding section). Some of these factors, such as age and genetics, are out of your control. But many of them aren't. Although a healthy way of life may not always eliminate high blood pressure, it almost always makes a difference. In fact, the small choices you make every day often mean the difference between taking one prescription drug versus two or three. When you factor in the costs and potential side effects of medication, the payoff is huge. The following sections take a closer look at the main risk factors for hypertension.

Diet

The food you eat is both fuel and medicine for your body. And though your body is remarkably good at turning just about any raw material into energy, it functions better when you feed it the good stuff. A diet that's loaded with saturated fat from red meat and high-fat dairy, fried foods, and high-sodium processed snacks and is low on fruits and vegetables is *really* bad medicine. A mad scientist couldn't have designed a diet more likely to cause hypertension, cardiovascular disease, diabetes, cancer, and dementia.

Doctors and dietitians have known for decades that food has a major impact on blood pressure. In the 1940s, before the advent of effective and safe medication for hypertension, one of the standard treatments was a diet of plain rice and fruit. As boring as it sounds, this strategy helped because it essentially eliminated salt while boosting potassium and magnesium levels.

Fifty years later, the clinical trial that resulted in DASH, which stands for Dietary Approaches to Stop Hypertension, tested the effects of nutrients in food on blood pressure. It was one of the first studies that approached food as medicine. The impressive results showed that eating a diet high in fruits, vegetables, and low-fat dairy and low in saturated fat and sodium can have the same effect on blood pressure as many prescription medications. (For more on the science behind the DASH diet, head to Chapter 2.)

Obesity

Obesity is a major risk factor for high blood pressure because it creates stress and inflammation in the body, both of which can lead to hypertension. In fact, fat tissue is a functioning organ, and when you have too much of it, it can produce chemicals and hormones that drive blood pressure up. Excess body fat may also have a directly toxic effect on the kidneys, which are critical in regulating blood pressure. And the heavier you are, the more sensitive you are to the blood pressure–raising effects of salt.

Obesity also makes you more prone to developing *sleep apnea*, a condition in which the airway temporarily closes off during sleep, causing heavy snoring and periods of no breathing at all. Sleep apnea itself increases blood pressure and also contributes to a range of heart conditions, including rhythm disturbances and heart failure.

TIP

As many as two out of every three cases of hypertension may be directly due to overweight and obesity. That's depressing, but here's the good news: Losing even 10 pounds can make a big difference in lowering blood pressure.

Exercise

The life of a couch potato is a fast track to hypertension. Whether you're watching TV, playing video games, or camped out in front of your computer, screen time ups the likelihood of high blood pressure. In fact, a British study found a 10 percent increase in hypertension risk with every hour of TV watched per day, and a study of kids and screen time found that watching TV slowed metabolism even more than simply resting.

Regular exercise can have a major impact on blood pressure. Simply adding two and a half hours of exercise to your week can lower blood pressure by 5 to 10 points, even if you don't lose a pound. This same amount of weekly exercise also cuts your risk of heart attack, stroke, and dementia by at least 30 percent.

If you're taking medication to lower your blood pressure, you may find that after a while of exercising just 30 minutes 5 times per week, you need less medication to keep your numbers in line.

Exercise doesn't have to be stressful, unpleasant, or even sweaty. Physical activity is any body movement that involves working the muscles and using energy. Activities such as walking, jogging, swimming, dancing, yoga, weight lifting, rowing, housework, and gardening all count, as long as you sustain the activity for at least 20 minutes. Find something, or a combination of activities, that you enjoy, and create goals to help you stay motivated. Shorter bursts of exercise are great for burning calories and improving muscle tone, but they don't have the same impact on your blood pressure or heart health. Nevertheless, there is nothing wrong with starting small and building up. If 20 minutes sounds overwhelming, start with 10 minutes and grow your habit as you feel able.

In general, make a habit of sitting less and moving more. But be sure to get your doctor's approval before you get started if you've been accustomed to a sedentary way of life or if you have existing health conditions.

Smoking

We bet you already know that smoking causes lung cancer and chronic lung disease. You may also be aware that the habit can increase heart attack risk by as much as three times (for men) or six times (for women) that of nonsmokers. What you probably don't know is that smoking can also raise your blood pressure.

In the minutes and hours after you light up, smoking just one cigarette can send your blood pressure soaring by as much as 20 points. Over the long term, smoking stiffens the walls of your arteries, which directly raises blood pressure. Smoking also has a toxic effect on the kidneys, which are involved in blood pressure regulation. That's one reason why smokers with hypertension are more likely to develop kidney failure than nonsmokers are.

Quitting smoking helps lower blood pressure, although it may take a few years after quitting for blood pressure to improve. For pointers on quitting, see the nearby "Kicking the habit" sidebar.

KICKING THE HABIT

No discussion of smoking is complete without a tip of the hat to quitting the habit. Surveys report that four out of five smokers wish they could quit, but if you're a smoker, you've probably found that task very hard to do. That's because tobacco of any kind is even more addictive than heroin.

The earlier in life you quit, the easier it will be to do so. Quitting in your 20s or 30s usually ensures that your body is able to overcome any damage you may have done. The older you are today, and the younger you were when you started smoking, the stronger and deeper the cravings.

It's never too late to quit! Within weeks, you'll experience measurable improvement in circulation and lung function, and after a year, your risk of a blocked coronary artery is about half that of a smoker. After five years, you've substantially reduced the likelihood of a stroke. Although cancer risk may take years to drop off, by ten years, your risk of lung cancer is cut in half, and your risk for other smoking-related cancers is also considerably lower.

Some people are able to quit by going cold turkey, but often the addiction can be too strong. Ask your doctor for help and motivation. Nicotine patches (available over the counter) can be very effective; so can hypnosis. Several prescription drugs are also available, though they all carry potential side effects, so your physician needs to monitor you carefully if you use them. Enlisting family or friends to help you stay on track and support your decision to quit is helpful. Even better, if your spouse, partner, or friends quit, you're more likely to stick to your goals.

Weight gain (on average, about 5 pounds) is a common side effect of quitting smoking. But remember that if you can quit smoking, you can also lose the weight and get healthier in the process. The harmful effects of smoking far outweigh a few extra pounds.

Alcohol

In moderation, alcohol appears to be protective for the heart and the brain, potentially cutting heart attack and stroke risk by a third or more. Although red wine appears to have extra health benefits because of its powerful antioxidant effects, any sort of alcohol appears to be beneficial to the heart and brain — again, as long as you enjoy it in moderation. Light to moderate drinkers also appear to have a lower risk for diabetes.

TIP

Here's the tricky part: What do we mean by moderation? For women, your limit is one drink per day. Fair or not, men can have up to two drinks per day because of their body composition and metabolism. And before you break out those giant wine glasses, know that "one drink" has defined limits. A standard one-drink pour means

>> 5 ounces of wine

>> 12 ounces of beer

>> 1 ounce of liquor

Drink more than the moderate limit on a regular basis, and bad things can happen. For instance, more than two drinks daily doubles your risk for hypertension. Binge drinking, such as abstaining all week and then pounding a six-pack on the weekend, also contributes to high blood pressure.

WARNING

Apart from its effects on cardiovascular health, excessive alcohol can increase the risk of liver disease, breast cancer, and cancers of the stomach, esophagus, head, and neck. (Head and neck cancers are especially high in smokers who drink.) Even in moderation, alcohol can raise the risk for breast cancer by 10 percent or more. Alcohol is also toxic to the developing fetus during pregnancy.

Stress

Stress can mean different things to different people. Some people thrive on the stuff, but for most folks, too much stress can have some pretty negative effects on health, including blood pressure. For one thing, when you're stressed, you may be more likely to make unhealthy choices, such as overeating, drinking to excess, and spending too much time in front of the TV. As a result, your blood pressure may pay the price, so working on stress reduction is a win-win for your overall health and well-being.

Also, stress can cause high levels of hormones such as adrenaline to pour into the bloodstream, immediately raising blood pressure and heart rate. With chronic stress, cortisol levels may rise, leading to higher levels of insulin and increased cravings. Overeating may cause weight gain, which also impacts blood pressure. Poor sleep and insomnia caused by stress may further compound these problems.

TIP

If you can reduce the stress in your life, why not give it a shot? Exercise is a great way to lower stress levels and drop blood pressure at the same time. Some people also find that caring for a pet helps bring their numbers into line, likely by lowering stress and nurturing unconditional love.

Family history

You have a say in a lot of things, but your genes aren't one of them. At least 200 genes are associated with hypertension, and combinations of these genes, along with diet and lifestyle, appear to be involved in its development. If you're lucky, you may even have *protective genes,* meaning you're less likely to develop high blood pressure despite other risk factors. If you're not so lucky and have a family history of developing high blood pressure before the age of 60, then you're twice as likely to develop hypertension as someone without this risk factor.

REMEMBER

Genetics are only part of the picture. Your family members may have high blood pressure because of their own lifestyle choices or because of health conditions that you won't necessarily inherit. At this point, no standard genetic testing is available to tell you whether you may be high or low risk. So keep your family history in mind, but know that it's only part of the puzzle.

Age

As you age, your blood pressure naturally tends to run higher. Take a look at the stats in Table 6-1 from the U.S. National Health and Nutrition Examination Survey (NHANES).

TABLE 6-1

Prevalence of Hypertension

Age	Percentage of Demographic with Hypertension
18–44	23%
45-64	57%
65 and up	77%

TIP

In general, the likelihood of high blood pressure increases about 10 percent with every decade over the age of 50, such that by the age of 90, about 90 percent of people are hypertensive. That's mainly because of stiffening of the arteries, which typically causes high systolic pressure with relatively normal diastolic pressure.

PREGNANCY-INDUCED HYPERTENSION

Pregnancy is another important, although still uncommon, cause of hypertension, affecting about 1 in 15 pregnant women. Obesity and the mother's age are both important risk factors; teenage moms and mothers over 40 are more apt to develop this problem. A twin (or multiple) pregnancy is another potential trigger.

Preeclampsia is the most dangerous form of pregnancy-induced hypertension (PIH) and is often associated with swelling in the legs and headaches. Left untreated, it can be fatal to both the mother and her developing fetus. Any routine office visit with your obstetrician usually includes a blood pressure check so that the problem can be identified and treated as early and effectively as possible.

In most cases of PIH, the blood pressure returns to normal within a few months after the delivery. However, scientists now know that PIH and preeclampsia are risk factors for essential hypertension and other cardiovascular problems later in life. (*Essential hypertension* is high blood pressure that isn't due to other underlying causes.)

WARNING

We're not saying that hypertension is inevitable, but you should know about the risks. People often accumulate more reversible risk factors for hypertension, such as excess body weight and a sedentary lifestyle, as they get older. However, many older folks experience hypertension even if they follow all the heart–healthy rules. The most important thing is to recognize the problem and get it treated before any harm is done.

Exploring the Medical Treatments for Hypertension

Eating the DASH way, exercising regularly, and generally living a healthy lifestyle doesn't always prevent hypertension in everyone. Many people with hypertension still need medications to keep the problem in check. The basic idea behind most blood pressure medications is to get the blood vessels to relax, but they all do it in different ways. Sometimes a combination of lower doses of two or three meds is better than a high dose of one. Everyone is different, and what works for some people may cause serious (or annoying) side effects for others.

TIP

Statistically, most people with hypertension need two or more drugs, although the DASH diet can help keep your pills to a minimum.

We're not going to get into the nitty-gritty of high blood pressure medications. That would be a book of its own! Instead, we've listed the classes of drugs commonly prescribed in Table 6-2.

TABLE 6-2 **Common Types of Blood Pressure Medicines**

Type	Action
Thiazide diuretics	Reduce blood volume by stimulating the kidneys to eliminate water and sodium. Also have a direct relaxing effect on the arteries.
Beta blockers	Slow your heart rate and open blood vessels, reducing the workload on your heart.
Angiotensin converting enzyme (ACE) inhibitors	Relax blood vessels by blocking the formation of natural chemicals that narrow them.
Angiotensin II receptor blockers	Relax blood vessels by blocking the action of the natural chemicals that narrow them.
Alpha blockers	Relax the blood vessel walls to open blood vessels, causing pressure to go down.
Calcium channel blockers	Relax the muscles of blood vessels. Some may also slow heart rate.

REMEMBER

No simple test is available to sort out what may work best for you in particular, although usually your doctor will try to choose a regimen that addresses your personal health issues. If you have trouble taking a medication or if you have questions or concerns, bringing that up with your doctor is critical. You're the one taking the medication, and your input matters. When you see your doctor, be sure to ask questions about anything you don't understand. Some sample questions:

>> What's my systolic number? What's my diastolic number?

>> What are my blood pressure goal numbers?

>> What's a healthy weight range for me? What's my body mass index? (We define BMI and provide a handy chart to determine your BMI in Chapter 8.)

>> May I see a dietitian to help me set dietary goals?

>> Is it safe for me to begin more physical activity?

>> What time should I take my medicine? Should I take it with food or avoid any particular foods?

>> What should I do if I forget to take my medication?

THEY ONLY WORK IF YOU TAKE THEM PROPERLY

If you require medication to keep your blood pressure in line, you need to be vigilant about taking your pills on schedule. Easier said than done a lot of the time, right? Here are some tips to help you remember:

- Take your medicine at the same time daily, as directed.

- Use a pillbox that has 7 slots — one for each day. If you take other medications at a different time of day, you may want a pillbox organizer that has 14 slots — one for a.m. and one for p.m.

- Put a "Don't forget!" reminder in a spot that you view frequently — on the refrigerator, the coffeepot, or your bathroom mirror.

- Ask your spouse, a friend, or a family member to remind you or call you about taking your medicine.

- Use technology. Program a daily reminder into your smartphone or computer.

Reducing Your Risk of Hypertension with DASH

In our professions as physician and dietitians, we've seen the good that can come of the DASH diet, particularly regarding blood pressure, as well as the harm that an unhealthy diet and lifestyle can wreak on the human body. DASH works to treat and prevent hypertension because

» Fruits and vegetables are high in antioxidants, potassium, magnesium, and fiber, all of which can help to lower blood pressure — but only when consumed as whole foods rather than supplements.

» Whole grains, nuts, seeds, and beans are also rich in antioxidants, fiber, and magnesium.

» Low-fat dairy products provide plenty of food-based calcium, which is known to help lower blood pressure.

» Moderate amounts of unsaturated fats from plant sources improve blood pressure compared to a diet high in saturated fat.

» Limiting fats and sweets helps with weight loss and reduces inflammation (inflammation in the arteries occurs as a defensive response against "injuries" such as smoking, high blood pressure, and high cholesterol).

» Cutting back on sodium is often a quick and easy way to lower blood pressure.

TIP

The DASH diet was expressly designed to lower blood pressure, but it's also a great way to take control of your daily calorie count. Thanks to an abundance of fiber-rich fruits and vegetables, DASH gives you that happily full feeling called *satiety*.

Chapter **7**

Reducing the Risk of Heart Disease and Stroke

ardiovascular disease — which includes heart attacks, strokes, and heart failure — is often referred to as "the silent killer." The moniker sounds cheesy until you really think about it. In the movies, the "silent killer" usually sneaks in when you least expect him, swiftly and efficiently doing his business before slipping out the back door without a trace. Cardiovascular disease can be kind of like that, except that, unlike hapless movie victims, you often have a chance to call the shots — as long as you can take control of the situation before it gets out of hand.

The path to cardiovascular disease often begins as early as the teen years, thanks to a toxic sludge of fast food, processed snacks, and sodas, combined with a sedentary TV and computer screen–driven lifestyle. Sounds a bit harsh, doesn't it? But the truth is that a typical, modern-day lifestyle is custom-designed to create cardiovascular disease. Never fear: We have faith that you can take control and turn this around. After all, science has proven that up to 80 percent of cardiovascular disease can be prevented with a healthy diet and lifestyle (along with medications when needed). In this chapter, we give you the specifics on heart disease and stroke and explain how sticking to the DASH diet can help you lower your risk for these problems.

REMEMBER

No matter what your age, what you do now can have an enormous impact on your health today and for years to come.

Introducing the Cholesterol Component of Cardiovascular Disease

Most heart attacks and many strokes are caused by damage to the protective lining of the arteries that feed your heart and brain. This (often self-inflicted) injury makes your blood vessels vulnerable to buildup of cholesterol deposits that can, over time, constrict and block blood flow. Cholesterol buildup in the arteries is known as *plaque* (or *atherosclerosis* if you want to sound fancy). The following sections clue you in to how plaque buildup actually occurs and reveal the ideal cholesterol numbers for avoiding cardiovascular disease.

Understanding how plaque happens

Unlike dental plaque, cholesterol plaque is a cheesy, thick substance that doesn't really sit on the artery's surface but actually takes root and becomes incorporated into the blood vessel lining, as you can see in Figure 7-1. That's one reason it's so hard to get rid of. Then again, cholesterol doesn't necessarily stick to any two people's arteries the same way. It may slide off one person's arteries while sticking to another's like superglue. Scientists don't fully understand the reason why, but the key seems to be inflammation. The more inflamed your arteries become, the more injured the lining, and the more vulnerable you are to plaque. High blood pressure can directly damage the walls of the blood vessels, which also makes you more vulnerable to inflammation. Genetics definitely play a role in terms of the body's inflammatory response and plaque formation, but diet, exercise, and whether you smoke have an even stronger impact. Diabetes and obesity are other important sources of inflammation.

Breaking down the ideal numbers

When it comes to cholesterol, the ideal numbers vary depending on your risk factors for cardiovascular disease. Doctors used to measure total cholesterol and leave it at that. As long as the number was under 200, everyone was happy. Now that LDL (the bad cholesterol) and HDL (the good stuff) are measured routinely, the total cholesterol number isn't very meaningful. Some people have a high total cholesterol simply because their HDL level is high; others may have a dismally low HDL count with a high LDL count and yet a seemingly normal total cholesterol level.

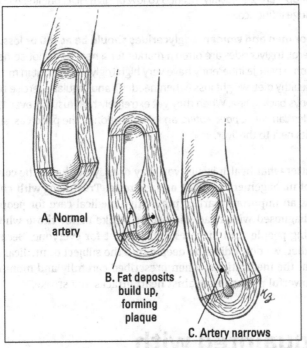

A. Normal artery

B. Fat deposits build up, forming plaque

C. Artery narrows

Illustration by Kathryn Born

FIGURE 7-1:
A normal artery before and after plaque develops.

TECHNICAL STUFF

Cholesterol is measured in milligrams per deciliter, but because scientific notation can get a bit tedious, we just refer to it by number.

Newer guidelines have made the idea of shooting for specific targets somewhat controversial, but it helps to have a framework to understand what goals are optimal for you.

REMEMBER

Here are what your individual cholesterol levels should be:

>> **For men and women, LDL should run around 100 or less.** If you have cardiovascular disease or diabetes or are otherwise high risk, under 70 is considered optimal. At these levels, you're less likely to have cholesterol buildup in your arteries. Yet the average American's LDL cholesterol is around 130. Contrast this with the LDL of 50 to 70 typical of native peoples who have to hunt and gather their food, and it's clear that the Western diet and sedentary lifestyle have really done a number on the typical American's cholesterol. The good news? You have room for improvement.

>> **For women, an HDL of 50 or better is considered ideal; for men, the target is at least 40.** In general, a high HDL is protective, but not always, so good cholesterol doesn't cancel out the bad stuff. Women naturally tend to run higher HDLs, in part because of the female hormone estrogen. Some people are genetically inclined to low or high HDL, but lifestyle and diet have a huge influence.

>> **For men and women, triglycerides should be at 150 or less.** Like cholesterol, triglycerides are often a marker for a healthy or not-so-healthy lifestyle. Some people inherently have very high triglycerides, but in most cases, a healthy diet, weight loss (when needed), and regular exercise bring these bad boys back in line. When they get extremely high (usually over 1,000), triglycerides can cause *pancreatitis*, an inflammation of the pancreas, an organ that sits next to the liver.

REMEMBER

No matter what health issues you may or may not have, the cornerstones of cholesterol management are diet and exercise. Treatment with cholesterol medications is an important part of preventive medical care for people who've already been diagnosed with heart disease or stroke or for those who are at high risk, including people with diabetes, but it's not for everyone. Because this is a book about diet, we don't dive too deeply into the subject of medical therapy, except to say that the medications, when prescribed carefully and monitored closely, provide powerful protection against heart attacks and stroke.

Getting Acquainted with Matters of the Heart

Your heart beats more than 100,000 times in a day (that's more than 35 million times in the course of a single year), pumping richly oxygenated blood to your brain and other vital organs. When you're exercising or stressed out and you need a little more blood flow, your heart senses that and picks up the pace. And while you're sleeping or resting, your heart slows down and takes it a little easier.

In truth, your heart is a miracle, and like many miracles, you can take it for granted pretty darn easily. But what happens when this miraculous organ falls down on the job? The following sections give you a deeper comprehension of the problems the human heart can encounter.

Palpitations: Heart rhythms gone haywire

Because your heart is not only a strong muscle but also an incredible network of electrical tissue, sometimes things can go a bit haywire. Heart rhythm problems run the spectrum from mildly irritating to life-threatening. Following are some common heart rhythm abnormalities:

>> **Premature atrial contractions (PACs):** These are irregular beats that originate in the *atria*, or top chambers, of the heart. Most people with normal, healthy hearts have a few of these every day. When they occur singly or in brief groupings, they can sometimes be uncomfortable but rarely harmful. Stress, fatigue, excessive caffeine, low potassium or magnesium, thyroid problems, and other hormonal changes are common causes.

>> **Premature ventricular contractions (PVCs):** PVCs originate in the *ventricles*, or bottom pumping chambers of the heart. Like PACs, it's normal to have a few PVCs over the course of a day. Some people feel them, but most people don't. The same triggers for PACs can also generate PVCs. However, PVCs are more common in people with weak or damaged hearts and in people with abnormal heart valves.

>> **Atrial fibrillation (a-fib):** A-fib is a potentially dangerous heart rhythm that usually requires medical therapy. It's caused by a continually erratic rhythm that starts in the atria. Usually, but not always, it causes a rapid, irregular heart rate that feels very uncomfortable. Doctors take a-fib very seriously, not only because it makes your heart work so hard but also because it's a leading cause of stroke. When the heart is in a-fib, blood clots can form in the atria. If those clots break free, they can travel to the brain and cut off blood flow, causing permanent damage to the brain tissue. Thankfully, blood thinners are available to prevent this from happening.

>> **Ventricular tachycardia (v-tach):** V-tach happens when a rogue bundle of electrical tissue in one of the ventricles takes over the heart rhythm. It often happens for just a few beats, but in more serious instances, it can go on for minutes and, rarely, even longer. It can temporarily drop blood pressure and reduce blood flow to the brain and other organs. Although v-tach can occur in healthy hearts, it's more common in people with weak or scarred hearts. If you've had a large heart attack in the past, you're especially at risk. V-tach is a potentially very dangerous rhythm because it can degenerate into *ventricular fibrillation*, a rhythm that's nearly always fatal without prompt treatment.

REMEMBER

The sensation of an irregular heartbeat is referred to as *palpitations*. The specific type of irregular heartbeat can be tricky to self-diagnose, although home monitoring devices can be helpful. If you suspect any change in your sense of heart rhythm, play it safe and visit your doctor.

WARNING

If you're experiencing frequent palpitations combined with dizziness or chest discomfort, contact your doctor or (in the case of severe or persistent symptoms) seek emergency care. The cause of your symptoms can usually be readily sorted out with an *EKG* (an electrical tracing of the heart rhythm) or a heart monitor.

Your doctor will probably order blood work and may also order an echocardiogram, or sonogram, of the heart. Treatment, if needed, typically involves medication, although in some more serious cases, electrical shock or a hospital procedure may be required.

Heart attack: When the flow of oxygen-rich blood gets blocked

Although it would seem logical, a heart attack isn't usually the consequence of slow and steady cholesterol buildup. It's often caused by inflammation, which causes the existing cholesterol plaque to become unstable. Your body, detecting an injury, tries to form a clot at the affected site. This process of clotting and sudden blockage of the artery is what leads to a heart attack.

This process explains why someone can have a normal stress test or EKG and then a few weeks later show up in the ER with a heart attack. The test didn't necessarily miss the problem, although that sometimes happens. Instead, the problem may not have been as severe at the time of the checkup.

REMEMBER

Because inflammation of already-diseased arteries is a key trigger of heart attacks, the key to reducing the risk of heart attack is twofold: Prevent plaque from forming in the first place and do everything possible to reduce inflammation of the heart arteries. That's where you can make a huge difference. In fact, up to 70 percent of heart disease is directly related to your lifestyle choices, including diet, exercise, weight, and smoking. Stress and sleep quality are also important contributors.

The following sections help you understand the difference between chest pain and a heart attack, recognize what a heart attack feels like, and know what to do in the case of a heart attack.

Distinguishing between chest pain and a heart attack

Cardiac chest pain, or *angina*, occurs with exertion or stress and generally resolves within a few minutes after stopping the activity. These symptoms may include unexpected shortness of breath and discomfort in the chest, back, arms, neck, or jaw. Angina usually indicates a narrowed artery. Although it can be a chronic, stable problem, if the symptoms are new, angina may be an early warning sign of a heart attack, requiring prompt medical attention. Angina is often treated by opening up a blocked blood vessel, but sometimes medical treatment is all that's required.

Pain or discomfort from a heart attack is similar to angina pain, but it doesn't go away with rest. That's because it's due to a complete, or nearly complete, blockage of a heart artery, such that little or no blood can get through. In most cases, the discomfort gets progressively worse and may be accompanied by nausea or sweating. These symptoms require urgent medical attention.

Recognizing heart attack symptoms

The symptoms of a heart attack can vary widely, but the following symptoms are typical and often occur together:

» Left-sided chest pain, sometimes radiating to the left arm

» Shortness of breath

» Breaking out in a cold sweat

» Nausea

Men are more likely than women to experience these typical symptoms, but nontypical symptoms are by no means limited to women. The following nontypical symptoms may happen in combination or you may have just one or two symptoms:

» Right-sided chest pain

» Back pain

» Arm pain alone

» Shortness of breath alone

» Jaw or neck pain

» Severe unexplained fatigue

Although many people experience brief, or less severe, symptoms with exertion in the weeks or months leading up to a heart attack, some people have no warning symptoms at all.

Knowing what to do if you think you're having a heart attack

When a heart attack strikes, we say that "time is muscle." What that means is that the longer you wait, the greater the amount of heart muscle that's likely to be permanently damaged. If you can get to help within a few hours (and ideally less than one hour), your cardiologist is more likely to be able to restore the life-sustaining blood flow to your heart.

Women are notoriously slow to get to the ER compared to men, and this is one reason why women's heart attacks tend to be more devastating.

WARNING

If you think you or someone else is experiencing a heart attack:

» Call 911.

» Don't attempt to drive yourself or a heart attack victim to the hospital, because a heart attack can cause sudden collapse, requiring immediate resuscitation.

» Unless you're allergic to it or unable to swallow, take a full-strength aspirin. If you can chew it, all the better, because it will get into your bloodstream sooner and help to limit any potential blood clot.

» If the individual collapses, start CPR until emergency responders arrive.

TIP

Don't know CPR? Stop everything right now and sign up for a class! It's easy, and you could save a life. (Don't be squeamish! Mouth-to-mouth resuscitation is no longer part of basic CPR.)

Heart failure: When the heart can't keep up

Heart failure is a pretty broad term that, generally speaking, means the heart is unable to keep up with the body's demands. It can be caused by the following:

» **Weakening of the heart muscle (known as *systolic heart failure*):** This can be the consequence of a heart attack but may also be due to a condition known as cardiomyopathy. In *cardiomyopathy*, the heart muscle is weakened as a result of one of a variety of conditions including viral illness, heavy alcohol use, chemotherapy, genetic factors, or even (in rare cases) pregnancy.

» **Stiffening of the heart muscle (*diastolic heart failure*):** Diastolic heart failure is often caused by high blood pressure. When caught early enough, it may be reversible with effective blood pressure treatment. Obesity, a sedentary lifestyle, aging, and genetic conditions can also lead to diastolic heart failure.

» **A chronically rapid heart rate:** If the heart rate is too fast for the heart muscle to keep up with, and if it persists for a long time (usually weeks or longer), it may fatigue and weaken the heart. Usually we're talking about heart rates of 120 beats per minute or more. Atrial fibrillation that isn't adequately controlled with medication, an overactive thyroid, and stimulant pills can cause this condition. It usually gets better after the heart rate comes down.

Symptoms of heart failure include shortness of breath, swelling in the legs, inability to breathe normally when lying flat, and waking up at night gasping for air. These symptoms may develop gradually, which means heart failure can easily be mistaken for a respiratory infection. To diagnose heart failure, your doctor will probably start with an echocardiogram and blood work. If a blocked artery is suspected, a stress test or *coronary angiogram* (a test to look directly at the heart arteries) may be the next step. Treatment of congestive heart failure depends on the cause but often involves *diuretics* (water pills) and medication to help strengthen the heart and control the heart rate.

Stroke, Otherwise Known as a "Brain Attack"

You already know that your brain is pretty impressive. It has billions of *neurons*, or nerve cells, with literally trillions of connections that allow it to communicate with itself. Your movements, your speech, your senses, and your thoughts all depend on the normal functioning of your brain. Like your heart, it's constantly on the job and absolutely dependent on blood flow for its life force.

Blood flow to the brain comes largely through the two *carotid arteries* (one on the right and one on the left), as well as the *vertebral arteries*, which come up the back of the neck (see Figure 7-2). When the blood supply to part of the brain is cut off, a *stroke* occurs. Just like a heart attack, if blood flow is restricted long enough, the tissue supplied by that artery dies. In the case of a stroke, that means the functions of the body or mind controlled by the affected part of the brain are severely — and possibly permanently — limited.

A stroke can be large, involving a major artery, or very small, if a small branch off of a larger blood vessel is affected. Although large strokes tend to be the most devastating, even very small strokes can have profound effects, especially if they involve a crucial segment of the brain that's involved in coordination of the neurons' messages. Strokes may cause paralysis of an arm, leg, or both. Speech may be affected, as can normal thought processes. Sometimes, the thought processes remain intact, but the individual loses the ability to communicate, either verbally or in writing.

REMEMBER

Most strokes are caused by the same things that contribute to heart disease: hypertension, diabetes, high cholesterol, smoking, obesity, and a sedentary lifestyle. In fact, hypertension accounts for about half of all strokes, and atrial fibrillation contributes to another 15 percent to 20 percent. Most strokes are preventable, but it's up to you to take control.

The following sections fill you in on the main facts regarding strokes and how to react if you think you (or someone else) is having one.

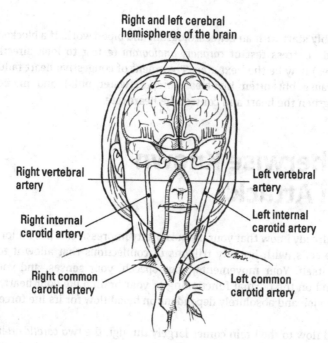

Right and left cerebral
hemispheres of the brain

Right vertebral
artery

Left vertebral
artery

Right internal
carotid artery

Left internal
carotid artery

Right common
carotid artery

Left common
carotid artery

FIGURE 7-2:
Blood supply to
the brain.

Illustration by Kathryn Born

Sifting through the facts on strokes

Stroke is the fourth-leading cause of death in the United States and a serious cause of life-changing disability. The World Heart Federation estimates that 15 million people worldwide will suffer a stroke each year. Although more aggressive treatment of risk factors such as hypertension and cholesterol and fewer smokers mean that strokes are declining in the Western world, it's estimated that over the next two decades, stroke mortality will triple in the developing world (such as Latin America, the Middle East, and Africa).

There are two general types of strokes, both of which can be equally devastating:

» **Ischemic strokes** happen when an artery gets blocked off, or plugged up, by cholesterol plaque or by a blood clot. Nearly 90 percent of all strokes are ischemic.

Transient ischemic attacks (TIA), sometimes referred to as *mini-strokes,* are a type of ischemic stroke in which the artery is only briefly blocked. The symptoms are similar to a stroke but typically last less than five minutes. TIAs are often a warning that a full-blown stroke is on the way and should be taken just as seriously as a stroke.

>> **Hemorrhagic strokes** are caused by the rupture of a blood vessel. In this case, blood leaks into the brain, causing compression and damage to the tissue. Hemorrhagic strokes are usually caused by aneurysms or other malformations of the blood vessels. Although less common, hemorrhagic strokes can be more devastating and account for about 30 percent of all deaths from strokes.

Although most strokes occur in people over 65, more than one in three occur in people who haven't yet reached Medicare age. The incidence of stroke in men and women under 50 has skyrocketed in the last two decades. This can be directly attributed to poor lifestyle choices, which are epidemic in younger folks. That is to say: Put down the double bacon cheeseburger, people!

The effects of a stroke can be mercifully minor or they may be devastating. Rehabilitation can help tremendously by retraining the healthy parts of the brain to take over the function of the damaged portion. Some people can make nearly miraculous recoveries, while others, generally those who have larger strokes or strokes affecting critical areas of the brain, are permanently and severely disabled. In truth, only 10 percent of people ever fully recover from a stroke.

Acting FAST if you suspect a stroke

WARNING

If you suspect that you or someone else is having a stroke, the National Stroke Association recommends that you take the FAST test:

>> **F for Face:** Ask the person to smile. If her face droops, it could be a stroke.

>> **A for Arms:** Can the person raise both arms? If one seems weaker, it could be a stroke.

>> **S for Speech:** Can the person repeat a simple sentence? If not or if the speech is slurred or seems strange, it could be a stroke.

>> **T for Time:** Time is crucial. Call 911 if you suspect a stroke.

Other symptoms that should get your attention include a sudden loss of vision, confusion, difficulty walking, loss of coordination, or a severe headache.

VASCULAR DEMENTIA

Vascular dementia accounts for 15 to 20 percent of dementia cases in the United States and is often mistaken for Alzheimer's dementia. It tends to occur in older people and can happen gradually over time. Unlike Alzheimer's, vascular dementia is caused by narrowing and blockage of the small blood vessels that feed the brain. It can happen after an obvious stroke, but it's often the consequence of multiple, very small strokes that sometimes go unrecognized. An MRI of the brain can generally make the diagnosis.

Vascular dementia, like stroke and heart disease, is usually caused by the usual suspects, including hypertension, diabetes, smoking, and high cholesterol. Regular exercise and a healthy diet can help reduce the risk.

Fighting Heart Disease and Stroke with DASH

The DASH diet is designed to lower blood pressure, which is the leading cause of stroke and a major contributor to heart disease. So it's no surprise that studies that have looked at dietary patterns of average Americans have found a nearly 25 percent lower likelihood of heart disease and a 20 percent lower incidence of stroke in people whose dietary patterns mesh most closely with DASH, compared to those whose diets are the least healthy.

Thanks to its high content of whole grains, fruits, and vegetables, inclusion of healthy fats, as well as limited red meat and saturated fat, DASH helps to reduce blood levels of inflammation, which is protective for both the heart and brain.

REMEMBER

People who choose DASH are 30 percent less likely to develop congestive heart failure, in part because of the lower salt content. In those with diastolic dysfunction, a lower salt diet has been shown to improve or even reverse the condition. On top of all that, DASH can help you maintain a healthy body weight, which in and of itself reduces your cardiovascular risk.

TECHNICAL STUFF

The focus on low-fat dairy foods isn't arbitrary. A Swedish study of more than 75,000 men and women found that, all other factors being equal, those who ate the most low-fat dairy (up to 4 servings per day) had a nearly 15 percent lower likelihood for stroke. The effect of full-fat dairy foods was basically neutral in this study.

IN THIS CHAPTER

» Seeing some of the health problems that being overweight can cause

» Discovering what factors put you at risk for weight gain

» Determining your BMI and waist circumference

» Using DASH to help you get to your healthy weight goal

Chapter **8**

Maintaining a Healthy Weight

No matter what your relationship with food is, it's probably a pretty personal matter. Maybe you find that the scale is a barometer of your stress level, or perhaps you just like eating good food but sometimes overindulge. Maybe you're struggling with your weight because you never really learned exactly how much and what kind of food is best for your body. Or perhaps you have a medical condition or problems with mobility that make maintaining a healthy weight a challenge.

If you're overweight, you're not alone. Over 70 percent of American adults are overweight, and nearly 40 percent meet the medical criteria for obesity. The World Health Organization (WHO) estimates that, since 1975, obesity levels have nearly tripled around the globe, affecting fully 13 percent of the world's adult citizens. These numbers don't mean that carrying extra weight is unavoidable or even okay. Instead, they point to a worldwide obesity epidemic.

This chapter helps you understand why the extra weight is such a serious concern and who's at risk for developing obesity. It also explains how to identify where you fall on the weight spectrum and how the DASH diet can help you lose weight if your risk is in the danger zone. We understand, however, that weight is a multifaceted issue and many people have a very difficult time managing it. We encourage you to contact a registered dietitian for personalized support.

Understanding the True Effect of Excess Weight on Your Health

According to the WHO, every year, obesity is directly responsible for nearly 3 million deaths worldwide and contributes to many more. In fact, overweight and obesity contribute to more deaths globally than being underweight does. Obesity is also a huge driver of disability and soaring healthcare costs. And it's often a very stigmatized condition. Because of the stigma, some people who struggle with weight avoid seeking help, and some health practitioners even respond negatively to patients who are overweight or obese. Treatment is challenging, but the following sections clarify the role excess weight plays on your health.

REMEMBER

No one ever said losing weight was easy, but understanding how and why excess body fat is so harmful can help you get on track to a healthier life. Even a modest weight loss can do that. The most important outcome is improved health.

Diabetes

The U.S. Centers for Disease Control and Prevention (CDC) estimates that nearly 90 percent of diabetes cases can be traced directly to being overweight or obese, and most cases of diabetes in the modern world are the type 2 variety (which we describe in detail in Chapter 9). Worldwide, more than 450 million people are currently living with diabetes. If the growth trend continues, more than 700 million people will have type 2 diabetes by 2045 — that's *seven times* the number affected in 1980.

REMEMBER

Extra weight raises your chances of developing diabetes. What you must understand is that diabetes is *not* just about sugar. The disease more than doubles your risk of heart disease and stroke. It also increases your chances of infections, amputations, blindness, and kidney failure. The real tragedy here is that all this misery comes from a largely preventable risk factor: excess weight.

Hypertension

That body fat that you carry around is complicated stuff. It does more than just annoy you by making your clothes feel tight. The visceral (abdominal) fat that is snuggled up against your vital organs creates a host of chemicals that can affect your health in a wide range of ways that medical science is only beginning to understand.

Fat creates a variety of hormones and other chemicals that can goose your sympathetic nervous system into raising your blood pressure. Fat also appears to have a direct effect on your kidneys, causing you to retain more sodium, which can elevate blood pressure and also cause fluid retention. Even worse, over time, obesity can cause damage to the kidneys — damage that isn't always reversible — that may in turn may raise your blood pressure.

REMEMBER

Losing just 10 pounds of excess body weight has the potential to drop your blood pressure as much as ten points. Lose even more and you have a good chance of getting off blood pressure meds altogether. That's because when all is said and done, 75 percent of hypertension cases in the Western world are due in part or in full to overweight.

High cholesterol, heart disease, and stroke

As we explain in Chapter 7, inflammation and cholesterol buildup in the arteries is the cause of most heart attacks and many strokes. Obesity and overweight can have a negative effect on all three components of cholesterol, raising overall cholesterol levels and boosting your risk of heart disease and stroke.

Even independent of these factors, being overweight (even if you're not obese) can increase your heart attack risk by 50 percent or more. Inflammation from that pesky belly fat is likely the key, as this can damage the lining of your arteries, making them more vulnerable to cholesterol buildup.

The risk of stroke is especially high if you're obese and under the age of 65, a demographic in which the incidence of stroke is rising rapidly. Obesity also increases the chances that you'll develop congestive heart failure, a condition associated with either weakness or stiffness of the heart muscle, along with fluid congestion in the lungs, belly, and legs.

Lung disease

Although you may not connect lung disease and asthma with obesity, the same inflammation that can hurt your blood vessels may also affect the health of your airways. In fact, overweight people are about 40 percent more likely to become asthmatic compared to those of normal weight, and obesity nearly doubles the risk.

Obesity also has a direct, mechanical effect on your ability to breathe normally. The effort required to expand the chest and take in a deep breath is much greater if you have more body mass to move.

Obesity also directly impacts your chances of surviving COVID-19. The likelihood of death and severe respiratory disease is far greater in obese individuals.

SLEEP APNEA AND OBESITY

Sleep apnea is yet another important consequence of obesity. People with sleep apnea often snore heavily, may stop breathing for seconds at a time while asleep, and usually don't get restful sleep. This condition is much more common in obese people than in those of normal weight. Sleep apnea itself can contribute to hypertension and is a commonly overlooked cause of atrial fibrillation (see Chapter 7). Treatment (often consisting of a mask-like device that pushes air into the lungs while you sleep) can be lifesaving. Weight loss will often improve or even cure the problem.

Intestinal issues

Gastroesophageal reflux (GERD) is a common problem in which food and stomach acid refluxes up from the stomach into the esophagus. It can cause abdominal and chest pain, as well as coughing. Symptoms may wake you up in the middle of the night, especially if you go to bed right after eating. In worse cases, it can cause aspiration of stomach contents into the lungs, setting you up for pneumonia. More than 40 percent of obese individuals suffer from GERD. Women with a body mass index (BMI) over 35 are more than six times more likely to suffer from GERD than women of normal weight.

If you're obese, you're also more likely to have gallstones. And though weight loss helps your health in general, if you lose weight rapidly, such as with severe calorie restriction or a liquid diet, you may be setting yourself up for a gallbladder attack. That's one reason that it's usually best to go slow and steady.

TECHNICAL STUFF

Fatty liver is a common finding in obese individuals. That's because the liver is one of the places in the body where excess calories are stored. In most cases, fatty liver doesn't cause any serious trouble. However, the disease can progress to a more severe condition known as *nonalcoholic steatohepatitis* (NASH). In the worst-case scenario, NASH can cause permanent damage to the liver. To treat NASH, diet and weight loss are key, because there are currently no approved or proven medical therapies for this condition.

Reproductive issues

Whether you're a mom or dad-to-be, your body weight can directly affect your fertility and your baby's health. Overweight women are more susceptible to *polycystic ovary syndrome* (PCOS). This condition is associated with infertility and connected to insulin resistance (pre-diabetes). Losing weight doesn't cure the problem, but it can help alleviate the symptoms and improve your chances of fertility.

Obesity may increase the risks of serious heart defects and miscarriage. Heavier moms tend to give birth to abnormally large babies, and if you're obese during your pregnancy, your child's future risk for obesity and diabetes is higher.

A growing number of studies have correlated obesity in mothers or fathers to autism in their offspring, although the exact cause or combination of factors remains elusive.

For men, obesity may put a damper on your libido and contribute to erectile dysfunction, likely due to the hormonal effects of that extra fat tissue. Some studies even suggest that changes in sperm quality (impacted by obesity and not necessarily genetics) cause an obese dad to pass along a tendency toward obesity to his offspring.

Arthritis

Extra weight puts a lot of stress on your joints. Osteoarthritis, the most common form of arthritis, is widespread in obesity not only because of the extra workload but also because of the inflammation created by the fat tissue. It's because of inflammation that even arthritis of the non-weight-bearing joints like the hands is more likely if you're overweight.

It's estimated that for every extra pound you carry, the relative stress on your knees increases by 4 pounds. That's why even a little bit of weight loss can make a big difference for people with arthritis. One study found that for every 11 pounds an overweight woman lost, her risk of knee arthritis dropped by more than 50 percent. On the other end of the spectrum, if your BMI runs above 35, you're 14 times more likely to have osteoarthritis of the knee than someone of normal weight.

Being obese or overweight also increases your chances of developing gout, a painful condition that commonly affects the big toe but can also occur in other joints.

Fibromyalgia, a chronic pain syndrome, is considerably more common in overweight people than in those of normal weight. So are other inflammatory conditions, such as lupus and rheumatoid arthritis.

Cancer

The food you eat has a lot to do with your risk for cancer, a topic we cover in depth in Chapter 10. Regardless of specific foods you eat, obesity itself raises your risk of this dreaded disease.

Cancers of the esophagus, pancreas, colon, rectum, kidney, thyroid, gallbladder, and uterus are clearly linked to obesity, as is breast cancer when it develops after menopause. Of course, you can be unlucky enough to develop any of these cancers regardless of your weight, but why stack the cards against yourself?

For cancer survivors, obesity may play an important role in quality of life, cancer recurrence and progression, and overall prognosis.

Mental health issues

Though many obese people live richly rewarding and happy lives, obesity increases your likelihood of developing a mood disorder such as depression by more than 50 percent. This may be because of the other chronic medical conditions that obesity can bring about, or perhaps for some people, the depression itself leads to overeating and obesity. Regardless of the cause, depression is a serious condition that should never be overlooked or underestimated. Treating depression may help with weight loss or vice versa.

REMEMBER

If depression is something you struggle with, ask your doctor for help. This is one condition that is not a do-it-yourself project.

Being obese or overweight also ups your chances of developing Alzheimer's dementia and vascular dementia later in life. Interestingly, being significantly underweight may also raise your risk of dementia.

Figuring Out whether You're Overweight

People come in all shapes and sizes. Where your weight falls is a combination of your genetics, your family life, your environment, your habits, and your conscious choices. Understanding what your weight means is important though. Your body mass index (BMI) number and/or your waist circumference can tell you whether you're crossing (or have already crossed) into an unhealthy weight category.

Determining your body mass index

Simply put, BMI is a number that correlates with how your weight may impact your health. BMI is an estimate of body fat based on a calculation using one's weight and height. With its wide range of normal numbers, BMI can be a valuable tool to help you understand where your weight falls, but it isn't perfect. And it's not the only tool that can be used to evaluate your disease risk. If your BMI is above 30, however, discuss the situation with your doctor and dietitian so that you understand how it fits into the context of your overall health.

We're not going to make you calculate your BMI. Instead, we've provided a handy chart in Figure 8-1. Simply find your height in inches on the left side. Then follow along that line until you see your weight. Move your finger up to the top row to find your BMI.

TIP

If you can't find your BMI on this chart, go to https://bit.ly/2GMRHqs and enter your height and weight to calculate your BMI. Or just search the web for "BMI calculator" and you'll find lots of websites where you can calculate it.

Now that you know your number, here's what it means:

>> A BMI under 18.5 is considered underweight.

>> A BMI of 18.5 to 24.9 is considered normal weight.

>> A BMI of 25 or more qualifies as overweight.

>> A BMI of 30 and above is considered obese.

>> A BMI over 40 qualifies as morbidly obese, which is especially harmful to your health.

REMEMBER

BMI is only one tool that can be used to evaluate your health, and it doesn't differentiate fat from muscle. If you're very muscular, the chart in Figure 8-1 may not apply to you. But for most folks, the BMI chart does a pretty good job of characterizing body weight as normal, overweight, or obese. Although we know obesity is a health risk in most cases, we also understand how challenging weight management is. It's not just about the numbers. An evaluation with a registered dietitian nutritionist (RDN) can help you set your personal weight goal and provide long-term support.

BMI (kg/m²)	19	20	21	22	23	24	25	26	27	28	29	30	35	40
Height (in.)	Weight (lb.)													
58	91	96	100	105	110	115	119	124	129	134	138	143	167	191
59	94	99	104	109	114	119	124	128	133	138	143	148	173	198
60	97	102	107	112	118	123	128	133	138	143	148	153	179	204
61	100	106	111	116	122	127	132	137	143	148	153	158	185	211
62	104	109	115	120	126	131	136	142	147	153	158	164	191	218
63	107	113	118	124	130	135	141	146	152	158	163	169	197	225
64	110	116	122	128	134	140	145	151	157	163	169	174	204	232
65	114	120	126	132	138	144	150	156	162	168	174	180	210	240
66	118	124	130	136	142	148	155	161	167	173	179	186	216	247
67	121	127	134	140	146	153	159	166	172	178	185	191	223	255
68	125	131	138	144	151	158	164	171	177	184	190	197	230	262
69	128	135	142	149	155	162	169	176	182	189	196	203	236	270
70	132	139	146	153	160	167	174	181	188	195	202	207	243	278
71	136	143	150	157	165	172	179	186	193	200	208	215	250	286
72	140	147	154	162	169	177	184	191	199	206	213	221	258	294
73	144	151	159	166	174	182	189	197	204	212	219	227	265	302
74	148	155	163	171	179	186	194	202	210	218	225	233	272	311
75	152	160	168	176	184	192	200	208	216	224	232	240	279	319
76	156	164	172	180	189	197	205	213	221	230	238	246	287	328

© John Wiley & Sons, Inc.

FIGURE 8-1:
A BMI chart.

Measuring waist circumference

Another way to assess health risk is to measure your waist circumference. Larger waist sizes are a good gauge of the more harmful type of body fat known as *visceral fat*. This is the fat that's tucked in around, and surrounding, your abdominal organs. So what's the harm of a little extra body fat? As it turns out, fat tissue is a highly active body organ which, when overgrown, can wreak havoc on your health.

Your optimal waist size depends on your gender and, to some extent, your race. Organizations vary in their advice depending on all risk factors, but these numbers will give you a general idea where you fall:

>> If you're a white or African-American man, your ideal waist size is less than 37 inches.

>> If you're male and Asian, South Asian, or ethnic South or Central American, your ideal waist size is 35.5 inches or less.

>> If you're a woman (of any ethnicity), your ideal waist size is less than 31.5 inches.

TIP

Your doctor may measure your waistline when you go in for a checkup, but if she doesn't, you can easily check it yourself. Wrap a tape measure around your belly, skimming the top of your hipbones and across your navel. Don't suck it in! You don't have to tell anyone your number, but you do need to be honest with yourself.

Who's at Risk for Obesity?

It doesn't matter who you are or where you're from: Under the right circumstances, you're apt to add on a few extra pounds. Ditch the idea that people only develop obesity if they have no self-control or the desire to change their behaviors. That's not always the case. For some people, obesity is not a result of behaviors but is a chronic disease in itself.

However, certain factors can tip the scales against you:

>> Hormonal conditions such as thyroid disease and adrenal abnormalities can affect your appetite and slow your metabolism, causing you to burn fewer calories. So can some diabetes medications. Your physician can test you for these problems.

>> Menopause and normal aging are associated with a drop in metabolism. It's a sad truth, but as people grow older, they simply don't need as many calories as they did in their younger years.

>> There's at least one "fat gene" circulating through the human genome. Up to 40 percent of Americans carry it. Some lines of evidence suggest that eating a diet high in saturated fat may make this gene more active. So can a sedentary lifestyle. A healthier lifestyle can lessen the genetic impact. So even if you have a fat gene, obesity isn't your destiny.

>> Fidgety people (calling all foot shakers!) tend to burn more calories, even when they're not exercising, whereas people who sit immobile for hours at a time burn fewer calories.

>> In the United States, obesity rates are higher for African Americans, Hispanics, and Native Americans than they are for Caucasians. People of East Asian descent tend to have lower BMIs than other groups. Variables in diet, lifestyle, and genetics all contribute to this. However, obesity levels are rising across the globe.

>> If your friends and family are heavy, you're likely to be overweight as well. But wait! Before you decide to diss the people you love, resolve to work as a team to lose weight and get healthier.

Eating Your Way to a Healthy Weight with DASH

The DASH diet was formulated to provide a structure for healthy eating, not as a weight-loss program. However, because it can be easily adapted to one's personal calorie goal and is steeped in good nutrition, it works for weight loss. The next sections explain how to lose weight and maintain loss by eating the DASH way.

Losing weight

Broken down to its simplest elements, losing weight is a matter of burning up more calories than you take in. Food brings calories in, and activity burns them up. The number of calories your body uses each day to maintain your current weight (before adding in exercise) is known as your *basal metabolic rate* (BMR).

TIP

That's all well and good, but how do you know how many calories you really need? It varies from person to person. Younger adults burn more calories than older adults do, and men generally burn more than women. The average woman needs 2,000 calories a day; the average man, 2,500. To lose weight, you'll have to take in less than that (say, 1,500 to 2,000 calories per day). Although your genetics may have a small effect on your BMR, your gender, age, and muscle mass are more important. This quickie calculation doesn't include that information, so if you want to get more precise, schedule a visit with your dietitian to determine your daily caloric needs. You can also find quick and easy BMR calculators online that take into account your age, gender, height, activity level, and goal weight.

After you're armed with your BMR, it's time to start tracking your calories. If you're serious about losing weight, it's a good idea to measure and record everything. After a while you may be able to eyeball it, but research shows that writing it down leads to more success. Also, most people underestimate the amount they eat and overestimate the number of calories they burn. After you see how your numbers line up, then you can set goals to make changes that support weight loss (we help you figure out how to make changes that support the DASH diet in Chapter 11).

DASH is easily adaptable to a weight-loss plan because it includes lots of volume with fiber, is balanced for protein, limits junk, and is moderately low in fat. The genius of DASH is that your food can be as simple or as complex as you want it to be. It's accessible to just about anyone, and although it wasn't designed or tested for vegetarians or those with dairy intolerance, you can easily modify it to suit your needs. We have loads of great recipes and tips for incorporating DASH into your life in Parts 3 and 4 of the book. Why wait to start feeling stronger and healthier than ever?

Maintaining a healthy weight

So you've lost some pounds, and now your weight is just where you want it. Congratulations! You deserve to feel proud of yourself, but now's not the time to give up your vigilance. Most people agree that maintaining a weight loss is the biggest challenge. To maintain your weight loss, you can't just go back to your old habits. That's why true, lasting weight loss is dependent on lifestyle changes.

DASH can help you maintain your ideal weight by giving you a healthy structure to work with that won't leave you feeling hungry or deprived. You can enjoy a treat every now and then and indulge in a special meal as long as you stay true to the healthy eating plan that helped you get to your goal.

MOVE IT AND LOSE IT

Exercise alone doesn't support weight loss without a calorie deficit, but it is important (and helps just about every other complication of obesity we describe in this chapter). For example, if you walk briskly for 30 minutes, you'll burn 150 calories. Considering that a pound of body fat equals about 3,500 calories, you'd have to walk for nearly 24 hours to see the scale budge by 1 measly pound. On the other hand, exercise boosts your metabolism because it builds muscle, which itself burns calories. The more vigorous the exercise, the more calories burned.

Exercise can be powerful medicine. No drug, supplement, or exotic ingredient pumps your cells full of vitality like a good, regular workout. Exercise lowers blood pressure, heart rate, cholesterol, and blood sugar. In fact, if you exercise as little as two and a half hours per week, you'll cut your risk of heart disease, stroke, and dementia by at least 30 percent compared to those who do nothing at all.

Remember: If exercise hasn't been part of your life, check in with your doctor before strapping on your sneakers, just to be sure you don't have any special restrictions.

TIP

We don't recommend daily weigh-ins. Weight fluctuates depending on hydration, hormonal changes, and salt intake, so don't let a couple of pounds up or down throw you off your game. We do recommend weighing yourself at least once a week, however, to catch yourself if you start to slip. Do this not only while you're on a weight loss plan but also as you maintain your new healthy weight. After you achieve your goal weight, you may just need to check in a few times a month.

IN THIS CHAPTER

» Taking stock of type 1 and type 2 diabetes, pre-diabetes, and metabolic syndrome

» Realizing how many health effects diabetes can have

» Recognizing your diabetes risk and monitoring symptoms

» Checking out medical and lifestyle treatments for diabetes, including the DASH diet

Chapter **9**

Reducing Diabetes Risk

Y ou may recall from your high school biology class that the human body requires sugar, also known as *glucose*, for energy in order to function normally. Without glucose, the body wouldn't have the energy it needs to feed your heart, lungs, brain, and other organs. So, does sugar really deserve its bad reputation? Not really, as long as the body processes glucose the way it was designed to do. It's when this natural processing system gets out of whack that diabetes can take hold.

Because having diabetes adds to your risk of heart disease, consider this chapter your primer on diabetes — what it is, why it's such a serious health concern, and whether you're in danger of developing it (or already have it). We also fill you in on how following the DASH way of eating can help reduce your risk of developing diabetes (or help improve the condition if you already have it).

Digging into Diabetes

The primary factors in diabetes are glucose and insulin. Whether the food you eat is gourmet gastronomic, down-to-earth with Mother Nature, or somewhere in between, your body breaks it down into the simplest of building blocks, glucose, which is the end product of almost all carbohydrate you consume. Glucose energizes the cells of your body and brain. You need glucose to live, but when you get too much of the sweet stuff, your health can take a dangerous turn.

Insulin is the critical hormone that helps keep the level of glucose in your body in balance. Your pancreas releases insulin whenever it detects glucose in your bloodstream. That insulin guides the glucose out of your bloodstream and into your cells, where it's put to work.

Diabetes happens either when your body makes inadequate amounts of insulin or when your cells are unable to respond normally to the effects of insulin.

Two main types of diabetes exist: the less common type 1 and the far more prevalent type 2. There's also *gestational diabetes* (see the nearby sidebar), which can happen with pregnancy and is a form of type 2 diabetes. In general, when we talk about diabetes in this book, we're referring to the type 2 variety, which accounts for 95 percent of diabetes cases today. Table 9-1 shows the differences between the two types of diabetes.

TABLE 9-1   **Looking at the Two Types of Diabetes**

	Type 1 Diabetes	Type 2 Diabetes
Problem	The pancreas stops producing insulin.	The body's cells become unable to process all the glucose in the bloodstream, even though plenty of insulin is available. The pancreas must increase insulin production to overcome the cells' resistance to insulin.
Cause	Most likely caused by an immune reaction gone wrong, causing the body to kill off its own insulin-producing cells.	The majority of cases are directly caused by unhealthy diet, lifestyle, and obesity, although genetics may play a role.
Who's affected	Usually begins in childhood (which is why it was previously known as "juvenile diabetes").	Usually occurs in adults, but can develop in overweight or obese children.
How diagnosed	Severely elevated blood sugar level.	A high fasting blood sugar and elevated hemoglobin A1C blood test.
Treatment	Insulin shots and very careful blood glucose monitoring.	Medications are usually necessary, although weight loss and lifestyle changes can sometimes cure the condition.

WHAT IS GESTATIONAL DIABETES?

Gestational diabetes is a form of type 2 diabetes that typically shows up around the 24th week of pregnancy. If left untreated, gestational diabetes raises the risk of miscarriage and heart and brain defects in the fetus. It can also cause the baby to have a higher-than-normal birth weight and an increased likelihood of becoming an obese child.

Pregnant women receiving routine prenatal care are typically tested for gestational diabetes early in the third trimester of pregnancy. The mother drinks a special drink that's high in glucose, waits for one hour, and then gets a blood draw. If her glucose numbers are beyond the acceptable range, she's called back in for a three-hour test and additional blood draws.

The good news about gestational diabetes is that it's often controllable with diet and tends to go away after the baby is born. The downside is that both the mother and the child have an increased risk of developing type 2 diabetes and heart disease in the future, especially if blood glucose is not well managed during pregnancy.

We can't possibly overstate the enormity of type 2 diabetes. This largely preventable disease affects more than 34 million Americans, including 8 million who have no idea that they have diabetes. By the year 2050, it's estimated that one out of three adult Americans will have diabetes. According to the World Health Organization, the number of individuals living with diabetes worldwide has quadrupled since 1980, affecting more than 400 million people. Unlike an infection or a broken ankle, type 2 diabetes doesn't just strike out of the blue. Rather, it develops gradually, even over several years' time, and may be preceded by one of the conditions we cover in the following sections.

Pre-diabetes

Pre-diabetes is when you have a high fasting blood glucose level that's generally between 100 and 125 milligrams per deciliter but haven't crossed over (yet) to fullblown diabetes. Doctors sometimes refer to it as *borderline diabetes* or *impaired glucose tolerance.* Whatever you want to call it, the condition is a problem of epic proportions, affecting more than one in three American adults. Worldwide, 350 million people are living with pre-diabetes, and by 2030, more than 470 million will likely develop pre-diabetes.

You're at risk of developing pre-diabetes if you

>> Are over age 45

>> Are overweight or obese

>> Are sedentary

>> Have a family history of diabetes

>> Are African American, Hispanic, Asian, Native American, or Pacific Islander

>> Have a history of gestational diabetes

>> Suffer from polycystic ovary syndrome

REMEMBER

You probably aren't surprised to hear that the risk factors for pre-diabetes are the same ones as for type 2 diabetes. The U.S. Centers for Disease Control and Prevention estimates that if no steps are taken to reverse individual risk factors, about 25 percent of people with pre-diabetes will develop diabetes within 5 years. Fortunately, simple lifestyle changes can reduce the likelihood of transitioning to diabetes by a whopping 60 percent. How simple? Losing as little as 5 to 7 percent of your body weight (that's only 10 to 15 pounds, if you weigh 200), and walking 30 minutes five days a week can do the trick.

REMEMBER

Pre-diabetes matters not only because it's a precursor to diabetes but also because it means you're more likely to develop a range of serious health conditions, even if you never actually develop diabetes. These conditions, which are also common in people with diabetes, include the following:

>> Heart disease

>> Stroke

>> Kidney disease

>> Visual problems

>> Nerve damage

Metabolic syndrome

Metabolic syndrome, which raises your risk for both diabetes and cardiovascular disease, is another growing problem globally. According to estimates from the International Diabetes Federation (IDF), between 20 and 25 percent of the world's population has metabolic syndrome. In the United States, a heart-stopping 50 percent of those over age 60 meet the criteria. So, what exactly is metabolic syndrome? The IDF defines it as central (abdominal) obesity or BMI over 30 plus any two of the following four risk factors:

>> High triglycerides (over 150)

>> Low HDL cholesterol (under 50 in women, under 40 in men)

> » Systolic blood pressure over 130 or diastolic over 85 (or a diagnosis of hypertension)
>
> » Fasting blood glucose over 100, or a diagnosis of diabetes

WARNING

If your BMI is under 30 (which is the cutoff for being considered obese), you're not off the hook. Although BMI is conventionally used to diagnose obesity, metabolic syndrome is more concerned with your waistline. Deep inside the belly is where the really bad fat hides, and that's the fat that's more likely to cause inflammation and raise your risk for heart disease and stroke. To assess this, your doctor will take a look at your waist measurement. For men, 37 inches is the cutoff (35½ inches if you're of Asian descent), and for women, a waist measurement over 31½ inches is risky.

REMEMBER

If you have metabolic syndrome but not diabetes, your risk for heart disease is two to three times higher than that of someone who doesn't have metabolic syndrome. You're also much more likely to develop diabetes as time goes on. If you're already living with diabetes *and* metabolic syndrome, your risk for heart disease is even higher.

If you have metabolic syndrome, wringing your hands and cursing your genes and your bad luck is no use. You *can* take control, and DASH can help. Stick with us, and we'll show you how.

TESTING BLOOD GLUCOSE LEVELS

Single glucose readings aren't always reliable because they provide a blood glucose level for that moment. To get more reliable results, your doctor may order a blood test called *hemoglobin A1C*. This test can give you an estimate of your average glucose level over the past three months. Here's what the numbers in the test mean:

Hemoglobin A1C range	Classification
Under 5.7	Normal
5.7–6.4	Pre-diabetes
Over 6.4	Diabetes

Because the A1C test can miss many cases of pre-diabetes (defined in the nearby related section), your doctor may decide that you need a glucose tolerance test. This test involves drinking a disgustingly sweet liquid and testing your blood sugar a couple of hours later to see how well your system has cleared the stuff. The test evaluates how well your body processes a large glucose load, so it gives your doctor a better idea how your body responds to glucose.

DIABETES: A DISEASE OF THE MODERN WORLD

In truth, your body is a miracle of efficiency. Up to a point, it's able to chug along quite well, doing its best to handle most of the stuff you put into it. However, your body evolved to process real food, not the disastrous processed, high-fat, starchy, simple diet that many have come to view as normal.

In addition, everyday life of ages past revolved around some sort of physical activity. Obesity was a rarity, and although folks had limited knowledge of nutrition, food was typically fresher and closer to nature. Meat came from leaner animals that ate a natural diet, and due to cost and convention, portions were naturally smaller as well.

Today's overly sweet, salty, and fatty foods are the result of modern food processing. The availability of convenience foods may, indeed, have an impact on how much people eat. People living in Western countries these days have all sorts of processed foods readily available, and the rest of the world is quickly catching up.

Modern medicine has also helped increase the number of people living with chronic illnesses, albeit unintentionally. By extending the human life span beyond what our ancestors dreamed of, people now live long enough for heart disease, diabetes, and other chronic diseases to become an issue. (Centuries ago, infectious diseases were the fear of the day.)

Examining the Not-So-Obvious Downsides of Diabetes

Perhaps you're wondering why you should be so afraid of a little extra sugar. Can't you just take a pill or shoot some insulin and make it all better? The simple answer is that although medications can help, diabetes deals some serious wallops to your health. Chronically high blood sugar levels, caused by insulin resistance in type 2 diabetes, can raise blood levels of inflammation and contribute to the dangerous effects of diabetes, including the following:

>> Heart disease (double the normal risk for men; five times the risk for women)

>> Stroke (more than double the usual risk)

>> Nerve damage (neuropathy), which can cause chronic pain and numbness and may also lead to unrecognized injuries, especially to the legs

>> Poor healing of wounds

>> Blockage of the arteries that feed the legs; when combined with nerve damage and poor healing, this blockage greatly raises the risk for infections severe enough to require amputation

>> Blindness

>> Kidney failure, sometimes requiring dialysis or transplant

>> Nerve damage to the stomach, causing slow transit of food through the gut

Having diabetes more than doubles an individual's healthcare costs. (Not to mention the fact that the aforementioned complications are all pretty miserable things to have to live with.) In the United States, one in four healthcare dollars goes to treating diabetes and its complications, to the tune of nearly $250 billion per year. That's a staggering amount of money to be spent on a largely preventable disease.

Determining Your Risk for Diabetes

Although some cases of diabetes are purely genetic, multiple risk factors, most of which are preventable, contribute to the disease. Not surprisingly, these risks are similar to those for pre-diabetes.

>> **Family history:** The likelihood that you'll develop diabetes is two to three times the normal rate if you have one first-degree relative (parent, sibling, or child) with diabetes; it's five to six times the normal rate if you have a history of diabetes on both sides of the family.

>> **Ethnicity:** The risk is higher for Asians, Hispanics, Pacific Islanders, Native Americans, and African Americans (although not necessarily Africans) than for Caucasians.

>> **Obesity:** Obesity may increase the risk as much as 20 fold.

>> **Belly fat:** More belly fat (also known as visceral fat; it's stored around the abdominal organs) means a greater likelihood of diabetes.

>> **Diet:** Even if your weight is normal, a diet high in simple carbs and sugar-sweetened beverages puts you at risk, while the DASH diet or a Mediterranean-style diet keeps your blood sugar (and thus your risk for pre-diabetes) lower.

>> **Sedentary lifestyle:** Aerobic exercise two and a half hours per week lowers your risk 50 percent; add in some weight training, and your risk drops 60 percent.

>> **Too much TV time:** Every two hours you spend per day in front of the tube raises your risk by 20 percent.

>> **Smoking:** Smoking raises your risk 40 percent on average and also increases belly fat.

>> **Sleep:** Regularly getting by on six or fewer hours of sleep may raise your risk.

>> **Gestational diabetes:** If your pregnancy was complicated by diabetes, you're more likely to develop type 2 diabetes later in life. (Head to the earlier sidebar "What is gestational diabetes?" for info on this condition.)

>> **Polycystic ovary syndrome:** This complicated but fairly common hormonal disorder is linked to infertility and high levels of testosterone; 10 percent of women with the syndrome will develop diabetes by age 40.

TIP

Could diabetes be in your future? If you're at risk, now is the moment to make the time and the effort to keep yourself healthy.

Watching for the Signs That You Have Diabetes

Type 1 diabetes is usually diagnosed in childhood. Symptoms, including weight loss, very frequent urination, and extreme thirst, can develop rapidly. If not treated promptly, the disease is life-threatening and may require urgent hospitalization to avoid diabetic coma or death.

WARNING

Type 2 diabetes, on the other hand, can come on gradually and with very little warning. That's why one in four people with the condition have no idea what trouble they're in. Warning signs of type 2 diabetes can be similar to (but less intense than) those of type 1 diabetes, including the following:

>> Excessive thirst

>> Frequent urination

>> Unexpected weight loss

>> Blurry vision

>> Tingling or numbness in the hands and feet

>> Frequent infections

>> Irritability and extreme fatigue

TIP

The best way to find out whether you have diabetes is to see your doctor and get a blood test. It's easy to do, and it could save your life.

Treating Diabetes

Doctors can offer multiple treatment options for individuals with type 2 diabetes compared to a single treatment method for those with type 1 diabetes because of the differences in the diseases (which we explain in the earlier "Digging into Diabetes" section). In the next sections, we walk you through the general progression of treatment options for type 2 diabetes.

Lifestyle

If you're overweight and have diabetes, losing just 5 to 10 percent of your body weight can have a huge impact on your illness. As many as 20 percent of people with type 2 diabetes can actually reverse the disease when they lose weight by following a healthier diet with fewer simple carbs and exercising at least two and a half hours per week. Some studies estimate that number to be as high as 70 percent, if you're fully committed to following the program for life. (Unfortunately, this doesn't apply to people with type 1 diabetes, who, while they may improve their health, will need insulin no matter what they do.)

Making big changes may seem daunting if your life has revolved around convenience foods, eating out, binge-watching your favorite shows, and surfing the Internet. The key is to take it one small step at a time, reminding yourself why it matters. It also helps tremendously if your friends and family are on board to support your efforts.

REMEMBER

Sometimes you can do everything right, but the diabetes just doesn't go away. When that happens, you're probably dealing with your genetics (thanks, Mom and Dad!). Even so, making healthy, smart changes will improve your health and your outlook on life and minimize the number of medications you require, so don't give up or give in.

Pills

The medical treatment of type 2 diabetes usually starts with pills (what doctors sometimes call "oral medication"), often a drug called *metformin*. The liver holds excess glucose in storage, and metformin reduces the amount of glucose the liver is able to produce. Metformin also increases the sensitivity of your cells to insulin.

It often causes a little bit of weight loss, which is a nice side effect for most people with diabetes. And unlike many other diabetes medications, it appears to lower the user's risk for heart disease.

A number of other pills can be prescribed for diabetes. Some stimulate the pancreas to churn out more insulin, some work through the intestine to slow down the uptake of glucose, and others make the cells more sensitive to insulin. A combination of drugs is often necessary to keep blood sugar in line.

Shots

Because people with type 1 diabetes produce zero insulin, they require daily insulin injections to stay alive. In type 2 diabetes, insulin is usually used later in the game, when pills are no longer effective because the pancreas just gets worn out and is no longer able to make enough of the stuff. Insulin may also be necessary when, regardless of the medication you're taking, the cells of your body are just so darn resistant to insulin that you need more than you're able to make.

You can also get some shots (including the drugs known as Byetta, Victoza, and Trulicity) that aren't insulin but that enhance the release of insulin, slow the emptying of the stomach, and prevent the liver from overproducing glucose. These medications aren't usually the first plan for intervention, and they're almost always given along with diabetes pills, but in complicated cases, they can be very helpful.

DASH and Diabetes: A Perfect Prescription

DASH is a terrific diet for people with diabetes or for those trying to lower their risk (like people with pre-diabetes and metabolic syndrome, conditions we cover earlier in this chapter). You may be surprised to learn that this is thanks in part to the fact that DASH features high-quality carbs — and we're talking complex carbs, not the stuff you get at the drive-through.

A study of more than 40,000 health professionals found that those whose diets most closely mimicked DASH had a 25 percent lower likelihood of developing diabetes. The researchers attributed this result to the complex (versus simple) carbohydrates, higher fiber, greater levels of magnesium, lower amounts of saturated fat, and substantial servings of dairy protein in the DASH-type diets. All these components of DASH have been connected to a lower risk for diabetes.

Even if you already have diabetes, adopting the DASH way of eating can really help. One study showed that individuals assigned to the DASH diet dropped hemoglobin A1C (a blood test described in the earlier "Testing blood glucose levels" sidebar) by a substantial 1.7 points after just eight weeks on the diet, even when calories were held steady, compared to the other group who ate a typical diet. As expected, lipids and blood pressure improved significantly in the DASH group, too.

REMEMBER

DASH is important for what it offers as well as for what it eliminates. The DASH diet limits sweets, as does any plan for eating well with diabetes. And we're not just talking about dessert. Sugar-sweetened beverages are one sneaky source of added sugar in the diet; some research suggests that drinking just one or two sugary drinks daily may increase your risk for diabetes, especially if your overall diet is less than ideal. Other than in cases of *hypoglycemia* (low blood sugar), sugar-sweetened beverages really have no place in a diet for someone with diabetes.

TECHNICAL STUFF

More recent research that builds on the DASH diet's foundation has suggested that adding more monounsaturated fats, such as olive oil and canola oil, can be especially helpful in diabetes. The OmniHeart study, which we describe in Chapter 2, took a DASH-style regimen and replaced just 10 percent of the daily calories originally assigned to carbs with heart-healthy monounsaturated fats. By making this minor but important change, insulin sensitivity improved. If you have diabetes, pre-diabetes, or metabolic syndrome, or even if you just want to stay well, DASH (with a dollop of olive oil) may be just what the doctor ordered.

Chapter 10

Keeping Yourself Healthy from Head to Toe

The DASH diet was designed to improve blood pressure, but it comes with bonus features. The food you eat sustains and supports your health in a variety of ways, each element working in synergy with the others. The same diet that supports normal blood pressure and heart health is also protective for your brain, kidneys, and other vital organs. Regardless of your age, gender, or ethnicity, good nutrition and regular exercise can lower the likelihood of a multitude of health conditions and improve your well-being and vitality. DASH can help keep your brain sharp, keep your kidneys healthy, and lower your cancer risk. How's that for special features?

Realizing How Food Affects Your Brain

In Chapter 7, we tell you all about how the brain gets supplied with blood, how strokes happen, and how cardiovascular risk factors such as hypertension and smoking can contribute to dementia. But what about the day-to-day function of a healthy brain? As it happens, a healthy diet is absolutely critical for critical thinking. The following sections detail two brain conditions that can be made worse through poor eating and reveal how DASH can help improve brain function.

Breaking down brain fog

Brain fog is a very unscientific term for something that affects everyone from time to time. Symptoms include the following:

» Difficulty following a thought through to its conclusion

» Distractedness

» Forgetfulness

» Losing everyday items such as your car keys

Sound familiar? Although brain fog is part of being human, it can also be seriously impacted by your sleep, diet, multi-tasking habits, exercise, and other daily choices.

» If you miss a night of sleep, you just expect your brain to be foggy. The problem usually goes away after you get a night of good shut-eye. Chronic sleep deprivation can cause more serious trouble and should be checked out by your doctor.

» The food you eat also has a tremendous impact on your ability to stay alert and to think on your feet. For instance, if you reach for a candy bar or a sugary drink when you feel the urge to snack, you may get a quick burst of energy, but what comes next can change the course of your whole day. To deal with the glucose rush of your sweet treat, your pancreas pours out a load of insulin. The insulin pushes the sugar into the cells, but there's often enough insulin left over that, a few hours later, it drives your blood sugar level down just enough below the normal range that you naturally start craving sweets all over again. This creates a dysfunctional cycle of fatigue on one end and agitation on the other. Instead, be sure your meals are balanced with carbs, protein, and good fats. Choose a DASH snack such as a small handful of nuts, a homemade yogurt smoothie, or the Crave-Worthy Toast in Chapter 17.

WARNING

That candy bar is also high in saturated fat, which may be another productivity killer. This type of unhealthy fat may make you sleepy and less able to concentrate fully on the job at hand. As a result, your brain may feel foggier than ever, you'll have a hard time staying focused, and you'll have less energy for family time or working out at the end of the day. In other words, you'll feel crummy with a capital *C*.

» Multitasking is another common brain fog culprit. Despite the best intentions and perhaps firmest convictions, for most people, focusing intently on more than one task at a time is impossible. Trying to do too many things at once is a recipe for brain fog.

TIP

Exercise is a great way to clear out brain fog. Research consistently shows that people who exercise regularly (generally at least 2½ hours per week) perform better on tests of clear thinking and also have as much as a 30 percent lower risk for dementia.

Mulling over mild cognitive impairment

Most of the time, brain fog is just a temporary state, but as you age, you run the risk of developing what doctors call *mild cognitive impairment* (MCI). MCI isn't exactly dementia, but it is a state of heightened forgetfulness and poor memory. About 20 percent of folks over the age of 70 have this condition, and people with MCI are more apt to go on to develop dementia.

Although you may think of MCI as part of normal aging, MCI is, like so many conditions that affect your health and well-being, often preventable. People with a history of heart disease or stroke are also more likely to develop MCI, and the condition affects men more than it does women. Risk factors include the following:

>> Diabetes

>> Hypertension

>> Obesity

>> Smoking

Are these risk factors starting to sound familiar? Makes the DASH diet sound like a keeper, right?

TIP

Moderate alcohol use (up to one drink per day for women and two or fewer for men) is associated with a lower MCI risk, whereas heavy alcohol use can take a toll on the brain.

Bettering your brain function with DASH

Whether you have simple brain fog or true MCI, the food you eat really does matter. If you want to keep your brain humming along like the beautiful miracle of nature that it is, you have to feed it well. That means saying no to the siren song of sausage muffins, pepperoni pizza, and cheeseburgers. Without a healthy start, middle, and end to your day, you can't possibly function at your very best.

REMEMBER

Fortunately, eating DASH–approved foods in the proper number of servings per day (noted in Chapter 5) can help support good brain health in a variety of ways:

>> Tests of memory, learning, and brain function have found that people with amped-up blood sugar levels do worse than those with normal levels, even in people who don't have full-fledged diabetes. By choosing DASH, you'll cut back on simple carbs that raise your blood sugar quickly, including sodas and processed snack foods, and you'll increase complex carbohydrates like vegetables and whole grains.

>> Artery-blocking saturated fats are abundant in fatty meats and tropical oils (such as coconut oil and palm oil). Saturated fats make up about 16 percent of calories in a typical Western diet. Studies of adults of all ages have found a strong connection between high saturated fat intake and poorer performance on tests of memory and mental skills. DASH cuts these harmful fats by nearly two-thirds.

>> A sub-study of DASH found that after just four months on the plan, those who were assigned to DASH versus a typical Western diet had sharper mental reflexes. Those who also participated in a weight-loss program, including aerobic exercise and reduced calories, tested even better, showing improvements in problem-solving and memory.

>> If you're 65 or older, DASH gives you the edge when it comes to MCI. An 11-year study of more than 3,800 seniors in Utah found that those whose diets were more like DASH scored higher on tests of brain function. The foods that researchers found to be especially brain-friendly were whole grains, nuts, and legumes. Studies of similar diets, particularly those including more olive oil, have also found a lower incidence of Alzheimer's dementia.

Maintaining Healthy Kidney Function

It's so easy to take your kidneys for granted, especially because they chug along day after day, working their magic without you having to lift a finger. And if you happen to lose a kidney because of infection, injury, or donating one, the remaining kidney just takes over the extra load and keeps on trucking. In fact, a healthy person who donates one of his kidneys has a life span equal to someone who has two normal, healthy kidneys.

So what does this amazing organ have to do with hypertension? Plenty. The following sections help you get a better understanding of these little gems, the role blood pressure plays in their functioning, and how the DASH diet can help keep your kidneys on track.

Getting a grip on normal kidney function

Your kidneys, two little bean-shaped organs (see Figure 10-1), continually filter your blood for toxins, flushing out waste products along with excess water. They also help keep your *electrolytes* — including sodium, potassium, and magnesium — in balance and prevent your blood from becoming too acidic or too alkaline. Because blood continually circulates through them, over the course of a normal day, your kidneys filter about 45 gallons of blood. But wait, there's more! The kidneys also function as *endocrine organs*, meaning they're responsible for the production of a variety of hormones that affect blood pressure, red blood cell production, and bone health. Those little guys work hard for you!

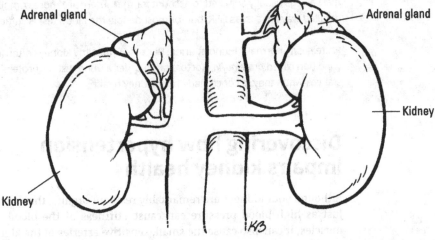

FIGURE 10-1: The kidneys are bean-shaped organs that play a huge role in your body's functioning.

Illustration by Kathryn Born

The large arteries that feed your kidneys, known as the *renal arteries*, are critical to maintaining kidney health. That stands to reason because these arteries bring the kidneys blood to filter and provide life-sustaining oxygen and other nutrients. These arteries also have nerves that detect blood pressure and signal the kidneys if something seems amiss.

TECHNICAL STUFF

Like all your organs, the kidneys are much more complex than they appear on the surface. Each of your kidneys is home to about a million tiny complexes called *nephrons.* Each nephron is made up of an intricate series of *capillaries* (the smallest of blood vessels), along with a complicated structure known as a *tubule.* Ultimately, all the urine filtered by these microscopic nephrons converges into the ureter, which takes it out of the kidney and into the bladder. The urine then exits the body through the urethra.

HOW IS KIDNEY FUNCTION MEASURED?

Doctors measure your kidney function through blood tests, including BUN (blood urea nitrogen) and creatinine tests. Higher levels usually indicate trouble with the kidneys, although dehydration may also cause abnormalities.

Glomerular filtration rate (GFR) is a more specific way to assess the health of the kidneys. This test, usually done as part of your routine blood work, takes into account your age and gender, along with your creatinine level. Because muscle mass can alter your creatinine level (even if your kidneys are working just fine), the test may underestimate kidney function in more muscular individuals. If you're black, you're genetically likely to be more muscular than people of other races, even if you don't exercise, so the test's normal value is usually adjusted to account for that. There are more complicated and detailed ways to assess GFR, but for most people the blood test is sufficient.

Protein isn't normally found in urine. Because unhealthy kidneys often leak protein, a condition called *proteinuria,* doctors often order a urine test for protein and other substances when they're concerned about kidney health.

Discovering how hypertension impairs kidney health

Although your kidneys are remarkably resilient organs, they're not indestructible. Just as high blood pressure can cause stiffness of the blood vessels and heart muscles, it can also cause the small, sensitive arteries of the kidneys to thicken up and become less functional. This starts out as a protective response, as the kidneys try to shield themselves from the relentless high pressure. When detected in time, controlling blood pressure can prevent any permanent harm. But eventually, without adequate treatment, the damage is often irreversible. African Americans and people with diabetes are especially vulnerable to the harmful effects of hypertension on the kidneys.

REMEMBER

Although diabetes is the leading cause of kidney failure requiring dialysis, hypertension is a close second, and the two often work in tandem to inflict damage on the kidneys. In fact, hypertension is a contributor to at least 85 percent of cases of chronic kidney failure in the United States and throughout the developed world.

WARNING

Kidney disease can itself cause hypertension, so it's important to have blood tests to check your kidney function if you're diagnosed with high blood pressure. See the nearby sidebar "How is kidney function measured?" to find out what tests your doctor will likely order.

Another factor that can influence blood pressure is the blood supply to the kidneys. If there's poor flow, often due to blockage from cholesterol buildup, then the kidney may "think" the blood pressure is low and send out signals to raise it. However, opening up the blockage doesn't usually improve blood pressure in people with long-standing hypertension. This is probably because people with blocked arteries are also likely to have multiple other risk factors for kidney disease and hypertension, and opening up a blocked artery doesn't make those other problems go away. In the case of new-onset hypertension, however, opening up a blocked artery may be helpful.

TIP

A long list of other conditions and toxins can influence your kidney function. If you want to know more, the National Kidney Foundation's website (www.kidney.org) offers a wealth of information.

WHAT YOU SHOULD KNOW ABOUT DIALYSIS

Dialysis, in which a machine artificially filters the blood, is usually recommended when the kidneys are down to about 15 percent of normal function. Dialysis is complicated and life-changing but also lifesaving. Some dialysis patients go on to receive kidney transplants, but many more commit to receiving dialysis for life. If you need dialysis and go without out it, you'll likely die within a matter of weeks as fluids and toxins build up.

There are two different forms of dialysis:

- **Hemodialysis:** This is the most common form of dialysis. It's usually done at a dialysis center, where the procedure is run on multiple people throughout the day. For most people, three to five hours three times a week are required, during which time they're tethered to the dialysis machine. Most dialysis patients have a *shunt* in their arm. This is a blood vessel that has been surgically enhanced, such that large volumes of blood can course through it. During dialysis, a large catheter is inserted into the shunt, through which blood is removed for cleansing in the dialyzer machine and then returned to the body.

- **Peritoneal dialysis:** A less common procedure, this type of dialysis is done through a large catheter inserted directly into the abdominal cavity (also known as the *peritoneum,* hence the name). Fluid is inserted into the catheter and then slowly removed, allowing the blood vessels that line the inside of the abdominal cavity to filter the blood. The advantage is that this can be done at home while you sleep. The chief disadvantages of peritoneal dialysis compared to hemodialysis are that it's less efficient and that it may predispose the patient to *peritonitis,* an infection inside the abdominal cavity.

Creating balance with DASH

DASH is designed to help your kidneys function at their very best. While a typical Western diet provides much more salt and far less potassium than your kidneys were intended to handle, DASH attempts to bring that balance back to a more natural state. It does so by greatly reducing added salt and by increasing potassium-rich fruits and vegetables. By bringing potassium and sodium levels back into equilibrium, blood pressure improves.

DASH can also help reduce your risk for kidney stones. These crystalline collections of minerals are created in the kidneys and then travel down the ureters, often getting stuck on the way, creating excruciating pain. Anything that may increase urinary excretion of calcium, oxalate, or uric acid increases risk for kidney stones. Risk factors for kidney stones include:

>> Dehydration

>> Excessive fructose (found in fruit juices, table sugar, high-fructose corn syrup, honey, agave nectar, and other added sugars in processed foods and sugary beverages)

>> A high-protein diet

>> Too much salt

>> BMI over 30 or increased waist circumference

REMEMBER

Though fructose is the sugar found naturally in fruit, it's best to eat more whole fruit and keep juices to small servings, such as 4 to 6 ounces.

Although some kidney stones are made up primarily of calcium, a diet high in dairy products actually reduces the risk of this type of stone, and the addition of more vegetables to the diet helps by keeping the urine more alkaline. A study from the Harvard School of Public Health found that people whose diets were most consistent with DASH had a 45 percent lower likelihood of developing stones compared to those whose diets were the least DASH-like.

Many popular diets encourage you to eat a lot of high-protein foods. Though DASH offers a healthy amount of protein (18 percent of calories are from protein-rich foods), it doesn't go overboard. That's important because a high-protein diet can make kidney disease worse.

REMEMBER

If you have kidney disease, check in with your doctor or dietitian before making any sort of drastic change to your diet. Your doctor can make individualized protein recommendations, and in some cases, you may need to limit potassium-rich foods. Alternately, if you successfully adopt the DASH lifestyle, your doctor may decide to adjust your medications to accommodate your healthier way of life.

Reducing Cancer Risk

Cancer kills more than 9 million people worldwide every year, including more than 600,000 in the United States alone. Over the next 20 years, new cases of cancer are expected to nearly double across the globe. Even though cardiovascular disease kills more people than all forms of cancer combined, most people identify cancer as their greatest health fear, and some recent statistics predict that cancer could soon be the number one cause of death.

Many people also believe cancer to be out of their personal control, but nothing could be further from the truth. Although some cancers are clearly inherited and many are simply bad luck, 40 percent of cancers can be directly traced to lifestyle factors, including diet, obesity, smoking, a sedentary lifestyle, and excessive alcohol. The following sections describe various types of cancers and explain how the DASH diet can help prevent them.

What you should know about cancer

Although many people with cancer don't die from the disease, a diagnosis of cancer is scary, and the treatment may take months or even years. In the United States, with proper treatment, two out of every three people with cancer are still alive and kicking at the five-year mark. But unlike heart disease, hiding a diagnosis of cancer is difficult, and therapy, including chemotherapy and surgery, can be painful and life-changing.

What is cancer?

The term *cancer* refers to a group of more than 100 separate diseases. In its simplest terms, cancer is a disease in which abnormal cells multiply without control, taking over and invading the surrounding tissue. This happens because of defective DNA (the body's genetic code) and may affect any organ or body part. Although the defective DNA may be inherited, in most cases the cause is either random chance or exposure to something harmful.

Following are the five major categories of cancer:

>> **Carcinoma:** Cancers of the skin and of tissues that line your internal organs

>> **Central nervous system cancers:** Cancers of the brain and spinal cord

>> **Leukemia:** Cancers of the blood cells

>> **Lymphoma and myeloma:** Cancers of the immune system

>> **Sarcoma:** Cancers of the muscle, bone, fat, or other connective or supportive tissue

Not all cancers respond the same way to treatment. Some are highly curable, while others carry a dismal prognosis. Many are somewhere in between. Regardless, cancer cells are very hard to kill because of their abnormal features and their rapid and unregulated growth. Treatment targets the bad cells, but killing them without damaging or killing some of the healthy tissue as well is difficult.

TECHNICAL STUFF

In some forms of cancer, the cells may gain access to the lymphatic system, which is designed to clear away toxins in normal, healthy individuals. By taking this route, they're able to spread to other organs of the body. This process is known as *metastasis*.

Who's at risk?

Although your genetic code and sheer bad luck can put you in cancer's sights, often cancer is a preventable disease. Tobacco is an obvious risk factor for cancer, contributing to 22 percent of cancer deaths worldwide. But in the United States, the combined effects of a poor diet, unhealthy lifestyle, and obesity account for even more cancers than smoking.

According to the American Institute for Cancer Research (AICR), of the 12 most common forms of cancer, about one-third can be prevented with an improved diet, exercise, and maintaining a healthy weight. Fully one half of cancer deaths can be prevented with a healthier way of life. The good news is that we are not helpless in our fight against cancer. By making a change right now, you can have an impact on your chances of developing this dreaded disease.

Here are some details about common forms of cancer:

» **Breast cancer:** Though sorting out which risk factors play the most important role in any individual woman's breast cancer is impossible, the AICR estimates that one in three cases can be prevented every year by choosing a healthy lifestyle. Obesity, in particular, raises the risk for breast cancer, especially after menopause, and likely contributes to the continued rise in cases of this dreaded disease. Some studies have found good evidence that a plant-based diet high in calcium with very little red meat or high-fat dairy foods may reduce breast cancer risk.

» **Colorectal cancer:** According to the AICR, one out of every two cases of this cancer is connected to lifestyle choices, including diet. Red meat, especially processed meats (like ham, bacon, and lunchmeat) and meat cooked over a flame, is especially risky. Obesity is clearly a risk factor, more so for men than for women, while exercise seems to lower risk. A high-fiber diet, including plenty of fruits and vegetables, is protective.

>> **Endometrial cancer:** Also known as *uterine cancer,* this is another cancer that has been linked to obesity. In fact, the AICR estimates that nearly 60 percent of cases can be prevented with a healthy lifestyle.

>> **Lung cancer:** The majority of cases of lung cancer are the direct result of tobacco, and there is good evidence that some cases of lung cancers may be due to lifestyle choices. In fact, a diet high in fruits and vegetables appears to lower your risk by as much as 50 percent, whereas a high-fat diet may raise the risk. For smokers, dairy products may somehow be protective. And for everyone, exercise is beneficial.

>> **Pancreatic cancer:** Although it's much less prevalent than breast, prostate, and colorectal cancer, this cancer is more uniformly devastating. At the five-year mark, despite the very best therapy, only 6 percent of its victims are still alive. A diet high in red meat, processed meats, and sugary foods and drinks is known to raise one's risk, as are obesity and diabetes. Fruits and vegetables may be protective.

>> **Prostate cancer:** Although the connection between diet and lifestyle isn't as strong for prostate cancer as it is for cancers that affect women, it does account for more than 10 percent of cases. This translates to over 25,000 men every year in the United States who could have prevented their prostate cancer through simple healthy choices.

A host of other cancers are strongly influenced by diet, exercise, and body weight. These include cancers of the gallbladder, esophagus, mouth and throat, kidney, liver, and stomach.

The American Cancer Society estimates that about 40 percent of people in the United States will develop cancer at some point in their lifetimes, but the numbers don't have to be that high. It's heartening to know that though it may not be easy, and you may not always be able to avoid a diagnosis of cancer, you have much more control over your own health and well-being than you may have believed.

DASH as cancer prevention

Although DASH was developed to help prevent and treat hypertension, the foods that make up the diet protect and sustain your health in many ways:

>> **DASH is low in meat.** In fact, you could cut out red meat altogether, but small portions of lean cuts can be worked into your eating plan. Note that a high intake of processed meats (hot dogs, ham, bacon, sausage, and some deli meats) has been associated with risk of cancers of the colon, rectum, esophagus, stomach, prostate, lung, and kidney. These choices are also high in sodium and higher in saturated fat, so you should limit them in general.

>> **DASH is rich in fruits and vegetables.** People who eat little in the way of fruits and vegetables double their risk of cancers of the lung, mouth, throat, esophagus, breast, pancreas, stomach, colon, rectum, cervix, and bladder compared with those whose intake of fruits and vegetables tracks closely with DASH.

>> **DASH emphasizes low-fat dairy products.** The impact of dairy foods on cancer risk is less clear than it is for other foods. There is evidence that eating a lot of high-fat dairy foods compared to choosing low-fat or nonfat dairy products may be associated with breast cancer risk. Other studies have found a lower risk for certain cancers with dairy foods.

When it comes to prostate cancer, the data gets rather murky. A high intake of whole-fat dairy products (more than 2½ servings per day) has been linked to a greater likelihood of developing prostate cancer, whereas the connection appears to be weaker with low-fat dairy. One study of men with prostate cancer found that those who ate the least amount of yogurt were more apt to have more aggressive cancers. Until the medical community knows more, men concerned about prostate cancer risk should probably limit low-fat dairy to 2 servings or fewer on average per day.

>> **DASH has plenty of whole grains.** Whole grains are great for the digestive tract, with good evidence of protection against colorectal, pancreatic, and stomach cancer. Although the connection isn't clear, some studies suggest that whole grains may help prevent breast cancer.

>> **DASH includes moderate amounts of nuts, seeds, and beans.** Beans may make you feel a little gassy, but they're nutrient powerhouses and will keep your colon happy, cutting your risk for cancers of the colon, pancreas, and breast. And although you may think of nuts and seeds as high-fat foods, they mainly supply healthy monounsaturated and polyunsaturated fats (including omega-3) and little in the way of the more harmful saturated fats. Studies of nut consumption have pointed to a more than 10 percent drop in cancer incidence, including colon, breast, and prostate, in people who enjoy nuts regularly. Of course, you don't want to go nuts with nuts. Those calories aren't freebies, so it's best to stick to the DASH guidelines that we provide in Chapter 5.

>> **DASH limits fats and oils.** A diet high in saturated fats, lard, bacon grease, and butter is clearly linked to cancer risk, including cancers of the breast, colon, and pancreas. Less is known about cancer risk and the saturated fats from tropical oils such as coconut oil and palm oil, so until scientists know more, you can't assume that tropical oils are safer. Trans fats, including those from solid margarine and vegetable shortening, appear to increase your risk for lymphoma.

>> **DASH keeps sweets to a minimum.** Although sugar itself doesn't appear to cause cancer, sugary foods tend to be low in healthy nutrients. By choosing a sugary snack rather than a piece of fruit or a handful of nuts, you simultaneously deprive yourself of something that's really good for you and fill your body with empty calories.

LOOKING AT OTHER PREVENTABLE RISK FACTORS FOR CANCER

An unhealthy diet, lack of exercise, and obesity contribute to a variety of cancers, but they're not the only important risk factors worth knowing about:

- **Alcohol** (especially when more than one drink per day for women and more than two for men) raises the risk for cancers of the mouth, throat, esophagus, liver, colon, and breast. Smokers who drink greatly increase their chances of developing cancers of the head and neck.

- **Infections** contribute to 22 percent of cancer deaths worldwide, although only about 6 percent in more industrialized countries. These include hepatitis A and B (liver cancer), human papilloma virus (cervical cancer), helicobacter pylori (stomach cancer), and HIV/AIDS (Kaposi's sarcoma and lymphoma).

- **Pollution** is a growing concern and is responsible for as many as 4 percent of all cancers worldwide, including 15 percent of lung cancers.

- **Radiation exposure,** including exposure to radon gas (found in soil and building materials) and medical procedures, is another important and often overlooked cause of cancer. Though many medical tests that involve the use of radiation (including CT scans, nuclear medicine tests, and angiograms) can be lifesaving, awareness of the potential for harm is growing in the medical community. If one of these tests is recommended, it's reasonable to ask your doctor whether an alternative form of testing is available and appropriate for you.

- **Sun exposure** causes basal cell carcinoma, squamous cell carcinoma, and melanoma. Though the first two forms of cancer are usually easily treated, melanoma can be deadly, and rates of the disease are rising worldwide.

- **Tobacco** is an all-around cancer player. It contributes to cancers of the lung, mouth, throat, stomach, pancreas, colon, kidney, bladder, and cervix. Leukemia is also more common in smokers. If you can't quit for yourself, quit for those you love. Secondhand smoke can also cause cancer, as well as heart disease and stroke.

Understanding Diet and Healthy Aging

Taking good care of your health is like putting money in the bank. Not only are you safeguarding your well-being for today and for the immediate future, but you're also giving your future self a leg up. Diet and lifestyle play an important part in numerous conditions that tend to catch up to us as we age, but DASH can help with some very specific issues that are especially important to older folks.

Frailty

As we age, we become more vulnerable to fatigue, chronic disease, and general weakness. Older people often lack the ability to fully bounce back from a health challenge in the same way that they did when they were younger, and they may be more likely to fall and suffer serious injury.

Researchers delved into the database from the large, ongoing Nurses' Health Study (www.nurseshealthstudy.org) and found that those whose diets most closely aligned with DASH were significantly less likely to suffer from frailty in their senior years. When their diets included less red meat and saturated fat, more monounsaturated fats (like olive oil), more vegetables, and alcohol in moderation, there was an even more positive affect.

Bone health

Aging is often associated with loss of bone strength and structure. This is one area where a DASH diet can really make a difference, likely due to multiple beneficial effects, including the higher calcium content of the diet, the lower acidity of the diet, and perhaps even the health-sustaining antioxidants that DASH provides. Plus, there is evidence that when you cut back on salt, the kidneys are able to hold onto more calcium, which may help to keep the bones stronger.

3
Enjoying Life the DASH Way

Discover how to adopt the DASH diet in the way that improves your odds of sticking with it: by easing DASH-approved foods into your meals and making yourself aware of common pitfalls so you can avoid them more easily.

Get yourself organized before heading to the grocery store by creating a menu-based list so you can focus on making informed decisions.

Stock your pantry, refrigerator, and freezer with DASH-friendly ingredients so that you can easily whip up meals and snacks.

Recognize the importance of planning ahead for mealtimes and arming yourself with a well-equipped and well-organized kitchen.

Bring your new DASH eating habits along with you on your next family vacation or to your favorite restaurant, and feel confident in your ability to make heart-healthy eating choices.

Start incorporating other positive lifestyle changes, such as living mindfully and building up a support system of family and friends, to complement your new DASH diet and help you stick with it.

IN THIS CHAPTER

» Planning your dietary changes for optimum success

» Finding ways of adding healthy foods to your daily eating

» Overcoming obstacles to your DASH diet plan

» Looking at a sample two-week meal schedule

Chapter **11**

Adopting the DASH Diet

When embarking on a new way of eating and living, you have to keep in mind that change takes time. You need to put a plan in place, and this chapter helps you do just that. This chapter also helps you realize how easily you can incorporate DASH diet principles into your everyday life and provides you with the tools you need to overcome setbacks along the way. Get ready to discover how simple (and tasty!) the DASH lifestyle can be.

Creating a Change-Driven Plan of Attack

It's one thing to know that eating more fresh fruit is good for you, but it's a completely different thing to practice this behavior consistently. The good news is that by creating a simple plan, you'll get from point A (thinking) to point B (doing). How, you ask? Just follow these steps:

1. **Start with a vision that's unique to you.**

   For example, if you're currently overweight and have high blood pressure, perhaps your vision is to lose some weight and lower your blood pressure. Or you may have an even more defined vision of a slimmer you that feels better and has more energy, exercises regularly, and feels more comfortable.

2. **Set one realistic goal each week and be patient.**

We don't expect overnight successes in our own lives, and neither should you. Eating well and being physically active are lifelong endeavors, and realistic goals set you up for that lifelong success. Also, because you don't want to bite off more than you can chew (no pun intended), we advise working on just one or two goals at a time (see Chapter 4 for tips on goal setting). When those goals become second nature, then you can move on to the next ones.

3. **Plan out most of your weeknight meals over the weekend.**

You'll find lots of meal planning ideas later in this chapter. Consider using Saturday or Sunday to think about your weekly meal plan. Often, the work-week can get hectic, so if you take an hour or so on the weekend to create a shopping list and some lunch and dinner ideas (breakfast isn't usually as big of a challenge), you'll set yourself up for success through the week.

TIP

Keeping a food and exercise journal can help you stay on track with your goals. Whether you write it down on paper or use an app on your mobile phone or tablet, recording what you eat each day can help you notice whether you're consistently making the best eating choices. Using a food journal may surprise you. Are you eating out of boredom or stress? Do you make poor snack choices when you don't have a plan? Are you drinking enough water? Similarly, writing down an exercise schedule helps ensure you fit in the amount of exercise that you're going for every week.

Inevitably, obstacles will arise on your path to lasting lifestyle change. Life happens, and rolling with the changes is challenging. So keep in mind that you'll want to reevaluate your plan now and then. We help you address the most common obstacles later in this chapter (see "Surveying Common Obstacles").

Easing Tasty, DASH-Friendly Foods into Your Diet

As we explain in Chapter 5, following the DASH diet means eating more fruits and vegetables, as well as low-fat dairy. The DASH diet doesn't call for you to drink your weight in green smoothies or stock up on hard-to-find vegetables and exotic ingredients. When you eat the DASH way, you can simply choose the foods you want to enjoy from the fruit and vegetable groups. So if you like tomatoes, mushrooms, and green peppers, focus on adding more of those at first. Our goal is to make them all taste good, so even if you don't think you like something, try one of Cindy's recipes and you may change your mind.

Add more of your favorite produce items to your diet and experiment with different ways of preparing them. After all, cooking foods a new way can completely change their flavor and texture into something even more delicious! The goal is to increase your vegetable intake, so if you're preparing a dish that calls for a vegetable you don't like, swap it for one you do.

When you start to feel better about your vegetable consumption, gradually add in new foods. Consider the recipes we provide in Part 4 as your gateway into a whole new world of preparing and enjoying various foods, from whole grains to new-to-you vegetables (and even previously unloved vegetables prepared in new ways).

Here are some tips to help you make sure that you succeed with the DASH diet:

>> Keep a few things on the running grocery list: low-fat milk, plain low-fat yogurt, low-fat cottage cheese or ricotta, apples, bananas, berries (and any other fruit you enjoy; look for store specials and frozen versions), melons, baby carrots, celery, onions, fresh romaine lettuce, bagged salad, green beans, bell peppers, garbanzo beans, sugar snap peas, frozen peas, and broccoli or cauliflower.

>> Keep nuts in the house for cooking and snacking. We know that nuts are expensive, but portions should be small — and a little goes a long way. Look for sales or try purchasing larger quantities at discount stores. Nuts are so nutritious, and you're worth the expense!

Use the tips in Chapters 12 and 13 to help you get the most out of grocery shopping and stocking your pantry.

Sneaking in fruits and vegetables

Keeping vegetables visible and ready for consumption, either on your kitchen counter or in your refrigerator, allows you to easily throw together some quick meals during the week.

Here are some of our favorite tips for sneaking fruits and vegetables into meals where you least expect them:

>> Add 2 tablespoons of cooked spinach to two or three eggs (use no more than two yolks and up to four whites) to make a quick spinach omelet.

>> Dip your eggs in salsa or fill a whole-wheat tortilla with scrambled eggs, salsa, and spinach leaves for a nutrient-packed breakfast wrap.

>> Add sliced tomatoes and fresh baby spinach leaves to your sandwich. Try thinly sliced bell peppers or roasted peppers on a sandwich, too.

>> Use leftover brown rice to make a quick salad to pack for lunch the following day. Add baby spinach, dried cranberries, slivered almonds, chopped apples, and chopped carrots to the rice. Toss with 1 tablespoon of vinaigrette dressing.

>> Try a simple peanut sauce to add spunk to a vegetable stir-fry. Stir-fry 4 servings of your favorite vegetables for 2 minutes. Whisk together 3 tablespoons natural peanut butter, 2 tablespoons water, and 1 teaspoon low-sodium soy sauce. Pour sauce over vegetables, and stir-fry for an additional 1 to 2 minutes.

>> Use carrots, cucumber slices, and pepper strips instead of crackers or pretzels for dipping. Substitute hummus for cheese as a snack to go with the vegetables and get two vegetables in one (hummus is made from chickpeas).

>> Sauté chopped onion with 2 tablespoons of tomato paste; then add to hot rice for a quick side dish with added lycopene (a naturally occurring and powerful antioxidant that gives tomatoes their red color).

>> Add a side salad to your business lunch. Side salads usually include more vegetables and are always lower in calories than Caesar salads, which really aren't a great choice because of all the salty croutons, dressing, and cheese.

Enjoying vegetables in new ways

Sometimes a simple steamed vegetable may work well with a more complex entree, but in general, plain, steamed vegetables are pretty boring. So what can you do? Start with the steamed vegetable, but then add chopped herbs, some olive oil, lemon zest, or some fruit and nuts — easy ways to reinvent that vegetable you thought you hated!

Steaming

You can steam a vegetable either on the stovetop with a pot of boiling water and a steam basket or in the microwave. Steaming on the stovetop takes about 3 to 7 minutes after the water has reached the boiling point. To steam in the microwave, place washed vegetables into a microwave-safe glass dish with a lid, add about ½-inch of water, cover, cook for 3 to 5 minutes on high, remove the lid, and drain the water. Either way, the steamed vegetable should be crisp-tender and have a bright, vibrant color.

TIP

To add some flavor to your steamed vegetables, try the following:

>> Drizzle fresh green beans with olive oil and a few shakes of Herbs de Provence.

>> When you steam broccoli, add a clove or two of garlic. After it's cooked, remove the garlic. Add 2 teaspoons of olive oil, a shake of red pepper flakes, and 1 tablespoon of chopped dried cranberries. You can also mix the broccoli into a cup of brown rice and make a pilaf.

>> Steam baby carrots until they're fork-tender. Drain and drizzle 1 tablespoon of pure maple syrup over the hot carrots. Sprinkle with a touch of dried tarragon.

Roasting

Roasting vegetables tends to bring out the natural sugars in the vegetable, offering you a whole new set of flavors. Try roasting or grilling vegetables you don't like — you may be pleasantly surprised!

TIP

Following are some suggestions if you're new to roasting vegetables:

>> Peel an eggplant and cut off the ends. Cut into ½-inch slices, and then cut each into four pieces so you have cubes. Wash and cut a bell pepper into small cubes. Chop a sweet onion and peel three to four garlic cloves. Add 1 cup of chopped portobello mushrooms and 1 cup of baby carrots. Toss the vegetable mixture with about 2 to 4 tablespoons of olive oil. Toss until coated and pour the mixture into a glass baking dish. Bake at 400 degrees for 35 to 45 minutes, turning twice during cooking (at around 15 and 25 minutes).

>> Rinse a bunch of asparagus and cut about 1 to 2 inches off the bottom ends (you can also just snip them by hand; the point where the end snips is the tough part). Place the asparagus in a shallow dish, drizzle with olive oil, and toss to coat. Sprinkle with a squeeze of lemon juice and a touch of garlic powder. Place the asparagus directly onto a hot grill, being careful not to allow it to slip through the slots (you can also use a grill pan). Grill for about 10 to 15 minutes, turning once.

>> Peel, cut, and cube a butternut squash (cut it into small cubed pieces, about ½-inch in size, or for convenience use precut frozen squash). Toss with olive oil (see a trend here?) and one clove of minced garlic, and sprinkle with chopped fresh or dried rosemary. Roast for 30 to 45 minutes, or until it's fork-tender.

Mixing and matching

TIP

Mixing different vegetables together, adding them to grain dishes, or adding in fruit, nuts, or seeds is another flavorful way to enjoy vegetables. Here are some fun and flavorful additions to common vegetables:

>> **Beets:** Crumbled goat cheese, walnuts

>> **Broccoli:** Toasted walnuts, raisins, slivered carrots

- >> **Green beans:** Slivered almonds, toasted walnuts, raisins, pearl onions

- >> **Spinach:** Sunflower seeds, butternut squash, onions

- >> **Squash:** Caramelized onions, small amounts of grated Swiss cheese

- >> **Zucchini:** Toasted walnuts, feta cheese

Going beyond plain ol' milk to get your daily dairy

As we explain in Chapter 2, DASH studies show that people who include dairy in their diets have a more significant drop in blood pressure than those who don't. Consequently, dairy — particularly low-fat dairy — is an integral part of the DASH diet.

TIP

Don't get stuck on milk when you think about dairy. Here are some easy ways to get your dairy servings every day, beyond drinking a glass of plain milk:

- >> Keep a quart of plain low-fat yogurt in your refrigerator and eat it topped with fruit at snack time or use it as a substitute for sour cream in cooking and baking.

- >> Prepare heart-healthy oatmeal with low-fat milk rather than water to add some dairy and more nutrition.

- >> Consider a spread of ricotta cheese over a slice of whole-grain toast in the morning or cottage cheese topped with fruit for an afternoon snack. You can use both of these cheeses in cooking as well, or add a dollop to a salad.

- >> Add oomph to your dishes with 2 to 3 tablespoons of shredded cheese for a lower-sodium cost than adding salt or other high-sodium seasonings. Just be aware of the amount of cheese you add to recipes.

- >> Use yogurt to create delicious smoothie bowls (like the Breakfast Smoothie Bowl in Chapter 17) or create your own on-the-run yogurt smoothie option for busy mornings.

- >> Flavor your milk with a teaspoon of coffee syrup, such as vanilla or hazelnut (adding your own sweetener controls the amount of sugar).

- >> Prepare your own latte at home by mixing plain brewed coffee with 4 to 8 ounces of low-fat milk and adding a touch of your favorite sweetener (a better option than fancy coffee shop drinks). Enjoy it hot or over ice.

Surveying Common Obstacles

Each and every day of your life, you make choices about what you're going to eat. Some periods of your life are more hectic than others, making it difficult to focus on your DASH diet. Be aware that other, more day-to-day obstacles, exist as well. Your best bet for not letting these obstacles throw you off track is to plan for them so you know how to react if they rear their ugly heads. In the following sections, we present strategies to deal with any obstacle.

REMEMBER

Having a plan in place to help you deal with common obstacles is a good idea, but don't beat yourself up if you occasionally slip up regardless. Just aim to do better at the next meal.

Forgetting about liquid calories

Liquid calories can be problematic because they aren't filling, so it's easy to drink too many of them without realizing it. Check out the following estimates to see how quickly liquid calories can add up:

>> A typical 16-ounce coffee drink from a coffee shop can rack up anywhere from 120 to 350 calories. Black coffee has zero, and coffee with one creamer has about 30. A 16-ounce frozen mocha has 550 calories — more than a small milkshake!

>> A 20-ounce pour of soda has about 250 calories. Sugary drinks can be less hydrating as well. Choose water with lemon or fresh mint instead.

>> That smoothie at the mall packs 300 to 450 calories.

>> A 16-ounce lemonade has 100 calories.

>> A 5-ounce glass of wine, a shot of liquor, or a 12-ounce beer? All have about 150 calories.

REMEMBER

Becoming more aware of the calories in the liquids you drink is the first step to controlling those calories. It's also worth noting that beverages such as coffee, soda, and lemonade aren't part of the DASH diet, and overall you want to limit added sugars in your diet. Moderate amounts of alcohol may be of some benefit, but you don't want to go overboard with these liquid calories, especially if you need to lose weight.

Craving junk food

Sometimes when your body is craving something, that craving is just your body saying, "I'm hungry. Feed me!" You may be able to satisfy that craving *without* turning to junk food if you follow these suggestions:

>> If you like crunchy snacks, then keep fresh-cut vegetables (think sweet bell peppers and celery) ready to grab in your fridge and serve them with a portion of hummus. Or serve up a bowl of high-fiber cereal with nonfat or low-fat milk for a great crunchy and nutritious snack.

>> Another go-to, crunchy, high-fiber snack is popcorn. Rather than relying on the light microwave type, consider investing in an air popper or make it over the stove with regular popcorn kernels and vegetable oil. You only need about a tablespoon of oil in a large pot (use a heart-healthy high-heat oil like canola or avocado). Heat the oil until it starts to sizzle, add a half cup of popcorn, and put on the lid. Watch the pot, shaking it occasionally, and when the corn stops popping, remove the pot from the heat and enjoy. Enjoy the popcorn as is or season it with salt-free flavored powders.

>> If you have a sweet tooth, first have a sliced apple or a bowl of strawberries. You can also try adding a scoop of cottage cheese and a sprinkle of cinnamon to some cantaloupe for a filling and refreshing DASH diet snack.

If the craving won't budge, drink a glass of water. Try infusing your water with fresh mint, muddled strawberries, or citrus. Sometimes you get hunger signals when you're actually dehydrated.

>> If you're eager for something savory, try slicing a plum tomato and sprinkling it with feta cheese and a drizzle of balsamic vinegar.

>> String cheese is an easy dairy choice and is packaged in the perfect, portable, 1-serving portion.

>> Though we prefer that you stick with fresh and mostly whole foods, having some packaged foods on hand — such as granola or fruit-nut bars — is okay as long as you compare labels. Look for low-sodium choices and check the ingredient list for the basics (oats, nuts, fruit), with few additives.

REMEMBER

We get it. Sometimes your craving means business. If nothing satisfies your craving for those potato chips, just be sure to practice portion control. Get yourself a 1-ounce single-serve bag. If you're dying to have ice cream, serve one scoop in a small custard cup or ramekin so you aren't tempted to eat the whole pint. Be mindful as you eat to get full enjoyment from these treats.

TIP

Think about the times you were drawn to particular, not-so-good-for-you food. Were you stressed? Bored? Anxious? Understanding when you tend to treat eating as an emotional response can help you deal better with cravings in the future. Small changes in your environment or routine can help, too. Do you take snacks to your couch when you watch TV? Is it because you're hungry, or is it just a habit? If you really are hungry, take the opportunity to make this snack well portioned and DASH-friendly (for instance, count out 15 almonds, and slowly savor them). Do you automatically pour a glass of wine after work? Try pouring sparkling water into a wine glass instead, and maybe you can skip the wine completely, or pour less of it.

Meeting resistance within your household

There's no reason that everyone in the household — no matter how young or old — can't adopt the DASH diet. It's not just a diet for hypertension; it's a healthy diet that provides the nutrients that everyone needs and may even protect against cancer and maintain heart health. It's also just fine for someone with diabetes.

CONSIDERING DIETARY RESTRICTIONS

Even though you probably either have a family history of high blood pressure or have been diagnosed with it, it's best to meet with a registered dietitian to discuss your specific dietary and medical nutrition needs. For the most part you can still follow the DASH diet even if you have other dietary restrictions to consider.

- If you have *celiac disease*, a rare autoimmune disorder that causes gastrointestinal discomfort and malabsorption issues because of an abnormal response to gluten, you can still follow the DASH diet because fruit, vegetables, and dairy are naturally gluten-free. You'll have to eliminate some grains (bread products made with wheat, rye, or barley), but you can still include oats, rice, and quinoa.

- While dairy proved to be a key factor in lowering blood pressure in the DASH studies, if you're vegan, you can follow a modified DASH plan without it. Because DASH focuses on lots of fresh fruits and vegetables and also includes whole grains, nuts, and seeds, it's not difficult to maintain a vegan lifestyle and reap the blood-pressure-lowering benefit. If you're a vegetarian who eats dairy, eggs, and/or fish, you'll have no trouble incorporating all the DASH diet guidelines.

- If you're lactose intolerant, you may still be able to tolerate small portions of certain dairy foods. Some research shows that exposure helps increase tolerance. Try consuming 1 or 2 servings per day of yogurt or milk with the lactase enzyme added to it and monitor your body's reaction. If you experience abdominal cramping, bloating, or diarrhea, eliminate all dairy for a few days, check symptoms, add a small portion back, and continue monitoring symptoms.

Despite all that, someone in your household may balk at the idea of following the DASH diet. It's really difficult to be the only person in a household who's trying to make healthier choices. So if you meet resistance, consider enlisting a friend, your doctor, or another person that the resister respects to offer her side of the situation. Handing over a few pages from this book (or reading aloud to the person) may even help get the resister on board.

TIP

If you aren't the primary grocery shopper, consider joining that person at the store next time and gently suggesting: "I want to try some new vegetables this week" or "I'm going to start having yogurt as a snack." Another tactic is to say nothing. Sometimes, when you put the idea into a person's head that "we're going to start cooking healthy dinners around here!" he or she may immediately shut down and protest! Just gradually start making these changes and add some new tasty recipes to the table. Use the recipes in this book to create a new shopping list, and the tasty dishes your create will make embarking on a new lifestyle that much easier.

Presenting a Sample 14-Day Meal Plan

There's no exact, day-to-day meal plan that you must follow to incorporate the basic dietary principles of the DASH diet into your life. Your goal is to focus on incorporating more fruit and/or vegetables, 1 serving of low-fat dairy, some whole grains, and smaller serving of lean protein into meals and snacks, while adding some healthy fats into your diet as well (vegetable oils, nuts, seeds, avocados, and so on).

Because many people like to have a visual plan to get them jump-started, the following 14-day meal plan offers you some examples of breakfasts, lunches, and dinners that adhere to the principles of DASH. Some of the items listed are recipes in this book; we list the chapter number for your convenience. This meal plan provides about 1,800 calories per day, which may be less than you require. Schedule an appointment with a registered dietitian nutritionist (RDN), who can provide you with a specific calorie level that meets your individual needs.

TIP

Drink water with all meals and throughout the day. Enjoy no-calorie beverages such as coffee or tea with a small amount of milk added to them if desired.

Day 1

Breakfast

One whole-grain English muffin, toasted

2 teaspoons olive oil spread

4 ounces Greek yogurt with ½ cup blueberries

Lunch

Chicken Wrap with Spicy Peanut Sauce (Chapter 18)

One sliced apple and six carrot sticks

8 ounces nonfat milk

Snack

One piece of string cheese and one clementine

Dinner

4 ounces baked fish with lemon

Microwaved green beans with almonds, 1 cup

Olive oil–roasted potato wedges, ½ cup

One scoop light ice cream topped with fresh raspberries

Day 2

Breakfast

Breakfast Smoothie Bowl (Chapter 17)

One slice multi-grain toast with 1 tablespoon peanut butter

Snack

1 orange

Lunch

Turkey breast (2 ounces) sandwich on whole-grain bread, with 1 ounce low-fat cheese, spinach leaves, and 4 tomato slices

12 to 15 grapes

8 ounces low-fat chocolate milk

Snack

20 almonds

Dinner

5 ounces grilled chicken breast

½ cup brown rice with 1 cup julienned vegetables

1 cup tossed green salad with 2 tablespoons vinaigrette dressing

Snack

Yogurt parfait (4 to 6 ounces nonfat plain yogurt topped with fresh sliced fruit and 2 to 3 tablespoons granola)

Day 3

Breakfast

1 cup oatmeal topped with sliced banana and drizzled with 1 teaspoon honey
8 ounces nonfat milk

Lunch

Hearty Southwest Slow-Cooker Soup (Chapter 22)

Tossed green salad (2 cups) topped with 2 ounces leftover sliced chicken breast; 1 tablespoon each of dried cranberries, sliced almonds, and sunflower seeds; 2 tablespoons guacamole; and vinaigrette dressing

Snack

¼ cup dried fruit and nut mix

Dinner

4 ounces pork loin

One medium baked potato with 1 to 2 tablespoons light sour cream or nonfat plain Greek yogurt

Roasted mixed vegetables (such as broccoli, peppers, zucchini)

1 cup tossed salad with 1 to 2 tablespoons vinaigrette dressing

2-inch square of pear crisp topped with ½ cup light vanilla ice cream

Snack

Green smoothie (made with spinach and green apple)

Day 4

Breakfast

Banana Nut Hot Oatmeal (Chapter 17)

Café latte made with 6 ounces nonfat milk

Lunch

Confetti Quesadillas (Chapter 18)

½ cup black beans garnished with 2 tablespoons nonfat plain yogurt

One sliced apple

Snack

½ cup canned peaches and one light piece of string cheese

Dinner

Bold and Beefy Instant Pot Stew (Chapter 22)

2-inch square of corn bread

Spinach salad (1 cup) with 2 tablespoons balsamic vinaigrette and 3 tablespoons shredded Swiss cheese

Sautéed apples with cinnamon, ½ cup

Day 5

Breakfast

2 vegetable omelet muffin cups (scramble eggs, add chopped vegetables, pour into oil-sprayed muffin cups, and bake for 20 minutes at 350 degrees)

One slice whole-grain toast with 1 teaspoon spread margarine

½ cup mixed fruit

8 ounces nonfat milk

Lunch

Lemon Pepper Tuna and White Bean Salad (Chapter 18)

½ cup canned pears or 1 fresh pear

TIP

MAKING YOUR OWN DRESSINGS

Making your own salad dressing is easier than you may think! Here are two go-to recipes for 1 serving:

- **Basic Viniagrette:** Mix 1 tablespoon extra-virgin olive oil, 1 teaspoon red wine or balsamic vinegar, ¼ teaspoon sugar, and ½ teaspoon dried herbs of choice.

- **Mustard Viniagrette:** Mix 1 tablespoon extra-virgin olive oil, 1 teaspoon white wine vinegar (or lemon juice or orange juice), and ¼ teaspoon Dijon mustard.

Snack

Six to ten grape tomatoes

One soft cheese wedge (1 ounce)

Dinner

Seared Scallops with Pistachio Sauce (Chapter 19)

1 cup green beans

½ cup brown rice

1 cup tossed romaine salad with 2 tablespoons homemade or vinaigrette-style dressing (see the nearby "Making your own dressings" sidebar)

Day 6

Breakfast

One slice whole-wheat raisin toast topped with ¼ cup light ricotta cheese and sprinkled with cinnamon

1 cup sliced melon

8 ounces nonfat milk

Snack

½ cup low-fat cottage cheese mixed with ½ cup sliced peaches

Lunch

Fruit and Nut Chicken Salad Lettuce Wraps (Chapter 18)

One orange

Snack

½ cup sweet bell pepper strips dipped in 2 to 3 tablespoons hummus

Dinner

Whole-wheat pasta (1 cup) tossed with 4 ounces salmon and ¼ cup peas and 1 cup butternut squash "noodles"

Mango Banana Soft Serve (Chapter 23)

Snack

¼ cup peanuts

Day 7

Breakfast

Banana Nut Hot Oatmeal (Chapter 17)

8 ounces nonfat milk

Snack

String cheese

Small apple

Lunch

Tuna fish in a whole-wheat pita pocket (½ cup tuna salad made with minced bell peppers, minced onion, minced celery, and low-fat mayonnaise)

1 cup tossed field greens with 1 tablespoon homemade vinaigrette dressing (see the nearby sidebar, "Making your own dressings")

Two clementines

Snack

20 almonds and 8 ounces low-fat chocolate milk

Dinner

Stuffed pasta shells stuffed with low-fat ricotta and spinach, three shells

2 cups tossed green salad with chopped carrots and 2 tablespoons balsamic dressing

1 slice whole-grain bread toasted with olive oil and salt-free Italian seasoning

Day 8

Breakfast

1 cup steel-cut oats with two chopped dried apricots or 2 tablespoons raisins, drizzled with 1 teaspoon maple syrup

8 ounces nonfat or low-fat milk

Snack

One fruit-and-nut bar

Lunch

Grilled chicken (3 ounces) topped with avocado and mango slices on two slices whole-grain bread

1 cup spinach salad with 1 tablespoon homemade mustard dressing (see the "Making your own dressings" sidebar, earlier in this chapter)

Snack

One piece low-fat string cheese and 1 cup cut raw vegetables

Dinner

Two fish tacos (2 corn tortillas, 4 ounces baked fish, chopped lettuce, tomatoes, and peppers)

Southwest Corn with Chipotle Peppers (Chapter 20)

2-inch brownie square (using brownie mix, substitute applesauce for oil)

Day 9

Breakfast

Two-egg omelet with spinach, onions, and bell pepper

One slice whole-grain toast with spread margarine

6 ounces orange-pineapple juice

Snack

Greek yogurt smoothie (8 ounces, made with plain yogurt and 1 cup fruit)

Lunch

Quick flatbread pizza (whole-wheat flax wrap topped with fresh sliced tomatoes or sauce, 2 to 3 tablespoons low-fat mozzarella, spinach leaves, and roasted peppers, microwaved or toasted in toaster oven)

One medium apple

Dinner

5 ounces roast pork tenderloin with dried cherries and onions

Moroccan-Style Farro with Kale (Chapter 20)

1 cup low-fat frozen yogurt topped with sliced bananas and a 1-teaspoon drizzle of caramel sauce

Day 10

Breakfast

Crave-Worthy Toast (Chapter 17)

One orange

Lunch

Butternut Squash Enchiladas with Avocado Cream (Chapter 21)

1 cup tossed salad with vinaigrette (see the "Making your own dressings" sidebar, earlier in this chapter)

Snack

Ten carrot sticks with 2 tablespoons hummus

Dinner

1 cup penne pasta with shrimp and broccoli, tossed with garlic and olive oil

1 cup mixed field greens with homemade vinaigrette (see the "Making your own dressings" sidebar, earlier in this chapter)

Berry compote, 1 cup

Day 11

Breakfast

One whole-grain frozen waffle topped with ¼ cup part-skim ricotta and chopped berries, sprinkled with wheat germ or 2 tablespoons chopped walnuts

6 ounces orange-mango juice

Lunch

Tossed salad topped with ½ cup tuna salad made with chopped celery and apple, shredded carrots, and chopped walnuts

1 cup of homemade or low-sodium vegetable soup

Vanilla Chia Seed Pudding with Toppings (Chapter 23)

Snack

1 small homemade whole-wheat blueberry-pecan muffin

4 ounces low-fat milk

Dinner

Herbed Baked Chicken with Artichokes (Chapter 19)

Smashed potatoes, ½ cup

1 cup green beans

One slice angel food cake topped with strawberries

Day 12

Breakfast

One slice toasted whole-grain walnut-raisin bread spread with part-skim ricotta cheese

8 ounces yogurt smoothie

Snack

Apples slices with 2 teaspoons peanut butter

Lunch

Open-Faced Roast Beef Sandwich with Horseradish Sauce (Chapter 18)

1 cup melon

Dinner

Grilled or broiled 4-ounce salmon filet topped with mango salsa

1 cup roasted vegetable mix (choose vegetables such as zucchini, eggplant, onions, mushrooms, and bell peppers; cube and roast them with 3 tablespoons olive oil at 400 degrees for 45 minutes)

½ cup brown rice

Strawberries with Peppered Balsamic Drizzle (Chapter 23)

Day 13

Breakfast

Open-Faced Egg Sandwich (Chapter 17)

Grapefruit half

Lunch

Bean burger on whole-wheat roll topped with sliced tomato and avocado

Baked sweet potato fries, ½ cup

½ cup Waldorf salad

Snack

Mini wrap with leftover roasted vegetables and a slice of provolone cheese or ¼ cup reduced-fat feta (or substitute a half whole-wheat pita for mini wrap)

Dinner

Easy Eggplant Parm (Chapter 21)

1 cup tossed salad with 2 tablespoons Italian oil-and-vinegar dressing

½ cup chocolate pudding

Day 14

Breakfast

Breakfast burrito (1 scrambled egg [add ¼ cup 1% milk], 2 tablespoons bean salsa, and 2 to 3 tablespoons low-fat shredded cheddar cheese wrapped into a small whole-wheat tortilla)

Sliced kiwifruit and strawberries, 1 cup

Lunch

Tossed salad (spring mix, chopped tomato, cucumber, peppers), 1 teaspoon sunflower seeds, topped with ½ cup cottage cheese and pouch tuna and 1 tablespoon of homemade dressing

15 grapes

8 ounces 1% milk

Snack

6 ounces plain Greek yogurt topped with 2 tablespoons granola and berries

Dinner

Lasagna Spaghetti Squash Bowls (Chapter 21)

Six to ten spears roasted asparagus

Wine Poached Pears (Chapter 23)

Chapter **12**

DASHing Successfully through the Grocery Store

t's no secret that cooking more balanced meals at home starts with making healthier choices at the supermarket. There's certainly no shortage of choices as you push your cart down the aisles of the sometimes confusing maze. It's easy to be seduced by the colorful boxes and fancy displays. By following a few basic planning tips, you'll discover what a painless process shopping can be even if circumstances have you shopping online. Most stores now have shop-at-home with delivery services that help save time and even money!

This chapter helps you understand how to make informed decisions at the grocery store by evaluating health claims and Nutrition Facts labels for foods that fit in the DASH diet plan for lowering blood pressure. It also explains how to stretch your food budget, navigate the center aisles without going off-track and find goodies around the perimeter of the grocery store, and how to keep food safe.

Getting Organized before You Go

Grocery stores are filled with tantalizing smells and mouthwatering displays designed to distract you. Don't let them! You stand a better chance of sticking to your new DASH eating plan — not to mention saving cash — by getting yourself organized before you head out to the store. Here's an easy way to get organized for grocery shopping:

1. **Create a weekly meal plan.**

   Planning ahead helps reduce stress and increases the likelihood of making healthy choices. The 15 minutes you spend planning meals can save you hours of wasted time throughout the week (not to mention money at the store). Decide how many meals you'll be shopping for, such as 3 meals a day for 5 days, or 15 meals. Don't forget to plan for snacks, too. Then take an inventory of the staples you already have in your pantry and refrigerator, such as oils and spices, dairy products, fresh fruit, vegetables, and grains.

2. **Make a menu-based shopping list and check it twice.**

   Entering the grocery store armed with a detailed shopping list makes your trip more efficient, helps you avoid impulse purchases, and keeps you on track with your heart-healthy eating goals. Use the recipes in Part 4 as a guide for ingredients. Organize your list by food categories and include food you typically buy in each category, keeping in mind the dietary goals of the DASH diet.

TIP

Consider downloading a phone app such as Grocery iQ, Out of Milk, Flipp, Meal Board, AnyList, GroceryPal, BigOven, Buy Me a Pie!, or Grocery Gadget to help you keep an organized list.

Try to focus your grocery list on the foods found along the perimeter of the store: fresh produce, dairy, poultry, meat, and seafood. Groceries that come from nature are always the healthier choice. They contain less sodium, fat, and sugar and have more flavor and health-promoting nutrients than prepackaged and highly processed foods. For example, buy fresh chicken breasts instead of frozen breaded chicken tenders, and buy fresh or fresh-frozen vegetables instead of frozen vegetables with sauces (even individually frozen chicken is often pumped with a sodium solution, so read labels).

WARNING

Never do your grocery shopping on an empty stomach. If you do, *everything* will look tempting, and you may overfill your cart or add too many unhealthy choices. So make sure to have a quick snack before you head out or go to the store shortly after eating a meal.

STRETCHING YOUR FOOD BUDGET ON DASH

If you grocery shop on a budget, you don't have to forfeit nutritional quality. You just have to shop a little smarter by following these tips:

- Scan grocery store ads and circulars in the local newspapers for specials and coupons. Use coupons only for foods that are on your list. Buy meats when they're on special, and freeze individual family portions in freezer bags.

- Compare prices and package sizes to make the best-value choices.

- Pre-chopped vegetables and fruit or shredded cheese cost more than chopping and shredding yourself.

- Plan one or two meatless meals per week. You can substitute one of the non-meat protein choices listed in the later sidebar "Where to find non-meat protein sources" for chicken, beef, or pork. (Refer to Chapter 21 for recipe ideas.)

- Choose produce that's in season. It will cost a fraction of the price and have a more complex and richer flavor.

Deciphering the Many Details and Claims on Food Packaging

Nearly every packaged product in the grocery store comes with an ingredients list and a mountain of nutrition information. But what does all that label lingo really mean? Are those nutrition claims grounded in the truth? Get ready to become a label sleuth by reading the helpful information we provide in the next sections.

REMEMBER

Your first lesson involves the ingredients list. Ingredients appear in the order of the amount the product contains, with the largest-quantity ingredient listed first, the second-highest quantity listed second, and so on. A longer list of ingredients can imply fewer nutrients and more additives, but this may not always be the case. When it comes to making healthy choices, the most nutritious foods are generally the least processed foods with the least additives. Fewer ingredients generally relates to lower-sodium foods as well. The less processed the food, the more natural vitamins, minerals, fiber, and phytonutrients it contains.

TIP

One claim you can trust is that a packaged food is heart-healthy if it bears the American Heart Association's heart check mark. This easily recognized icon was created by the American Heart Association's Heart Check Food Certification Program that helps you make informed choices at the grocery store. The program helps you take the guesswork out of reading Nutrition Facts and considers the amount of saturated fat, trans fat, sodium, and other nutrients in approving products. You can shop by looking for the heart check mark or use the online Heart-Check Certified Product List at `www.heart.org/en/healthy-living/company-collaboration/heart-check-certification/heart-check-in-the-grocery-store/certified-foods-in-the-grocery-store`.

Analyzing the Nutrition Facts label

The U.S. Food and Drug Administration (FDA) updated the standardized Nutrition Facts label on packaged food and drink to help consumers make more informed choices. It's an excellent tool that helps you verify which foods fit into your healthy DASH diet. The new label tells you how many calories, minerals and vitamins, milligrams of sodium and cholesterol, and grams of fat are in a serving. It also shows you the Daily Values for these amounts. The label is designed to highlight more realistic serving sizes; display calories in larger, bolder print; and point out the amount of added sugar in the product.

Just what is a serving size? Serving size is based on the amount of the food eaten but not necessarily a recommendation of how much to eat. It also depends on the manufacturer. The average person may then consume much more than the serving size listed on the package, doubling or tripling the nutrients (good and bad). For example, a serving of 10 tortilla chips may provide 140 calories and 126 milligrams of sodium, which may seem like a modest amount. If you eat them out of the bag instead of portioning a 10-chip serving, though, the calorie and sodium counts quickly climb to an unhealthy amount. Be sure to do the math (and never eat from the bag or box; use a small bowl to portion out). If you eat twice the amount of the serving size listed, then you need to double the amount of calories and nutrients.

All the other information on the Nutrition Facts label is presented in terms of the percent daily value, which is based on a 2,000-calorie intake. Your personal calorie budget may be fewer than 2,000 calories per day, so you need to modify the nutrition information per serving accordingly.

TIP

To estimate your personal energy needs, check out Chapter 4 or the Mayo Clinic's calorie calculator at `www.mayoclinic.org/healthy-lifestyle/weight-loss/in-depth/calorie-calculator/itt-20402304` (or just search the web for "Mayo Clinic calorie calculator"). Set up an appointment with a registered dietitian nutritionist (RDN) for a full evaluation of your nutritional needs.

The following sections delve into the remaining components of the Nutrition Facts label. To see where these components fall on the actual label, see Figure 12-1.

FIGURE 12-1:
A sample
Nutrition
Facts label.

Nutrition Facts	
8 servings per container	
Serving size	**2/3 cup (55g)**

Amount per serving	
Calories	**230**

	% Daily Value*
Total Fat 8g	**10%**
Saturated Fat 1g	**5%**
Trans Fat 0g	
Cholesterol 0mg	**0%**
Sodium 160mg	**7%**
Total Carbohydrate 37g	**13%**
Dietary Fiber 4g	**14%**
Total Sugars 12g	
Includes 10g Added Sugars	**20%**
Protein 3g	
Vitamin D 2mcg	10%
Calcium 260mg	20%
Iron 8mg	45%
Potassium 240mg	6%

* The % Daily Value (DV) tells you how much a nutrient in a serving of food contributes to a daily diet. 2,000 calories a day is used for general nutrition advice.

Illustration courtesy of U.S. Food and Drug Administration

Calories and calories from fat

Nutrition facts labels list how many total calories are in the specified serving size. *Calories* provide a measure of how much energy food provides. Your body needs energy to move and support bodily functions (such as respiration and digestion), and you burn additional calories when your body is active. The calorie information on the Nutrition Facts label helps you determine how much of a food can fit into your overall diet to maintain a healthy weight.

FACTS UP FRONT

In 2011, the Grocery Manufacturers Association and the Food Marketing Institute released Facts Up Front, a labeling system designed to help consumers choose healthy foods. Facts Up Front appears on the front of packaged foods in a rectangular box and can serve as a quick reference to help you lower your intake of saturated fat and sodium. This labeling system highlights four main data categories: calories, saturated fat, sodium, and sugar. However, you may also see the amounts of potassium, fiber, protein, vitamin A, vitamin C, vitamin D, calcium, and iron per serving. For more information on Facts Up Front, go to www.factsupfront.org.

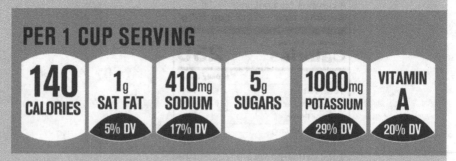

Illustration courtesy of the Grocery Manufacturers Association

The calories from fat give you an idea of how high in fat the food is. The closer the calories from fat number is to the total calories, the greater the percentage of fat. A high-fat food is one that provides more than 30 percent of its calories from fat. For a heart-healthy diet, most of the foods you consume should have a percent daily value of less than 30, but not all. Some foods may have a high percentage of calories from fat, and this doesn't necessarily mean you should avoid them. For example, a 1-ounce stick of low-fat string cheese contains approximately 60 calories, 2.5 grams of fat, and 9 grams of protein. Although 37 percent of the calories are from fat, this is still a healthy, lower-fat option compared to a regular mozzarella cheese stick, which has 8 grams of fat and 72 calories.

Total fat

The total fat line of the label describes the total fat per serving (which is the combined total of saturated, trans, and unsaturated fats). The American Heart Association (AHA) and the National Heart, Lung, and Blood Institute (NHLBI) recommend getting 25 to 30 percent of total daily calories from fat. You should limit saturated fat to 7 percent of total calories, and trans fat should be less than 1 percent of total calories.

Saturated fat and trans fat are key players in raising your blood cholesterol and increasing your risk of heart disease. Saturated fat comes mostly from animals. Trans fat is an unsaturated (plant-based) fat that has been processed to change its chemical composition, resulting in a fat that acts like a saturated fat. Look for foods that have 1 gram or less of saturated or trans fat per 100 calories (preferably 0 grams of trans fat). *Note:* The amount of trans fat will only be listed if the food has more than 0.5 grams per serving.

Unsaturated fat comes from plant sources. Polyunsaturated fats actually help lower LDL (bad cholesterol), and monounsaturated fats help increase HDL (good cholesterol). Manufacturers aren't required to list the amount of unsaturated fat, but you can estimate it by subtracting the saturated and trans fat from the total fat. Because the Nutrition Facts label features round numbers, the numbers don't always add up, but you can still get a rough idea.

Cholesterol

Cholesterol comes from animal products, and according to the 2010 Dietary Guidelines for Americans, you should consume less than 300 milligrams of cholesterol per day.

REMEMBER Although limiting your dietary cholesterol intake is important when following a heart-healthy eating plan, monitoring your saturated fat and trans fat intake is probably more important. Cholesterol is found only in animal products, but trans fats can be plant-based.

Sodium

Because a lower-sodium intake is a part of the DASH diet plan for lowering blood pressure, it's important to note the sodium content on the Nutrition Facts label. The percent daily value for sodium is based on 100 percent of the recommended amount of sodium, which is less than 2,300 milligrams per day. If you're over 50 years old or have high blood pressure, the limit should be 1,500 milligrams per day. Most of the sodium consumed comes from packaged and prepared foods, not necessarily from salt added to food in cooking and eating. As a guide, 5 percent of Daily Value or less of sodium per serving is considered low and 20 percent of Daily Value or more of sodium per serving is considered high.

TIP You can also check the front of the food package to quickly identify foods that may contain less sodium. Look for these claims:

>> **Salt/sodium-free:** Less than 5 milligrams of sodium per serving

>> **Very low sodium:** 35 milligrams of sodium or less per serving

>> **Low sodium:** 140 milligrams of sodium or less per serving

>> **Reduced sodium:** At least 25 percent less sodium than in the regular product

>> **Light in sodium or lightly salted:** At least 50 percent less sodium than in the regular product

>> **No salt added or unsalted:** No salt added during processing but not necessarily sodium-free; check the Nutrition Facts label to be sure

Total carbohydrate

The total carbohydrate entry on the Nutrition Facts label refers to all types of carbohydrates — sugar, complex carbohydrate, and fiber. The total carbohydrate entry is especially important to refer to when counting carbs, such as in diabetic meal planning, because all types of carbohydrates affect blood glucose.

Dietary fiber is important in weight control and can also help lower blood cholesterol levels. Unlike sodium and fat, you want to add *more* fiber to your diet when following the DASH eating plan. The best approach to adding fiber to your diet is to consume more fresh fruits and vegetables. These foods add fiber and all-important phytochemicals. A half-cup serving of a fruit or vegetable provides you with 3 to 5 grams of fiber, and black beans provide a whopping 8 to 10 grams of fiber per serving. If you follow the DASH diet guidelines of 8 to 10 servings of fruits and veggies daily, you'll easily consume 20 to 30 grams of fiber per day.

TIP

For packaged foods, the Whole Grains Council has created special stamps to help consumers identify products that are whole grain (see Figure 12-2):

>> **The basic stamp** displayed on a product means that it contains at least 8 grams of whole grain but contains primarily refined grain.

>> **The 100% stamp** displayed on a product means that all its grain ingredients are whole grain, and a full serving of the product has at least 16 grams of whole grain.

WARNING

Packaged foods touting "good source of fiber" may also carry too much sodium, sugar, fat, or calories.

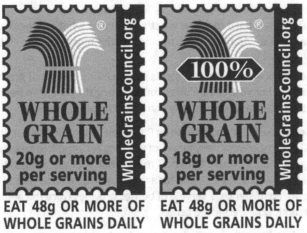

FIGURE 12-2:
The Whole Grain
Stamps, basic
(left) and 100%
(right).

Whole Grain Stamps are a trademark of Oldways Preservation Trust and the Whole Grains Council, www.wholegrainscouncil.org.

Protein

The protein entry on the Nutrition Facts label simply lists the amount of protein in 1 serving of that food item. Protein sources in your diet primarily come from meat, poultry, fish, cheese, dry beans, milk, and milk products (vegetables provide small amounts of protein also). Most Americans get plenty of protein but don't always get it from the healthiest sources or balance it with other foods. When choosing protein for the DASH diet, make choices that are lean, low-fat, or fat-free. In general, you're shooting for just 2 to 3 servings of low-fat dairy and 2 servings (or 6 to 8 ounces total) of lean meat or a meat alternative per day.

Vetting nutrient claims

Nutrition claims on food packaging are often classified as "health halos" — claims that mislead, usually over-promising and under-delivering. Just think of a bag of organic rice chips that boasts of having zero trans fat but is still highly processed with fat or salt. Or think of an embellished bottled water that has an insignificant quarter teaspoon of antioxidant added.

In the United States, health claims must be approved by the Food and Drug Administration, and claims stating that a certain food or components of a food may affect or reduce the risk of certain diseases must be supported by strong scientific evidence. Nutrient claims are far less regulated. If you're not well versed in the regulations, it's hard to know what's truth and what's hype. We spell out the difference for you when it comes to some of the more popular claims:

>> **Contains omega-3's:** Omega 3's get top billing on a lot of products, from milk to eggs. But you may be better off following the American Heart Association's recommendation to eat fatty fish at two meals per week.

>> **Good source of antioxidants:** Packaged foods only have to include 10 percent of your daily intake of vitamins A, C, and E to be considered a "good source." You're better off making half your plate vegetables and fruit, not only to meet your need for antioxidants but also as part of your DASH goals. For instance, 1 serving of berries provides twice the antioxidants of an antioxidant-enriched cereal.

>> **High in fiber:** Research shows that foods with naturally occurring fiber can reduce the risk of heart disease. Many of the products that promote a high-fiber content sometimes have added fiber from man-made sources or fiber extracted from plants. To meet your daily fiber needs, stick with whole grains, beans, oats, fresh fruit, and fresh vegetables.

OTHER LABEL LINGO TO KNOW

Even though the United States has the safest and most abundant food supply in the world, Americans must be diligent in making safe food choices. The FDA regulates packaged foods, drugs, and infant formula. The United State Department of Agriculture (USDA) regulates fresh produce and meats.

Here are the dates to be aware of when you're shopping:

• **Pack date:** The date the food was manufactured, processed, and packaged. For example, frozen food must be used a few months from this date. Canned goods are good for up to a year after the date.

• **Sell-by date:** The date is included on meat and dairy products and is the last day the product should be sold.

• **Best-if-used-by date:** This date represents the best quality of this product. Eating the product after this date may affect freshness but won't hurt you.

• **Expiration or use-by date:** The last date food should be eaten or used. This date is determined by the manufacturer.

For more information on food safety and storage, visit www.foodsafety.gov.

Focusing on the Perimeter of the Store for Wholesome Food Choices

The foods you can find along the outer walls of the grocery store — fruits and vegetables, whole grains, fresh lean meats, and low-fat dairy — are at the heart of the DASH diet. As an added bonus, the more whole foods like these that you eat, the more nutrients (and likely fewer calories) you pack in. The following sections guide you along the perimeter of the grocery store to help you start filling your cart with the foods that will help you lower your blood pressure.

Checking out the produce aisle

You can't go wrong in the produce section. It offers a world of flavor and a rainbow of colors that provide a wide assortment of vitamins, minerals, antioxidants, and phytochemicals that you need to maintain vibrant health and prevent disease. We recommend picking up a variety of fresh fruits and vegetables each week. Look for specials and sale items and alternate from one favorite to another. Buy only what you can use within a few days, though, because long storage times diminish quality, nutrient levels, and taste. Because some produce items have a longer shelf life than others, plan to make at least one additional trip to the grocery store each week. At least you know you'll be in and out in a flash!

TIP

For the best flavor and price, buy firm, brightly colored, blemish-free produce in season. Visit www.fruitsandveggies.org for resources on nutrition, storage and how to handle fruits and vegetables.

TIP

Are you wondering whether you should purchase organic produce? USDA-certified organic foods are grown and processed according to federal guidelines that address how animals are raised, soil quality, pest and weed control, and use of additives. Foods must not be genetically modified or irradiated and must be grown without synthetic fertilizers and pesticides (however, they *can* use natural pesticides). Organic meat, poultry, dairy, and eggs are produced without the use of antibiotics or growth hormones. A systematic review of research from various studies concludes that there is no significant difference in the nutritional value between conventional grown and organically produced food. For good health and to get all the nutrients needed for the DASH Diet Plan, it's important to eat fruits and vegetables. We believe that the value of consuming more fruits and vegetables far outweighs the benefits of choosing organic produce exclusively.

REMEMBER

Regardless of what type you buy, remember to follow food safety practices. According to the FDA, choose produce without obvious bruising. Washing fruits and vegetables before preparation is the best way to remove visible dirt and harmful pathogens that may be on your produce. Follow these tips for best cleaning practices:

>> Clean and sanitize your sink and other food contact surfaces and utensils.

>> Wash your hands for 20 seconds with warm water before and after preparing fresh produce.

>> Rinse the produce before you peel it to prevent transfer of bacteria from your knife to the produce.

>> Gently rub the produce under plain tap water. For firm produce, like cucumber and melons, use a clean veggie brush to scrub under tap water.

>> Dry the produce with a paper towel.

>> For leafy greens, remove the outer leaves.

>> Store produce in the refrigerator at 40 degrees or below.

TIP

On food labels, the organic labeling requirements apply to raw, fresh, and processed products. Products are labeled according to the percentage of organic ingredients they contain:

>> **100% organic:** Contains only organic products and ingredients. The organic seal is visible on products.

>> **Organic:** Must contain 95 percent organically produced ingredients. The organic seal is visible on products.

>> **Made with organic ingredients:** Can be used if products contain at least 70 percent organic items. The organic seal is not allowed on the label but must specify which ingredients are organic.

For more information about organic labels, go to www.ams.usda.gov.organic.

You may also see the term *natural* used on labels. For meat and poultry, the USDA defines *natural* as containing no artificial ingredients or added color and minimally processed. For all other products, there is no legal definition of this term. It's just a feel-good term used in marketing products.

EMBRACING HERBS AND SPICES

One of the easiest ways to incorporate more variety and flavor in your food is through the use of herbs, spices, and condiments. Herbs are also arguably the easiest of all edible plants to grow, whether in a backyard garden or in a pot. Fresh herbs can turn any dish from ho-hum to yum (more about that in Chapter 13). If you're not interested in growing your own herbs, you can always buy fresh ones from your grocery store's produce section. You can also pick up tubes of some herbs, such as basil. Visit http://na.gourmetgarden.com/us to figure out where to find herb tubes in your area.

Dried herbs and spices are available in the grocery store, many ethnic markets, and by mail order. Companies that manufacture herbs and spices (www.mccormick.com and www.penzeys.com) have created simple packets and blends to help inspire home cooks to add variety and flavor to their everyday cooking. If you want to start out slow and not invest in a large number of jars, you can always buy some spices in bulk and get just what you need for a recipe. *Note:* Be sure to read labels because many of the seasoning blends at the grocery store have salt as the main ingredient.

Sorting through the bread and grains

When selecting bread (or rice, pasta, or cereal), look for the 100 percent whole-grain variety. A *whole grain* is a grain that has the bran, germ, and endosperm intact. The bran forms a protective inner covering and is an excellent source of fiber. The germ is the embryo of a new plant and is a source of protein, vitamins, and minerals. The endosperm supplies most of the carbs, mainly in the form of starch. Refined grains, on the other hand, are whole grains that have been stripped of their outer coating, bran, and germ during the milling process, leaving only the starchy endosperm. That's why food manufacturers are mandated to fortify with the nutrients that have been stripped away.

Whole-wheat bread should list *whole-wheat flour* as the first ingredient on the list. Check bread, pasta, and cereal labels for fiber and sugar content too. Include some cereals in your pantry that supply at least 3 grams of fiber and less than 8 grams of sugar. If you can find some with more than 5 grams of fiber and less sugar, even better.

REMEMBER

It's still okay to consume some refined grains such as white rice, regular pasta, quick-cooking oats, or Italian or French bread. Just try to add some whole grains into the mix and be adventurous. Try something new like quinoa, farro, or whole-wheat couscous, which are very simple to prepare.

Protein pointers

When choosing meats on the DASH diet, the key words are "fresh" and "lean," and portion-controlled. Choose lean cuts of beef and pork, and a variety of poultry and fish. Poultry with the skin on is often less expensive, and you can simply remove the skin when you get home (on the other hand, you may be paying for the skin, so compare prices of skin-on versus skinless poultry). Flash-frozen chicken breasts often have added sodium, so a better choice is to buy fresh chicken, clean it, and freeze it yourself.

WHERE TO FIND NON-MEAT PROTEIN SOURCES

Plant-based foods such as legumes, peas, beans, and lentils are a super protein source, are low in sodium and saturated fat, and contain no cholesterol. They're inexpensive and versatile nutritional gems. You have many options, like using dry beans, which are lowest in sodium content, or canned beans. Canned varieties are available in reduced sodium, no added salt, and regular. If you choose the latter, rinse them thoroughly to remove as much of the sodium as possible.

Unsalted nuts and seeds are also good protein sources and supply a variety of nutrients, including monounsaturated and polyunsaturated fats. All plant proteins also have a high soluble fiber content that helps reduce blood cholesterol. Nuts and seeds are portable, low in saturated fat, and ideal for snacking. You can also add them to other foods for a protein kick. Choose unsalted nuts or seeds for cooking, and look for lightly salted or unsalted nuts for snacking.

Eggs are yet another excellent non-meat source of protein. They're relatively low in calories and saturated fat, although the egg yolk is a main source of cholesterol. Your recommended total cholesterol intake should be about 200 milligrams per day, roughly the amount in one egg. There's no limit to how many egg whites you can eat, so use more egg whites in your cooking, substituting two egg whites for one whole egg in most recipes.

Grains also provide protein in addition to carbohydrates, fiber, vitamins, and phytochemicals. Quinoa and amaranth are called *pseudo grains* because they look and taste like grains but are technically seeds. They contain all the essential acids to form a complete protein like meat. Other grains are missing an essential amino acid lysine, so when eating grains, be sure to include lysine-rich foods, such as lentils, beans, or quinoa to balance the proteins. Good examples are beans and rice or beans and corn tortillas. (See Chapter 21 for recipes using quinoa.)

All fish counts as lean meat (even fattier types of fish, because their fat content is mostly unsaturated fat). Eating fish twice a week can reduce risk of heart disease. Fish and shellfish have the same wonderful protein as meat and chicken plus the added benefit of omega-3 fatty acids. Oily fish such as salmon, sardines, and mackerel are especially high in omega-3. Whether you eat meat, chicken, or seafood, a 3-ounce portion, or the size of a deck of cards, is recommended twice a day. For more advice about eating fish check out www.fda.gov/food/consumers/advice-about-eating-fish.

WARNING

Although you can choose some leaner cuts of deli meat on occasion (such as low-sodium turkey breast, baked ham, and lean roast beef), avoid cuts such as bologna, corned beef, pastrami, salami, loaf meats, and pepperoni, which are not only loaded in sodium but also high in saturated fat. Check out our lunch ideas in Chapter 18 for fresh alternatives.

Also, pregnant women should avoid certain types of fish (shark, swordfish, king mackerel, tilefish, bigeye tuna [not canned tuna], marlin, and orange roughy) during pregnancy due to higher mercury content. For more information about safe seafood consumption, check www.seafoodnutrition.org/faqs.

Browsing the dairy case

As we explain in Chapter 5, the DASH diet encourages 2 to 3 servings of low-fat or fat-free dairy products per day. Whenever possible, choose low-fat or fat-free milk and yogurt. For cheeses, choose low-fat ricotta, part-skim mozzarella, or the many varieties of reduced-fat cheese now available. Buying bulk cheese and shredding yourself is a good option. Pre-shredded cheese is convenient and has ingredients that prevent clumping. Although these ingredients are safe, pre-shredded cheeses may differ in quality and taste.

TECHNICAL STUFF

When you include dairy in your diet, you get a wonderful supply of calcium and vitamin D. Calcium strengthens bones and teeth, but it also has many other health benefits. Vitamin D is very important to help your body absorb the calcium. Studies report that people who include more calcium in their diets tend to have lower blood pressure.

If you can't drink milk or consume milk products because of *lactose intolerance* (the inability to digest lactose, the natural sugar present in milk), simply look for lactose-free milk, cheese, and yogurt. Or purchase dairy products that contain lactose-digesting enzymes. Another option is calcium-fortified soy milk, which is naturally lactose-free. (For more on soy milk and other nondairy alternatives, see the nearby sidebar.)

EXPLORING NONDAIRY (PLANT-BASED) ALTERNATIVES

The standards of identity for milk are based on cow's milk. Several kinds of milk alternatives are available in grocery stores these days, but keep in mind that low-fat cow's milk is what provided the blood-pressure-lowering effect in the DASH trials. These alternatives don't supply adequate calcium and other valuable nutrients that milk provides and shouldn't be considered an equivalent to milk. Some studies question how well the added nutrients are absorbed. Following are the main categories:

- **Nut milk:** This nondairy beverage can be made from crushed almonds, hazelnuts, cashews, and so on that have been steeped in water and strained, with the liquid extracted. Many have added sweeteners to balance bitter tastes. They have little protein and added calcium and other key nutrients.

- **Rice milk:** Made from water and brown rice, rice milk has few nutrients on its own. Some have added vitamin D, calcium, and vitamin B12. Rice milk also contains oils, salt, rice syrup, evaporated cane juice, and other sweeteners.

- **Soy milk:** This naturally lactose-free milk alternative is made from soybeans that have been ground, cooked, strained, and fortified with additional nutrients. Lower-fat varieties may be lower in protein, calcium, vitamin D, and vitamin B12.

- **Hemp milk:** This is made from pressed seeds of the cannabis plant mixed with water and drained. It contains some protein and other nutrients.

Although many of the nondairy alternatives are fortified, these beverages do not necessarily supply the valuable nutrients that milk provides. Their cooking properties may also vary depending on the product.

Choosing wisely in the freezer section

The freezer section of the grocery store can be a mixed bag. On the one hand, it's a great place to find wholesome foods that have been flash-frozen so you can cook them as needed, seasoning to your own preferences and/or dietary requirements. On the other hand, it's stocked with tons of fast, convenient, pre-portioned meals that sound great to anyone running low on prep time. It's no surprise they're so popular. The challenge in this case is to find healthy frozen meals that taste good, satisfy your hunger, and won't sabotage your DASH eating goals. Following are our tips for making the most heart-healthy choices in the freezer section:

>> Look for entrees that are 300 to 500 calories per serving and low in fat and sodium — less than 30 percent of calories from fat, less than 10 percent of calories from saturated fat, and less than 600 milligrams of sodium per serving.

>> Skip frozen meals with cream sauces, gravies, or fried food.

>> With meat, poultry, and fish, choose plain and flash-frozen instead of breaded and fried items that have been frozen.

>> Choose the plain-frozen variety of vegetables, without sauces or added fats such as butter or nuts. Buy loose-pack plastic bags so you can use the amount you need and save the rest for another time.

>> Select flash-frozen fruits with no sugar added.

Buying fats and oils

Fat isn't the evil villain; it's an important nutrient necessary for good health. An important energy source, fat provides essential fatty acids and partners with fat-soluble vitamins to fully nourish the body. But not all fats are created equal. They differ depending on the amount of fatty acids they contain. All fats are a combination of fatty acids, but they're categorized by the fatty acid that is present in greatest amount. You should consume beneficial fats regularly, particularly monounsaturated fats. These fats are liquid at room temperature and found in some vegetable oils such as olive, canola, avocado, and peanut (as well as nuts, avocado, and olives). You don't need to avoid these fats. Fats that contain mostly polyunsaturated fatty acids are also usually liquid at room temperature; they include safflower, sunflower, grapeseed, corn, and soybean oils.

When it comes to saturated fat, we recommend proceeding with caution. There's quite a bit of historical research linking saturated fat and elevated blood cholesterol levels. Saturated fatty acids are usually solid at room temperature and come mostly from animal products, such as butter, ghee, stick margarine, shortening, and the fat in cheese and meat. They're also found in tropical vegetable oils (coconut, palm kernel, and palm oils), which are used in products to extend shelf life and add creamy texture. Researchers conclude that partially hydrogenated vegetable oils that create trans fat promote heart disease and may be even more detrimental than tropical oils (nonetheless, despite the popularity of coconut oil, we don't recommend it).

Fats and oils are available in many different forms and can make label-reading confusing. Grain and seed oils like grape seed oil (canola) and soybean oil can also be sold as spreads and stick margarine. How much saturated fat a margarine or spread contains depends on which vegetable oil it contains and how it was processed.

Look for a product with at least twice as much polyunsaturated as saturated fat. The softer or more fluid a margarine is, the less saturated it's likely to be. For this reason, liquid squeeze and spray margarine or tub margarine are almost always better than the stick type. Margarine with water listed as the first ingredient has one-third to one-half less fat than the average margarine. Many blends are now available as well, such as butter blended with olive or canola oil to form a soft spread. They provide the flavor of butter with less saturated fat. The sodium content can vary depending on whether the product is salted. There are also cholesterol-lowering spreads available that tout lowering total blood cholesterol by an average of 10 percent when eaten in sufficient quantities.

Bottom line: Choose soft, trans-fat-free spreads instead of butter or stick margarine. Choose blends with the least amount of saturated fat and zero trans fats.

REMEMBER

Use small amounts of monounsaturated liquid oils in cooking and either soft margarine or small amounts of butter.

Treading Carefully in the Center Aisles

The center aisles of the grocery store are where you're guaranteed to find the vast majority of processed foods. All the snack foods (chips, crackers, packaged cookies, and snack cakes) are found here, as well as salty condiments and sauces. Some processed foods, however, can play a role in a healthy diet. For instance, grains such as basic pasta, rice, and barley are found here, as well as nutritious canned beans and low-sodium tomato products. You'll also find whole-grain cereals made with oats and whole wheat. And for people with food allergies, sensitivities, or digestive diseases, there are some gluten-free or specialty foods available. In addition, being able to keep some foods available on the shelf or freezer by limiting spoiling and waste is a nice advantage for busy families.

On the other hand, some of the ingredients used to lengthen shelf life, improve food safety, and so on, are the very ingredients someone with hypertension needs to reduce in his diet (think sodium, sugars, and trans fats). In addition, many processed foods contain additives that are used purely to enhance the color or flavor of a food or to change or maintain its texture.

REMEMBER

When following the DASH diet, reading labels is key to navigate best choices. You're better off moving away from highly processed foods and toward more fresh whole foods, but you can still rely on some packaged foods as long as you become an informed shopper. Foods such as rice, pasta, canned or frozen vegetables and fruits, boxed cereals, oatmeal, some crackers, and breads, are all okay as long as you monitor the info on the nutrition labels. The secret to choosing healthier packaged foods is reading the Nutrition Facts label rather than blindly believing whatever claims the food's advertisers make on the package.

WARNING

Manufacturers use front-of-package labeling as a way to sell their products. For instance, the front of a package may claim that a product has no high-fructose corn syrup (a form of sugar), and although this is true, the product may still contain several other forms of sugar. Products touting that they're cholesterol-free may still be very high in trans or vegetable fats (cholesterol is only derived from animal fats). Although regulations are in place for what sort of claims manufacturers can make, we encourage you to use the Nutrition Facts label and the ingredient list to evaluate products. When you're short on time, focus on serving size, calories, saturated fat, trans fat, and sodium.

TIP

Consider these guidelines as you decide which processed foods to keep on the grocery list and which ones to skip:

>> **Don't assume "all-natural" or "organic" equals the best choice.** Packaged organic foods can be highly processed as well. Check the labels for excessive salt and sugar.

>> **Remember that your daily sodium goal is 1,500 to 2,300 milligrams per day.** Consider those numbers as you read labels for sodium.

>> **Look for reduced-sodium alternatives.** They're typically available for foods such as condiments, soups, canned tuna, and canned vegetables. Just be sure to rinse canned vegetables under fresh water to remove even more of the sodium.

>> **Don't rely on fiber-added processed foods that normally wouldn't contribute fiber to your diet, such as yogurt or water.** Get your fiber from fresh fruits and vegetables and from whole grains such as oats, barley, brown rice, and whole-grain bread.

>> **Check labels for sugar.** Sometimes when a manufacturer lowers fat, it adds sugar. For instance, a reduced-fat peanut butter may have only a few less grams of fat but have 2 added grams of sugar or more sodium compared to the full-fat version. You're better off using a smaller amount of the regular type. Added sugars may have a role in heart health and definitely contribute too many unneeded calories to the diet.

Keep in mind that sugar masquerades under many names — fructose, sucrose, high-fructose corn syrup, agave nectar, honey, brown rice syrup, and maltose, to name a few. The type doesn't matter as much as the amount. Less is best. A moderate amount of sugar is okay in the diet, but many processed foods contain more than you need. The new Nutrition Facts labels includes "added sugars" to help guide you.

>> **Watch out for the sodium content of condiments.** You can still buy ketchup, mustard, hot sauce, salsa, pickles, and relish to add flavor to your foods, but try to pick lower-sodium versions. If those aren't available in your grocery store, buy what you usually do but use it in moderation.

Some groceries to purchase only occasionally are refined grains such as sweets, bakery items, crackers, and cookies. These are low in fiber and/or high in sugar, void of many nutrients, and sometimes packed with unwanted trans fat, saturated fat, and salt.

Heading Home and Storing Your Food with Care

Good planning and organization carries through from shopping to transporting food safely. In the summer or if you plan to visit several grocery stores, put a cooler with ice or gel packs in your car to keep cold foods cold. *Note:* If the outside temperature is 90 degrees or higher, be sure to get cold foods home within one hour, even if you're using a cooler.

Now that you've made it home with the freshest, healthiest food, you need to store it correctly so it stays fresh and maintains its flavor and nutritional value as long as possible. Follow these tips:

>> Refrigerate perishable foods such as meat, poultry, seafood, and dairy within two hours.

>> For large packages of meat that you don't intend to use within a day or two, wrap them in zippered freezer bags and freeze for later use. Or portion out the meat into portioned-size bags that suit your family (2 servings or 4 servings perhaps). This way, when it comes time to defrost, you can defrost the portion you need and leave other packages frozen.

>> Don't wash produce until you're ready to use it, especially berries.

>> Store most fruits and vegetables in the suitable refrigerator crisper drawers. For zucchini and other small squash, try wrapping them in a paper towel before storing them in the fridge.

>> You can store almost all produce in the refrigerator except for bananas, tomatoes, potatoes, lemons, limes, garlic, and onions. These can be stored on the counter or in the pantry or other cool dark place. Potatoes and onions should not be stored together because onions emit a gas that causes potatoes to sprout faster.

Chapter 13

Setting Up a DASH-Friendly Kitchen

What best describes your cooking style? Are you a kitchen warrior, practical and straightforward, going into culinary battle armed with whatever ammunition you need to win over the mealtime? Or are you a kitchen explorer, always seeking new recipes or a twist on an old favorite? Maybe you're a kitchen procrastinator, and last-minute ideas catch your attention. You can be health-conscious no matter what your cooking style!

This chapter highlights the importance of organization in your culinary world. You may think your kitchen is nothing more than the mess hall, but this healthy kitchen makeover will help you create an environment that makes cooking as easy and seamless as possible. If you don't have what you need in the kitchen, you won't be able to create one of the top weapons in your hypertension-fighting arsenal: healthy meals!

We help you set up your pantry, fridge, and freezer (also known as your three go-to spots for ingredients). We also list basic cookware and kitchen gadgets that will transform the cooking experience for you. With some new inspiration and handy tips for developing flavor and modifying recipes, you'll soon be cooking our low-maintenance recipes and realizing that home cooking is oh-so-easy — and oh-so-delicious!

Creating a Healthy Pantry

A big part of following the DASH diet is eating more whole foods as opposed to prepackaged, highly processed foods that are often incredibly high in sodium and low in nutrients and fiber. You stand a better chance of making DASH-friendly food choices consistently when your pantry, refrigerator, and freezer are filled with healthy options and basic ingredients. The following sections break down what to keep on hand to make cooking easier.

TIP

Keep track of the staples you use most often so you can develop a running grocery list. When you start running low on, say, olive oil, add that to the list so you remember to buy a backup bottle before the current bottle runs out completely.

Pantry staples

To make cooking stress-free, you want to have several recipe ingredients on hand at all times, including the following:

» **Canned goods:** Although canned vegetables are higher in sodium than fresh or frozen ones, they have a long shelf life, so it's okay to keep some on hand for a quick meal. (After all, a home-cooked meal is still lower in sodium than most any restaurant meal.) Look for low-sodium and no-salt-added versions of items such as canned tomatoes, beans, broths, and vegetables. Canned salmon, canned tuna, and tuna pouches are economical and heart-healthy choices.

» **Condiments:** Dijon and other fancy mustards, chutneys, chipotle peppers in adobo sauce, low-sodium soy sauce, capers, and salsa are good flavor boosters to use in recipes. Although these contain more sodium than fresh ingredients or salt-free spices, a small spoonful goes a long way in salad dressing or main dish recipes. You can divide that spoonful among 4 to 8 servings, so your sodium intake is minimal and the flavor is maxed.

» **Grains and rice:** Quinoa, wild rice, brown rice, farro, barley, bulgur, and whole-grain rice blends are all good, high-fiber, antioxidant-rich choices.

» **Lentils and dry beans:** These nutrition powerhouses are a great substitute for animal protein. Lentils cook in 20 to 30 minutes — no soaking needed.

» **Nuts and seeds:** Walnuts, pecans, peanuts, hazelnuts, and almonds make wonderful additions to salads, stir-fries, and vegetable dishes and are a portable snack food. Sunflower and sesame seeds add flavor and texture to salads or pilaf dishes.

>> **Olive oil:** Consider buying two varieties, a lighter version for cooking and extra-virgin oil for salads, salad dressings, or to drizzle on veggies or whole-grain bread.

>> **Other vegetable oil:** Maintain a supply of soybean, corn, avocado, grapeseed, or canola oil. You may also consider oil blends and a small bottle of peanut oil, which is good for stir-frying. Sesame oil is a great finishing oil for Asian-inspired dishes.

>> **Pasta:** Whole-wheat couscous, penne, spaghetti varieties, bow ties, spirals, and orzo are good go-to's for quick meals.

>> **Pizza crusts:** Stock a couple of the ready-to-eat, whole-grain variety for quick last-minute meals. Don't forget to pile on the veggies!

>> **Potatoes:** Sweet and any white or yellow-fleshed or fingerling potatoes are pantry essentials.

>> **Seasonings:** Dried herbs and spices are great for adding flavor to dishes. Basil, cayenne pepper, chili powder, cumin, ginger, oregano, paprika, Herbs de Provence, and rosemary are common staples worth stocking up on.

>> **Vinegars:** Buy a couple varieties of vinegar for making marinades and salad dressings. We like keeping apple cider, rice, red wine, and balsamic vinegars on the shelf.

Refrigerator staples

Just like the pantry, your refrigerator begs to be consistently stocked with ingredients for home cooking. Keep these staples in your fridge:

>> **Fresh fruit:** Fruit makes a great healthy snack. Fruit is also delicious chopped or sliced and added to yogurt, salads, pilaf, or stuffing, or cooked with pork or poultry. Of course, it's terrific served as a dessert.

>> **Aromatic vegetables:** Onions, garlic, scallions, shallots, chives, and leeks add a distinct flavor and aroma to any food without the addition of sodium.

>> **Bell peppers:** Like onions, you can slice or dice bell peppers and add them to meat, egg, or vegetable dishes or mince them into appetizers.

>> **Butter:** Although butter is higher in saturated fat than liquid vegetable oils, using small amounts in recipes offers great flavor. By reducing the butter in traditional recipes by ½ or ¾, you can achieve the desired flavor with minimal saturated fat.

>> **Carrots:** Combine them with onions and celery and you have *mirepoix* (French for the combination of these vegetables sautéed), often used in soups, stews, stocks, or sauces.

>> **Cheeses:** Although high in saturated fat and sodium, a little bit of cheese can go a long way. A small amount of Parmigiano-Reggiano, Gruyère, goat, or mozzarella freshly grated into recipes provides a complex, sharp flavor.

>> **Citrus fruits:** Lemon, lime, and orange rinds help spark the flavor of many dishes. We recommend washing fruit thoroughly before zesting.

>> **Cream cheese, low-fat (light or Neufchâtel):** Cream cheese is useful for lightening up and thickening sauces and spreads.

>> **Dried fruits:** Dried apricots, cranberries, and cherries are tasty additions to stuffing, salads, and vegetable dishes. We recommend purchasing options with no added sugar.

>> **Eggs:** A staple for both baking and cooking, eggs can also star as the main dish for a quick and easy meal.

>> **Liquid spray or tub margarine:** Part of a heart-healthy lifestyle, tub margarines that are olive-oil based, yogurt based, or vegetable-oil based have less saturated fat than stick versions. Look for "light" vegetable oil spreads. Check the Nutrition Facts labels for 0 grams trans fat and a higher amount of polyunsaturated and monounsaturated fats.

>> **Mayonnaise, low-fat:** This staple serves as a base for sauces and toppings.

>> **Milk, 1%:** Yes, you can still enjoy creamy sauces by using low-fat milk.

>> **Salad greens:** Whether it's green leaf lettuce, spinach, Swiss chard, or kale, keeping some sort of green in the fridge enables you to add a nutrient-rich base to meals.

>> **Tofu and tempeh:** These are both good sources of plant protein and low in saturated fat. You can use tofu in a breakfast shake, for a quick and easy stir-fry, or to make a chocolate mousse. Unopened, they'll last for months in the refrigerator.

Freezer staples

Using the freezer to stock up on key ingredients such as meats, poultry, fish, seafood, and vegetables helps save time. If you don't have to run to the grocery store, you can have dinner on the table in a flash. Keep your freezer filled with the following:

» **Berries:** Frozen strawberries, blueberries, and raspberries often come in handy for smoothies, sauces, and toppings for yogurt and angel cake.

» **Meats:** Buying a variety of meats, plant-based meat items, and poultry, and cleaning and prepping if needed before you freeze them, can be a real timesaver when it comes to getting dinner on the table. Be sure to trim the skin from poultry and any visible fat from lean cuts of beef and pork before freezing. Store your meat in any or all of the following ways:

- Package 2 to 6 portions (depending on the size of your household) in individual freezer bags.

- Package extra-lean ground beef in 1-pound portions for use in recipes.

- Cut some meat for use in recipes (strips for stir-fries and fajitas, cubes for stews and soups, and so forth).

» **Seafood, shrimp, mollusks, fresh, frozen, or precooked:** These item are easy to use and make a quick meal or snack; shrimp heat in just 2 to 3 minutes. Be cautious if the seafood meal has sauces, it may be higher in sodium.

» **Vegetables:** Keep plain frozen corn, a bell pepper and onion mixture, spinach, and peas on hand to mix into recipes. Edamame are shelled green soybeans and a great source of protein. Frozen veggies go from freezer to recipe with no washing or chopping — a huge benefit.

WARNING

Some plant–based meats (such as ground beef or sausage substitutes) are loaded with sodium. Read labels carefully, and account for the extra sodium. Because you should only be consuming 3 to 5 ounces of meat a day, the health benefit of some of the plant substitutes is minimal.

Arming Yourself with the Right Kitchen Supplies

Having the right ingredients to whip up delicious breakfasts, lunches, and dinners is only half the battle. You also need to have the right kitchen equipment. The following sections help you figure out what you absolutely need and what would be helpful if you have the room for it.

Cookware basics

Good cookware can make a big difference in your end results in the kitchen. Purchase heavier pots and pans made from cast aluminum, copper, or stainless steel because they distribute heat evenly. You won't have to cook at high temperatures, so you'll lower your chances of burning dinner!

TIP

Pots with nonstick surfaces are easy to clean and can be used with little or no oil for healthy cooking. If you don't already have quality cookware, consider shopping for these items at name-brand discount stores or start a "cookware" fund to get just what you want.

Following are the basic pieces of cookware we recommend keeping in your kitchen:

>> **Sauté pans with lids, 6- and 12-inch sizes:** Use these pans to sauté onions, mushrooms, bell peppers, garlic, eggs, and more, and to cook chicken or fish.

>> **A large stockpot with a steamer insert:** A stockpot is great for cooking soups and big batches of sauces and for boiling water for pasta. You can cook corn on the cob and steam veggies in it, too.

>> **Saucepans, 2- and 4-quart sizes:** These pans are good for sauces and small batches of pasta and rice.

>> **Oven-safe nonstick pans, 8- and 10-inch sizes:** These pans have the same uses as sauté pans, but because they're nonstick, you don't need to add much fat to them.

>> **A large roasting pan:** A good roasting pan will last for years and is perfect for roasting a large pork or beef roast or a whole chicken or turkey. Look for one with a rack insert; this allows fat drippings from the meat to fall to the bottom of the pan and also allows you to easily remove the roast from the pan.

>> **A Dutch oven with a lid:** This pot has a handle on each side and can be used on the stovetop or in the oven. It works well for roasts and stews.

>> **A grill pan:** You can use this pan for anything you'd cook on an outdoor grill, such as hamburgers, chicken breasts, steaks, or fish.

>> **A stainless steel or plastic colander:** Both work well for draining pasta and rinsing or washing fruits and vegetables.

>> **Two or three mixing bowls (small, medium, large):** These are useful for mixing dry ingredients, holding measured and chopped vegetables before cooking, and mixing up meatloaf, among other uses.

>> **Glass baking dishes:** The 8-x-8-inch and 9-x-13-inch sizes come in handy. Glass pans hold up to high temperatures, are easy to clean, and don't warp like metal pans can.

>> **Two baking sheets:** Many times you may need to use two cookie sheets at once or you may choose to include a smaller one and a larger one in your cupboard.

>> **A round pizza pan or a pizza stone:** Both work well, but the advantage of a large rectangular stone is that you can make one large pizza or two smaller round ones on it.

>> **Chopper/dicer:** Makes meal prep quick and easy.

>> **Digital scale:** Helps with tracking food intake and precise measurements.

>> **Food processor and blender:** If you're uncertain about your knife skills and you want to save time with labor-intensive tasks, these versatile appliances can save time and money. Plus, a DASH smoothie is a great way to add fruits and veggies to your day!

>> **Instant Pot:** This all-in-one appliance is a combination pressure cooker, slow-cooker, rice cooker, steamer, and yogurt maker. It's nice to have but not necessary.

>> **Air fryer:** Using an air fryer is a quick, efficient way to crisp and brown frozen or fresh food without much oil.

>> **Spiralizer:** An inexpensive tool that can turn vegetables into veggie noodles to up your veggie intake and reduce carbs and calories. Nice to have but not necessary.

Essential knives

A good set of knives is the best investment in a well-equipped kitchen. Even the most basic cooking methods require the use of knives. Many kinds of knives exist, but you only need a few to start slicing and dicing:

>> **Chef's knife, 8-inch:** Probably the cook's most important tool. Use it to chop, slice, or mince vegetables or herbs. The best knives are forged from a single piece of steel that runs the entire length of the knife.

>> **Paring knife:** Usually about 3 to 4 inches long, this knife is handy for trimming fruits or vegetables.

>> **Santoku knife:** The blade of this Japanese-inspired knife works well for mincing and paper-thin slicing.

>> **Serrated bread knife:** As its name implies, this type of knife is used for slicing bread.

>> **Steak knives:** Use these knives to cut beef, pork, or chicken. They also work very well for slicing tomatoes!

>> **Utility knife:** A utility knife is a mid-sized knife, usually from 5 to 7 inches long, that's easy to use for multiple purposes.

TIP

Have your knives sharpened professionally at least once a year. Sharp knives actually minimize accidents. Learning to use them properly saves time and prevents loss of fingers.

Helpful kitchen tools and storage supplies

Like any good workspace, your kitchen requires good tools. To make your kitchen an enjoyable and easy place to work, make sure your tools are in good working order.

We recommend making sure you have these essential kitchen tools for easier cooking:

>> **Meal planner:** A simple pad will do but a formal planner or digital meal planner can help you succeed (see Chapter 12).

>> **Can/bottle opener:** Whether hand-crank, battery operated, or electric, make sure to buy one that will stand up to repeated use. After each use, wash and dry thoroughly to prevent bacteria buildup.

>> **Cutting boards:** Polyethylene plastic or acrylic boards are inexpensive, durable, and easy to clean. Wooden boards are less desirable because they're naturally porous, providing perfect hiding spots for bacteria. See the nearby sidebar for some helpful cutting board tips.

>> **Instant-read thermometer:** Use this important item to make sure your meat is cooked properly. Look for one that includes a chart with proper cooking times and temps.

>> **Measuring cups and spoons:** A set of metal or plastic measuring cups is useful for measuring dry ingredients; glass, silicone, or plastic measuring cups are good for liquids. Measuring spoons help you parcel out seasonings, thickeners, and more. Most sets come with a variety of sizes, usually from ⅛ teaspoon to 1 tablespoon.

>> **Utensils:** The right utensils are invaluable in the kitchen. Make sure you have heat-resistant nonstick spatulas, a vegetable peeler, a meat mallet, slotted spoons for draining, a wire whisk, tongs, an assortment of wooden spoons, a pastry brush, a ladle, and kitchen shears.

>> **Stackable glass containers with airtight lids:** Containers that come in a variety of sizes are perfect for batch cooking and leftovers.

>> **Reusable food bags:** Bags made from silicon are a great substitute for plastic and are dishwasher and microwave safe.

>> **Bee's Wrap food wrap:** These wraps are a sustainable and reusable natural wrap and a good substitute for plastic.

>> **Mason jars:** Economical and easy to use, mason jars are great for storing and meal prepping salads in a jar.

>> **Salt jar:** A salt jar, sometimes called a "salt pig," is a jar that you fill with salt and usually keep by your stove or cooking area. It makes it easier to "pinch" or measure salt because it allows you to see how much you're using.

The following tools and gadgets aren't as critical to own as those in the preceding list, but they sure do make life easier:

>> **Garlic press or garlic chopper:** Chopping garlic with a knife is a little time-consuming. You can save yourself some precious moments by investing in a garlic press or a garlic chopper (see the difference in Figure 13-1), both of which do the hard work for you so you can have fresh garlic for adding to your recipes. (Plus, pressing releases allicin, garlic's antioxidant and anti-inflammatory compound.)

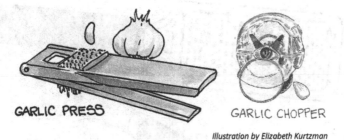

GARLIC PRESS   GARLIC CHOPPER

FIGURE 13-1:
A garlic press and
a garlic chopper.

Illustration by Elizabeth Kurtzman

- **Immersion blender:** Also known as a *stick blender,* this tool is a small kitchen appliance used to blend ingredients or purée food in the container in which it's being prepared. It's handy for blending soups in the pot — just be sure to remove the pot from the heat before you start blending!

- **Mandolin:** This tool cuts lots of uniform slices in a short period of time. Most mandolins have several different blades to vary the thickness of the slices and options such as matchstick slices, waffle slices, crinkle cuts, and julienne strips. A hand guard is an important feature for safety reasons.

- **Microplane grater and zester:** These are one-handed tools with tiny, razor-sharp holes that scrape slim strips from food (see Figure 13-2). A zester can grate citrus just far enough into the rind to get the most flavor. You can also use a zester or microplane grater to shave off a small amount of hard cheese for a huge punch of flavor.

- **Oil mister:** Ideal for adding a wee bit of fat, this non-aerosol mister ensures a precise amount of oil gets on your food. The top regulates the air pressure inside for easier spraying.

- **Rotary cheese grater:** This tool is a cinch to use. Compared to a traditional metal grater, a rotary cheese grater (see Figure 13-3) is easier to clean, and it can go right to the table for a finishing touch to soups or pasta dishes.

- **Salad spinner:** This gadget is great for washing and removing excess water from leafy greens and herbs. You'll never want to wash greens by hand again!

- **Steamers:** You can place a metal or silicone steamer on top of a pot of boiling water to cook fresh vegetables without losing nutrients. Steamers with an accordion-fold design fit in several pan sizes and make steaming veggies a snap.

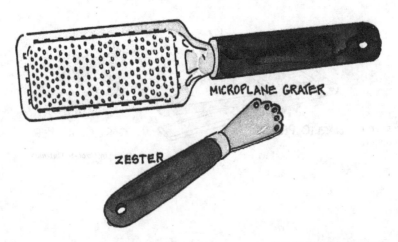

FIGURE 13-2:
A microplane grater and zester.

Illustration by Elizabeth Kurtzman

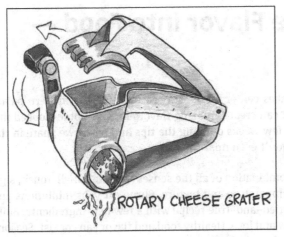

FIGURE 13-3:
A rotary cheese grater.

ROTARY CHEESE GRATER

Illustration by Elizabeth Kurtzman

LET'S CUT TO THE CHASE: CUTTING BOARD TIPS

Cutting boards are a critical piece of kitchen equipment, but not everyone knows how to choose the best ones for the job. Here are our tips on selecting, using, and maintaining cutting boards:

- Choose a board with a smooth, hard surface that is approved for contact with food.

- Replace cutting boards that become deeply scratched, carved, or grooved.

- Use separate cutting boards for raw vegetables and raw meat, poultry, and seafood. Always use a clean, separate cutting board for fresh vegetables, fruits, breads, and other foods that you don't cook prior to eating. Consider using color-coded cutting boards to help you keep them separate. That's one good way to minimize your chances of a food-related illness.

- Scrape off food, oils, and residue and scrub all cutting boards completely with soap and hot water after each use. You can put boards made from dishwasher-safe material in the dishwasher; do this whenever possible.

- Sanitize cutting boards periodically with a mixture of 1 teaspoon of chlorine to 1 quart of water. Pour the mixture over the board and let it stand a few minutes. Then rinse completely with fresh water. Let the board dry completely. Always sanitize cutting boards after cutting raw meat, poultry, and seafood.

Infusing More Flavor into Food — without Salt

Salt often takes center stage as a seasoning in the modern palate, but it doesn't have to. You can create amazing flavors in your home-cooked meals without any salt. After a few weeks of using the tips and tricks we share in the following sections, you won't even miss the salt.

REMEMBER

Flavor is a combination of all the senses — taste, smell, touch, sight, and sound — as well as temperature and texture. Shrug off your inhibitions and experiment by tweaking a tried-and-true recipe with a few new ingredients. Build from what you already know and love. Healthy food and flavor can coexist. Seasonings and flavorings replace the missing ingredients in low-sodium cooking. Citrus is your friend when it comes to brightening the flavor in a dish. Keep aromatic vegetables such as onions, chives, garlic, or shallots on hand in your kitchen. Finding how to use some simple tools and techniques allows you to immerse more flavors into your recipes. Even different cooking methods can change the flavor profile of foods. Your creativity is up to you. Refer to Chapter 25 for tips on elevating flavor with less salt.

Spice blends

Herbs and spices can be the backbone of many recipes, providing a wonderful flavor, visual appeal, and even antioxidant value. The use of herbs changes the flavor direction to whichever herb is prominent, and there's no end to the combinations. Many ethnic blends are very popular:

- **Asian:** ginger, five-spice powder, garlic, green onions
- **French:** tarragon, shallot
- **Indian:** ground nutmeg, coriander, cinnamon, curry powder
- **Italian:** garlic, onion, basil, oregano, thyme
- **Latin American:** ancho chile, paprika, cumin, Mexican oregano
- **Pumpkin pie spice:** cinnamon, nutmeg, ginger, cloves
- **South American:** chile peppers, lime juice, garlic, cilantro

The following blends are a little more exotic but still quite tasty:

- **Egyptian:** toasted hazelnuts, sesame seeds, coriander, cumin
- **Jamaican jerk:** red and black pepper, allspice, cinnamon, thyme
- **Middle Eastern Baharat:** black pepper, cinnamon, cloves, cumin

REMEMBER

When purchasing premade herb or spice blends, be sure to check the salt and sugar content. Look for salt-free blends.

Coulis

The French word *coulis* refers to a sauce made by puréeing cooked vegetables or uncooked fruit. The consistency is that of a thin tomato sauce. A coulis is one of the simplest "sauces" you can make. It can be made so easily and then simply stored in the refrigerator for a few days. Freezing is another option if you don't plan to use it right away.

>> **For a sweet coulis:** Add a half pint of raspberries and a tablespoon of orange juice in a deep cup and use an immersion blender to whiz those berries into a luscious, low-calorie sauce for your morning whole-grain pancakes.

>> **For a savory coulis:** Purée a roasted red bell pepper with a tablespoon of vegetable or chicken stock and a small amount of cooked rice or potatoes for a sauce to go with grilled fish. Because roasting caramelizes a vegetable, roasting the pepper first brings out the natural sweetness, perfect for making a complementary sauce.

Salsas

Salsas are chunky mixtures of fruits and/or vegetables. They're versatile, they have wonderful visual appeal, and they add a variety of nutrients to any dish. A traditional salsa is made with tomatoes, but you can use your creativity and use whatever you like, such as fresh mango for a fruity salsa! Take the tomato and mango up a notch by adding a strong flavor such as a chile or onion and a pop of fresh herb such as cilantro or parsley. You can also roast or grill chilies or vegetables before chopping them and adding them to the salsa, offering a smoky flavor.

TIP

For a nice dash of flavor, use seasonal veggies and fruit, such as fresh spring-ripe mango cut into bite-sized pieces, one-quarter to one-half of a jalapeño pepper, a few tablespoons of minced red onion, a handful of chopped cilantro, and a squeeze of fresh lime. Your family will be doing the Mambo Mango dance for more.

Making Over Recipes So You Can Indulge without Guilt

Nutritious recipes that include lots of veggies and low-fat dairy are the foundation of the DASH diet. Chances are some of the recipes you use every day already have healthy components. Others may need some tweaking, whether that's reducing the amount of sodium, saturated fat, and/or sugar or adding more fiber and nutrients to help prevent high blood pressure like calcium, potassium, and magnesium.

There are many ways to make over a recipe. You may want to reduce the caloric content or modify the type of fat. You can do this by changing the cooking method or the type and amount of ingredients, as we describe in the following sections.

Either way, start by examining a favorite recipe and deciding how you want to change it. Imagine what the recipe will look like if you alter it. Will it still taste similar? Will the texture be similar? Be sure to evaluate the product of your experimentation. Ideally, you'll enjoy it at least as much as the original.

REMEMBER

Healthy cooking is more than just limiting ingredients. To make a recipe healthy you also want to add ingredients so you get more beneficial nutrients. An example for the DASH plan may include adding a more colorful variety of vegetables to an already healthy tossed salad and, of course, going light on the dressing. You can add more dark greens like romaine, spinach, kale, and arugula or other raw vegetables and fruit like cherry tomatoes, carrots, beets, and berries, which contain significantly more vitamins A and C and phytonutrients. You can also add healthy fats such as an avocado slice or 2 teaspoons of sunflower seeds. Balance and portion are the key!

TIP

You can always change the presentation of recipes to reflect your new heart-healthy eating habits. For example, if you're trying to reduce the amount of meat you serve your family, and they fuss at the idea of smaller meat portions, think outside the traditional plated presentation of the meal. Why not cut the meat into 1-inch and ½ -inch cubes and alternate the meat on skewers with a variety of colorful veggies? Instead of a 6- to 8-ounce piece of meat on a plate, you can get by with 2 to 4 ounces of cubed meat per serving when adding the veggies. They may not notice the portion difference in this presentation! You can still marinate the meat for full flavor, and you're still offering red meat, but the finished product is a nutrition gold mine.

Changing cooking methods

Because DASH requires moderate fat intake and smaller portions of meat, you want your cooking methods to provide both the right amount and the right kind of fats. Using flavorful ingredients to begin the cooking process allows your cooking method to deliver moist, delicious food. Simple techniques such as using high-quality, nonstick cookware allow you to reduce fat yet deliver the great taste you love in your favorite recipe (and make cleanup easier!). Cooking methods such as grilling or broiling result in a reduced-fat product, but you must take care to prepare the food properly and not overcook it, so meats remain moist. Applying proper cooking methods and adding heart-healthy fats to vegetables helps you create dishes that will spur everyone to take second helpings.

Keep these simple tips in mind as you embark on your new cooking adventure:

» Consider an original recipe for juicy, breaded, deep-fried fish. Ask yourself whether this is a good candidate for a makeover. Recipes often rely on fat for the flavor and texture, such as deep-frying, but "oven-crisping" is often a good option to obtain a similar texture with a fraction of the fat. (See the Curry-Crusted Roasted Salmon recipe in Chapter 19.)

» Instead of pan-frying with a lot of butter, use a nonstick skillet with a smaller amount of butter or extra-virgin olive oil. (Check out the Seared Scallops with Pistachio Sauce recipe in Chapter 19.)

» Roasting or grilling vegetables brings out their natural sugars, which may make them more appealing to the family. (See the Roasted Broccolini with Toasted Sesame Seeds in Chapter 20.)

» Grilling or broiling may allow you to omit the fat that sautéing requires.

» When making a meatloaf, you can use a double meatloaf pan with a drip section to separate the excess fat from the meat or add chopped mushrooms to expand the meat portion.

» When using ground beef for tacos, spaghetti, or casseroles, be sure to drain the meat in a colander for easy fat removal or substitute lean ground turkey or chicken.

WALK THE PLANK!

TIP

Another awesome way to flavor food is with plank cooking. It's easy, and the mess ends up on the wood instead of in your grill. Alderwood and cedarwood are the most commonly used woods for plank cooking. You can purchase them at specialty shops and grocery stores. Hickory, mesquite, cherry, pear, pecan, and oak are all good choices, too. To plank cook, follow these steps:

1. **Completely submerge the wood and soak it in warm water or another liquid such as wine, beer, or apple cider for at least an hour (but preferably longer, to ensure complete saturation).**

2. **Dry the plank with a paper towel and lightly coat the top surface with olive, canola, or any flavored oil.**

3. **Preheat the plank on the grill until it starts to smoke and crackle just a little.**

4. **Place your fish or other meat onto the plank, cover, and grill.**

The cooking time will vary depending on the amount of food item you're grilling, its thickness, and your personal preference. Use an instant-read thermometer to get the right temperature. *Remember:* The food will continue to cook after you take it off the grill.

Modifying ingredients

You may be able to change up an existing recipe simply by modifying the ingredients. To do this, consider what you can do to keep the wonderful flavor profile of your favorite recipe. Then think about the function of the ingredients in the existing recipe. What happens if you use less of certain ingredients? What happens if you introduce a new ingredient?

The suggestions in Table 13-1 offer easy-to-use recipe substitutions, but we aren't suggesting that you never use butter, whole eggs, or cream cheese. These are just options to help you make your favorite recipes more DASH-friendly. Note that if an amount isn't listed in either column, then the substitution is equal. So if you want to change out 2 cups of whole milk for an option with less fat, use 2 cups of low-fat or nonfat milk.

TABLE 13-1   Recipe Substitutions

In Place of . . .	Use . . .
Whole milk	Low-fat (1% or 2%) milk, nonfat (skim) milk, nonfat milk powder, or evaporated skim milk
Butter	Tub margarine (light, low-fat) or oil; for heat conduction: defatted stocks, water, wine, or vegetable or fruit juice (limit to 1 teaspoon per serving); for pan preparation: nonstick spray or a light brush of liquid oil
1 cup fats for baking	1 cup applesauce or 1 cup fruit purée
1 cup buttermilk	1 cup skim milk less 1 tablespoon, plus 1 tablespoon lemon juice
Heavy cream	Evaporated skim milk (can be thickened with a fruit or vegetable purée)
Sour cream	Light sour cream, nonfat sour cream, plain nonfat yogurt, or low-fat cottage cheese puréed with skim milk
Cream cheese	Neufchâtel cheese, light cream cheese, or a fat-free cheese substitute
Whole eggs	Egg whites or egg substitutes
1 ounce baking chocolate	3 tablespoons cocoa and 1 tablespoon vegetable oil
Mayonnaise	Light or fat-free mayonnaise or nonfat plain yogurt
1 cup white flour	½ cup whole-wheat flour and ½ cup white flour
1 cup chopped nuts	½ cup toasted nuts
1 tablespoon fresh herbs	1 teaspoon dried herbs
Regular soy sauce	Light soy sauce

Here are a few actual recipe makeovers to show you just how easy it is to modify your favorite recipes with a pinch of a few extra spices or ingredients substitutions. We promise that if you make the homemade version once, you'll be hooked, and your heart will be glad you made the switch!

	Store-Bought Spicy Pizza Sauce	Homemade Spicy Pizza Sauce
Ingredients	1 cup pizza sauce from a jar	One 8-ounce can no-added-salt tomato sauce
		2 garlic cloves, minced
		1 teaspoon basil
		½ teaspoon oregano
		¼ teaspoon black pepper
		¼ teaspoon crushed red pepper

	Store-Bought Spicy Pizza Sauce	Homemade Spicy Pizza Sauce
Directions		Combine all ingredients in a small saucepan. Simmer gently over low heat for 10 minutes.
Yield	1 cup	1 cup

	Taco Soup	Taco Soup Redux
Ingredients	1 pound ground beef	½ pound lean ground beef
	½ cup chopped onions	1 medium onion, chopped
	One 15-ounce can tomatoes, undrained	One 15-ounce can no-added-salt crushed tomatoes
	One 15-ounce can kidney beans, undrained	One 15-ounce can no-added-salt kidney beans, drained
	One 15-ounce can whole kernel corn, undrained	2 cups plain frozen corn, thawed
	One 8-ounce can tomato sauce	One 8-ounce can no-added-salt tomato sauce
	1 package taco seasoning	2–3 teaspoons chili powder
	3 cups crushed tortilla chips	¼ teaspoon cayenne pepper
	6 tablespoons sour cream	½ teaspoon cumin
	6 tablespoons shredded cheddar cheese	¼ teaspoon garlic powder
		Few dashes hot sauce
		1½ cups crushed no-salt tortilla chips
		6 slices avocado
		6 tablespoons reduced-fat shredded cheddar cheese
Directions	Brown ground beef and onions. Add tomatoes, beans, and corn with their liquids; stir in tomato sauce, taco seasoning, and hot sauce. Bring to boil; reduce heat and simmer for 30 minutes. Serve with bowls of crushed tortilla chips, sour cream, and shredded cheddar cheese.	Brown ground beef and onions; drain fat. Add tomatoes, corn, beans, and tomato sauce. Stir in chili powder, paprika, cayenne pepper, cumin, garlic powder, and hot sauce. Bring to a boil; reduce heat and simmer for 30 minutes. Serve with bowls of crushed tortilla chips, avocado, and reduced-fat cheddar cheese.
Yield	6 servings	6 servings

	Store-Bought Tomato Spaghetti	Roasted Tomato Spaghetti
Ingredients	12-ounce box spaghetti 32-ounce bottle spaghetti sauce	12-ounce box whole-wheat spaghetti 6 ripe Roma tomatoes, cut in half, cored ½ onion, cut into chunks 1 tablespoon extra-virgin olive oil 2 tablespoons chopped fresh basil 1 teaspoon garlic powder Black pepper to taste
Directions	Cook spaghetti according to package directions. Drain and reserve in colander. Heat sauce in the microwave on high for 2 to 3 minutes. Serve over pasta.	Cook spaghetti according to package directions. Drain and reserve in colander. Preheat oven broiler. Place tomatoes and onion on a lined baking sheet and broil on both sides about 10 minutes per side. Place the tomatoes and onion, olive oil, and seasonings in a food processor or blender and blend on high until consistency is smooth. Heat sauce and serve over pasta.
Yield	4 servings	4 servings

Chapter 14

DASH Meal-Planning Strategies

M enu planning is a simple and effective way to prepare healthier meals, maximize your free time, save money, and minimize food waste. Whether you delight in creating an exceptional meal or dread the possibility of it, planning and preparation are two necessary skills that will help you succeed in eating the DASH way. This chapter provides practical tips for anyone responsible for putting food on the table. It gives you basic meal-planning guidance as well as specific guidance for the three main meals of the day — breakfast, lunch, and dinner.

Getting a Grip on How Meal Planning Works

After a tough day at the office or a harried day spent with the kids at the park, it's so much easier to order take-out if you don't have a plan in place. Having a plan saves you the stress of worrying about what to cook and means that you'll be eating really DASH-friendly meals, not just what's convenient.

Break the meal-planning process into small steps:

1. **Assess your situation, food habits, needs, and schedule.**

Are you cooking for one or a family of six? Do you have a demanding family schedule? How many nights will you cook meals? Considering your schedule and everything that's going on in your life right now helps you create a meal plan that works for you. Batch-cooking a few ingredients can save time. Consider cooking a double batch of lentils or barley, for instance, and either using it in two days or freezing it to save time at a future meal. Determine how many people you're feeding, how many meals per week, and a rough budget.

2. **Do your research.**

Sort through recipes, cookbooks (like the one you're holding!), and the Internet for tasty new meal ideas. Find inspiration from recipes or individual ingredients in your pantry. That's the purpose of developing a varied pantry for those go-to meal ideas. Keep your cooking style in mind. If cooking is a real chore for you, choose recipes with few ingredients or little prep time. Think seasonally when choosing recipes that include fruit and veggies.

3. **Write down five or six entrees you want to prepare for the week, making sure the meals correspond to specific days.**

For example, if you know you'll be busy on Wednesday, plan to use the slow cooker or a fast-cooking or no-cook meal that night. Don't forget to add a side dish or two to each day's menu so you can ensure you're making healthy, balanced meals (see Chapter 11 for meal plan ideas).

TIP

Designate at least one night a week as leftover night and be creative about how you use those leftovers. For instance, grill salmon one night and save the rest to top off a garden fresh salad another night. Save the ambitious undertakings when you have plenty of time to spend in the kitchen.

4. **Break down each of your planned meals into ingredients lists.**

When you know how many meals you're shopping for and which ingredients you need, one substantial shopping trip each week should be sufficient. Don't forget to include the necessary spices and little extras in addition to the main ingredients!

5. **Assess your pantry, freezer, and fridge.**

Now that you have your ingredient lists, it's time to see what you have on hand and what you may need to buy at the store. What meals can you make using the foods you already have? This is when your actual grocery list is created. Use a premade grocery list or make your own.

6. **Clip coupons and pick your stores.**

If you're trying to stay within your budget, clip coupons from the newspaper or online from various products' websites. Also, choose the one or two stores you shop the most and review their weekly circulars to look for deals. Often, items that are buy-one-get-one-free (such as berries) can be frozen for later use. (Note that some stores offer additional savings and specials around the holidays.)

7. **Head to the grocery store with your list and coupons.**

Refer to Chapter 12 for information on savvy shopping.

8. **Get food ready to use before you store it in your refrigerator and freezer to save time later.**

Portion meats into freezer bags in the portion you need. If cooking for two, use quart-size bags. Remove skin from poultry, pat dry, and freeze. Portion ground meat into 1-pound or ½-pound packages. Most produce is packaged in ways to preserve freshness, so don't wash it until you're ready to use it.

REMEMBER

Spending 30 minutes or so to prep some food after you return from the grocery store can save you an hour or more when it's time to cook. Plus, having foods frozen and ready for recipes saves you even more time. See the later "Prepping ingredients ahead of time" section for advice on getting foods ready in advance to make the dinner rush easier to handle.

TIP

Clean up as you do your preliminary prep work. Keep a bowl nearby to collect all your scraps and food particles for composting and rinse empty cans and containers that go to the garbage can and recycling. Clean up the little spills and load up the dishwasher as you go. Maintaining a clean kitchen is important for your health and safety.

If that isn't enough to make your life simple, always reserve the right to declare a "cook's night off"! In that case, adopt some basic rules for take-out or dining out. Chapter 15 guides you through the process!

The following sections explain how to use the U.S. Department of Agriculture's MyPlate tool to plan balanced meals and how to keep appropriate portion sizes in mind in your meal planning and plating.

MEAL PLANNING APPS TO THE RESCUE

Looking for digital help with planning meals? You're in luck. A variety of mobile apps exist. Some allow you to type in the DASH diet ingredients you have in your pantry and find time-saver recipes and grocery lists. Others help you plan and freeze a month's worth of meals for the family. Still others allow you to store favorite recipes, make shopping lists, create meal plans from them, and keep track of your pantry inventory. Keep in mind, however, that some of these apps may not always be encouraging you to follow DASH. Here are some of the apps we like:

- **Allrecipes Dinner Spinner:** http://dish.allrecipes.com/mobile-apps

- **Mealime:** www.mealime.com

- **Menu Planner:** http://menu-planner.com

- **Paprika:** www.paprikaapp.com

REMEMBER

As a basic rule, it may be best to try to take one substantial shopping trip per week. Doing so works well for weekly meal plans and ensures that your fruits and veggies stay fresh, that you have time for new ideas, and that you can take advantage of sales. Your approach will vary depending on your schedule, location, and lifestyle. If you're an overscheduled parent, you may need to think about a month-long schedule of meals or pay special attention to stretching your budget. Keep a running list on the fridge so you can write down items as you think of them. If you're cooking for two or just you, you may focus on a single elaborate meal per week and shop more frequently. Regardless of how you approach it, meal planning is a simple and effective way to avoid hassles and disappointments in the kitchen. It's a road map of sorts to get you to your healthiest you.

Using MyPlate to plan DASH-friendly meals

A healthy meal is based on a balance of food groups, a wide variety of foods, and proper portions. A healthy DASH meal is a plate that's half full of veggies and fruit (which means lots of color); one-quarter full of lean protein such as beef, pork, chicken, turkey, beans, tofu, or seafood; and one-quarter full of whole-grain foods (which have more nutrients and fiber than refined grains). It also includes the dairy group, which provides the extra calcium important in the DASH diet. Plan your meals to include yogurt or fat-free or low-fat milk.

TIP

We recommend using the MyPlate consumer education tool (www.choosemyplate.gov) as a guide for planning DASH-approved meals. As you can see from Figure 14-1, the proportions shown in MyPlate match up with the DASH diet guidelines for a balanced, heart-healthy meal. Download the free MyPlate app (www.choosemyplate.gov/startsimpleapp) onto your phone to set specific DASH goals and track them. You can track your fruits and vegetables with specific goals.

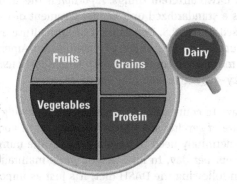

FIGURE 14-1: MyPlate proportions line up with those recommended for the DASH diet.

Using the MyPlate app, keep the following tips in mind:

>> **Set simple goals to include enough fruits and vegetables.** Be specific about how and when (include fruit or vegetable at breakfast or lunch, snack on fruit, add fruit to salads, include a leafy green, add more veggies to dinner, and so on).

>> **Set goals for protein.** Vary your protein and include beans and other plant proteins. Be sure to choose lean cuts and small 3- to 4-ounce portions.

>> **Choose visually stimulating foods.** That way, you'll ensure a broad source of nutrients and all-important phytochemicals. Aim for three to four colors for an interesting plate.

>> **Set goals to include dairy.** Look for ways to include your dairy servings into your meal plan. Beyond a glass of milk, use plain yogurt.

>> **Include enough whole grain to allow for 1 serving (about ½ cup).** Go for 2 servings of whole grains a day.

>> **Include more vegetables, some whole grains, and lean protein, your meal will be *nutrient-dense* (without solid fats and added sugars).**

>> **Pay attention to the size of your plate.** Does it correspond to your weight goals? Use a smaller plate at meals to help with portion control.

The app provides serving sizes for each food group. It also helps you track goals, especially for the fruit, vegetable, and dairy groups.

Putting portions into perspective

You may not realize this (and if you don't, you're not alone), but a *portion* of food and a *serving* of food are two different things. A *portion* is the amount you pile on your plate. A *serving* is a standardized unit of measurement of foods; it can be a cup or an ounce, as used in the U.S. Department of Agriculture and U.S. Department of Health and Human Services' Dietary Guidelines for Americans. Research shows that people eat more when confronted with larger portions. And if the food you're eating is sensory-attractive, you may eat more.

Although you don't have to count calories per se when following the DASH diet, you do need to be aware of serving sizes for a few reasons. If you're working on weight loss, then you definitely need to have an idea of the number of servings you need per food group, per day, to lose weight while maintaining a balanced diet. In addition, when following the DASH diet, it's just as important to ensure you eat *enough* of some groups (namely fruits, vegetables, dairy, and healthy fats). Table 14-1 gives you a general idea of what that looks like.

TABLE 14-1   **DASH Eating Plans**

Food Group	1,200 Calories	1,600 Calories	2,000 Calories	2,600 Calories
Grains*	4–5 servings per day	6 servings per day	6–8 servings per day	8–10 servings per day
Vegetables	3–4 servings per day	3–4 servings per day	4–5 servings per day	5–6 servings per day
Fruits	3–4 servings per day	4 servings per day	4–5 servings per day	5–6 servings per day
Fat-free or low-fat dairy	2–3 servings per day	2–3 servings per day	2–3 servings per day	3 servings per day
Lean meats, poultry, fish	3 ounces or less per day	3–4 ounces or less per day	6 ounces or less per day	6 ounces per day
Nuts, seeds, legumes	3 servings per week	3–4 servings per week	4–5 servings per week	5–6 servings per week
Added fats and oils	1–2 servings per day	2–3 servings per day	3–4 servings per day	5 servings per day
Sweets/ added sugar	3 servings or fewer per week	3 servings or fewer per week	4 servings or fewer per week	4 servings or fewer per week

* Half of these should be fiber-rich whole grains.

REMEMBER

A healthy meal consists of the right number of servings for your calorie needs. Less active women and older adults generally need about 1,600 calories a day; children, teen girls, active women, and less active men need about 2,200; and teen boys and active men need about 2,500. There are no rigid rules except to balance food choices over the course of the day. Three meals a day plus a planned snack is a good way to start. A registered dietitian nutritionist (RDN) can help you figure out exactly what's best for you. Foods with less saturated fat, sugar, or salt are balanced with foods in meals and snacks that are high in vitamins, minerals, healthy fats, and fiber. It's about balance. Low-fat and nonfat dairy are suggested, but it's okay to include some full-fat dairy portions, too. Meals and snacks should contain foods from all the food groups. To achieve success, it's crucial to plan ahead!

So, now you may be asking yourself: What is a serving exactly? Good question, and an important one! The amount of calories and nutrients you get from the food you eat depends on the serving size you choose. Doubling up on portions of some higher-calorie foods (like meats and fats) has a greater impact on calories than doubling up on your vegetables. Use the serving guidelines in Table 14-2 when planning and meeting your meal-plan goals.

TABLE 14-2   **Serving Sizes for Each Food Group**

Food Group	Serving Size Examples	DASH Contribution
Grains	1 slice of bread 1 ounce dry cereal (½–1 cup) ½ cup pasta, rice, grain, or cooked cereal	Source of fiber and energy
Vegetables	1 cup raw or leafy ½ cup cooked ½ cup juice	Source of potassium, magnesium, and fiber
Fruits	1 medium apple, pear, or peach 1 small banana ½ cup mixed fruit cup 1 cup berries or melon ¼ cup dried fruit	Source of potassium and fiber
Fat-free or low-fat dairy	8 ounces milk or yogurt 1½ ounces cheese	Source of calcium and protein

(continued)

TABLE 14-2 *(continued)*

Food Group	Serving Size Examples	DASH Contribution
Lean meats	1 ounce cooked meat, poultry, or fish 1 egg	Source of protein, zinc, and magnesium
Nuts, seeds, legumes	⅓ cup or 1½ ounces nuts 2 tablespoons peanut butter 2 tablespoons seeds ½ cup legumes or beans	Source of protein, magnesium, and fiber
Fats & oils	2 teaspoons soft margarine 1 teaspoon vegetable oil 1 tablespoon mayonnaise 2 tablespoons oily salad dressing	Less than 27% of calories from fat effective in DASH study
Sweets/sugars	1 tablespoon sugar 2 tablespoons jelly or jam ½ cup sorbet or gelatin 8 ounces lemonade or soda	Sweets should be limited, especially sugary drinks

TIP

In these times of super-sizing, it's easy to misjudge a standard serving size. Here are some comparisons to keep in mind so you stay on track:

>> 1 cup is the size of a baseball.

>> ½ cup is the size of a standard light bulb.

>> 1 ounce or 2 tablespoons is the size of a golf ball.

>> 3 ounces of protein is the size of a deck of cards.

Starting the Day off Right

Research shows that people who eat breakfast are more likely to maintain a healthy body weight and be physically active, both of which are so important in preventing high blood pressure. Eating in the morning also helps you get focused and energized for the day ahead.

Breakfast is a good opportunity to increase your nutrient and fiber intake. Hot and cold cereals have been the foundation of breakfast for generations, and they're a quick and easy way to add fiber to your diet. The thing to be aware of is added sugars — look for cereals that contain less than 9 grams of sugar per serving. Think about creative ways to vary the usual cereal and milk or shortcuts to the typical breakfast classics. Adding fresh fruit to your cereal bowl is a great way to add a fruit serving to your day.

Think about ways to include lean protein in your morning, too. Because you digest protein at a slower rate than refined carbohydrates, your blood sugar remains steady, which helps keep you satisfied longer. In the following sections, we show you just how easy it is to whip up the most important meal of the day with simple no-cook options and make-ahead ideas.

Grab-and-go breakfasts

Have little or no time in the morning? No sweat! The following grab-and-go options fit into a portable cup. You can even start enjoying them as you're heading out the door. They're that convenient!

>> Whip up a quick smoothie using 4 to 5 ounces of plain, low-fat Greek yogurt, and a banana or 1 cup of your favorite fruit. Pulse in the blender, pour into a travel cup, and go. You can portion out single servings of fresh fruit for the week so they're ready to grab and add to your blender for your morning smoothie. Or why not try the Breakfast Smoothie Bowl in Chapter 17?

>> Make a quick parfait by adding a dollop of Greek yogurt, cut fruit or berries, and 2 tablespoons of granola-type cereal in a portable cup to pack in your bag before you leave for work.

>> Make a to-go version of a peanut butter and banana sandwich. Spread a whole-grain, cinnamon-raisin English muffin with 2 tablespoons of peanut butter and banana slices.

>> Hard-boil your own eggs on the weekend and eat them throughout the week with a slice of whole-grain toast. If you're short on time, you can purchase hard-boiled eggs at the deli.

>> Portion out ½ cup of quick-cooking oats (*not* the instant kind), 1 tablespoon chopped walnuts, and 1 to 2 tablespoons of dried fruit into a cup. Add 1 cup of milk, zap in the microwave for 2 minutes, and stir it up.

>> Try the Open-Faced Egg Sandwich recipe in Chapter 17.

>> Stuff a whole-wheat tortilla with an ounce of turkey, chopped tomatoes, spinach leaves, and an ounce of low-fat cheese. Zap in the microwave for 10 to 20 seconds until the cheese melts and roll it up like a burrito for a hot breakfast-in-hand.

>> Make an open-faced bagel half topped with part-skim ricotta cheese. For a savory breakfast, add dried basil, fresh-cracked black pepper, fresh baby greens, and a sliced hard-boiled egg. For a sweeter breakfast, add ground cinnamon and a sliced nectarine.

Make-ahead morning fixings

If you have time and energy the night before, try your hand at one of these make-ahead options. All you'll have to do in the morning is reheat your dish of choice in the microwave.

>> Make your own breakfast egg sandwiches and freeze them. Lightly toast a whole-wheat English muffin. Cook an egg or two egg whites and place the cooked egg(s) on the toasted muffin. Wrap your sandwich in plastic wrap and place it in a freezer bag. When you're ready to eat, take out one sandwich at a time and microwave it for 30 to 60 seconds on medium-high or high (depending on the power of the microwave). Add fresh salsa and enjoy!

>> Make your own frittatas with any leftover ingredients you have in the refrigerator (don't forget the veggies!). The great thing about frittatas is that they usually create anywhere from 4 to 6 servings, so you'll have breakfast for several days after making one. You can also do these in muffin tins and bake in a 350-degree oven for 20 to 25 minutes.

>> Enjoy oats? Try a cool variation of muesli by mixing a packaged whole-grain oat mixture (or regular oats, not instant) with plain yogurt overnight. Or try the Banana Nut Hot Oatmeal recipe in Chapter 17.

>> Scramble egg whites or whole eggs with a variety of veggies and store them in the refrigerator. In the morning, heat 'em up, add a little of your favorite salsa, and wrap them in a whole-wheat tortilla. Or try our Easy Shakshuka recipe in Chapter 17.

>> Mix together a few tablespoons of nonfat refried beans with a tablespoon of your favorite salsa. When you're ready to head out the door, spread the bean mixture on a toasted, whole-wheat English muffin, top with shredded, low-fat cheese, and microwave on high until the cheese is melted, about 30 to 40 seconds.

» Make overnight oatmeal in the slow cooker! Place 2 cups of old-fashioned oats with 6 cups of water in a slow cooker. Set to low and cook overnight. In the morning, serve with dried raisins, cranberries, or blueberries; some chopped walnuts; and a drizzle of maple syrup.

» Line six ramekins or muffin tins with lean turkey or low-sodium ham. Crack an egg into each dish and sprinkle some freshly ground pepper and a dash of your favorite no-salt seasoning on top. Bake at 350 degrees for 25 minutes, or until the egg is done to your liking. Place your egg "muffins" in the refrigerator (or freeze them) and reheat them in the morning for a quick breakfast.

Packing Your Lunch to Avoid the Takeout Trap

For a far more flavorful and heart-healthy lunch, skip the drive-through and bring your lunch from home. You'll save money, have a better idea of how much sodium you're consuming, and be able to add more fruits and vegetables to your plate. The following sections provide ideas for homemade lunches that will be the envy of your coworkers.

Embracing the bento box

If the idea of bringing a sad ol' paper-bag lunch is holding you back, you're in luck. A bento box can keep your organized, and encourage that all food groups are met! They have compartments in each container to hold various foods. It's kind of like a throwback to 1960s TV dinners but with healthier, fresher components that offer a lot of variety — is in full swing for kids *and* adults. Bento boxes are a perfectly portioned and creative way to utilize leftovers and finger food. Here are some simple ideas for filling up a bento-style lunch container:

» **Caprese salad in a box:** Put marinated bocconcini (egg-sized mozzarella cheese balls; marinate with balsamic vinegar, olive oil, garlic, and chopped fresh basil) in the main compartment and cherry tomatoes in the second compartment. Add whole-grain crackers to the third. For a more substantial meal, add thinly sliced chicken to the fourth.

» **Chicken tender pockets:** Marinate and grill up some chicken tenders and fill the main compartment with two mini pita pockets with chicken tenders and baby spinach. Add a small Greek yogurt with grated cucumber and garlic clove to make a Greek tzatziki sauce in the third compartment, and add juicy Asian pear slices in the last compartment.

>> **Marinated tuna and bean salad:** Marinate a lemon-flavored tuna packet with olive oil, fresh squeezed lemon, minced red onion, and drained and rinsed cannellini beans and place in the two main compartments. Add whole-grain crackers in the third and a mixture of fresh berries in the last compartment.

>> **Quinoa lettuce wraps, edamame, and sliced veggies:** Mix cooked tricolor quinoa with sautéed shallots, dried cherries, a dash of ginger, garam masala (a spice mix), and turmeric and fill one compartment; fill the second compartment with Boston lettuce leaves. Add frozen, thawed edamame to the third and sliced raw veggies like carrots, celery, and jicama to the fourth.

>> **Turkey roll-ups, fresh fruit, and slaw:** To make turkey roll-ups, wrap two pieces of cracked-pepper turkey around a cube of cheddar cheese and spear with a toothpick. These make up the two main compartments. Fresh red and green grapes make up the third compartment, and an easy slaw of cabbage, carrots, and green onions with a drizzle of cider vinegar and oil make up the fourth.

TIP

Many kinds of bento-style lunch containers are available. Ziploc makes Twist 'n Loc containers that are good for packing liquids safely. LunchBots and Brandenburg Stainless have stainless-steel boxes for serious bento aficionados. Fit & Fresh has lunch totes, containers with compartments, removable lids, and built-in ice packs for keeping food cold.

Going beyond PB&J

A smashed peanut butter and jelly sandwich will do for lunch in a pinch, but you can easily get a little more creative with fairly minimal do-ahead effort. Putting together healthy weekday lunches is a snap when you have a plan. Use these ideas to plan easy lunches that incorporate ingredients you have on hand or allow you to recycle leftovers:

>> Mix together a garlic-and-herb-flavor fresh tuna pouch with a chopped, large, marinated artichoke heart, a tablespoon of sundried tomatoes in olive oil, and baby spinach leaves. Stuff inside a whole-wheat pita pocket.

>> Toss leftover shredded rotisserie chicken with a tablespoon of barbeque sauce and stuff into a whole-wheat slider bun.

>> Mash up canned and rinsed cannellini beans with 1 teaspoon of chopped chipotle peppers and a ripe avocado. Portion out (about ½ cup) and wrap in a whole-wheat tortilla.

>> Mix up some cooked tricolor (or plain, or pearl couscous) quinoa with a half cup of low-sodium black beans, drained and rinsed; a half cup of frozen thawed corn; cherry tomatoes, cut in half; and half an avocado, cut into chunks and drizzled with light ranch-flavored dressing mixed with chipotle salsa.

>> Trade a traditional shrimp cocktail for a mix of chopped, precooked shrimp; chopped tomatoes, peppers, onions, and cilantro; and a splash of fresh lime with whole-wheat pita chips. Add an apple on the side.

>> Stuff seeded tomatoes with chicken salad made with rotisserie or leftover chicken, chopped celery, green onions, apples, and walnuts.

>> Swap ordinary hot tomato soup for a cold shrimp gazpacho with blended tomatoes, green bell pepper, onions, cucumbers, and plump, cold, boiled shrimp.

>> Layer roast beef and baby spinach in a whole-wheat tortilla with a shredded cabbage and carrot slaw, mixed with prepared horseradish and plain Greek yogurt. Fold or roll.

>> Try an open-faced egg salad sandwich on half of a toasted, whole-grain English muffin.

Taking Shortcuts to Dinnertime

"Dinner is now being served." Don't you wish for a butler to ring the dinner chimes and have dinner ready while you enjoy the hammock after a long day at work? It's really as easy as having a meal plan and a little organization.

Use our quick tips to put together easy meals that use food-prep shortcuts and simple cooking techniques.

Prepping ingredients ahead of time

When you work ahead, ingredients become much easier to toss into your recipes on busy nights. We promise that even just a little bit of prep goes a long way toward getting DASH-friendly dinners on your table. The first step is knowing what you plan to do with your groceries so that when you unpack you can get some pre-prepping out of the way to help the cooking process for the week go a lot faster. Next, try these techniques for cutting down on the amount of time you spend preparing to cook each day:

>> Wash and core fresh bell peppers when you know you'll be using them within two days. Remove the core, stem, and seeds, and store them in a zipper storage bag in the vegetable bin of your refrigerator. When you need them, you can simply slice or dice them per your recipe.

>> Have vegetables ready for salad fixings or a veggie tray. Clean and slice cucumbers, bell peppers, carrots, and celery so they're ready to munch on before dinner or to use in a salad recipe. Place them in airtight containers or zipper storage bags.

>> Chop a medium-sized onion and store it in either a zipper storage bag or an airtight container in the vegetable drawer of your refrigerator for seven to ten days. Having chopped onions on hand saves time on recipes that call for them. If the recipe requires minced onions, you can easily chop them further. You can also freeze them in recipe portions (usually about ½ cup) and then take them out of the freezer and just toss them into the pan.

>> Take a few minutes in the morning to prep some of the food you plan to have for dinner that night. Chop vegetables and fruit and make a marinade or salad dressing as needed. Store them in the refrigerator to save time later when you prepare the meal.

>> Cook a little extra of staples such as meats, veggies, and grains; you can use these in meals over the next couple days. For example, if you're preparing a grilled chicken recipe, grill two extra boneless breasts to save for dinner in a day or two. Or if you cook rice or quinoa, make double and put half in the fridge for another day's salad mixture or lunch.

Stocking up on freezer-friendly staples

You can use your freezer to help you keep recipe items in stock, saving you additional or more frequent trips to the grocery store. You can purchase foods such as meats, fish, poultry, fresh herbs, and vegetables fresh and freeze them for later use. When you prepare a homemade tomato, pesto, or other sauce, you can divide and freeze it in sealed, freezer-safe containers. Here are some additional helpful ideas:

>> Roast a whole chicken or just chicken breasts or boneless, skinless thighs. Chop or shred the meat, and store it in 1- to 2-cup quantities in freezer bags. You can even simply poach boneless chicken breasts in boiling water with a few herbs added. This keeps the chicken moist, and it's easy to shred or chop.

You can even purchase a rotisserie chicken and pull all the meat off the bones and store the same way for future use (keep in mind these are higher in sodium).

» Freeze grilled chicken breasts or chicken breast tenderloins. You can use them in a garden fresh entree salad, chop them up for soup or a chicken salad, or make a panini sandwich using the already cooked chicken.

» You can freeze beef, chicken, or vegetable stock in any amounts, such as a tablespoonful in ice cube trays or a half or full cup.

» Brown and drain ground turkey or lean ground beef. When thawed, you can use these to make tacos or add to spaghetti sauce.

» You can make marinara sauce, spaghetti sauce, pizza sauce, and salsa in batches and freeze the sauce in various sized containers. It's best to make these recipes when tomatoes are ripe and in season.

» Other quick shortcuts: Freeze a backup carton of milk, grated cheese, bread, parboiled potatoes, and even whole sandwiches, minus the lettuce and tomato.

REMEMBER

To prevent your freezer from becoming a frozen wasteland, wrap everything properly to prevent freezer burns, and label and date the food so you know when it was prepared. Trust us: You can't always rely on your memory when safety and freshness matter. Rotate the inventory using the FIFO method (first-in, first-out). Note that most dishes will last about three to four months.

Freezing meats

Purchasing fresh meats, fish, and poultry for same-day preparation is great, but few people's schedules allow for that. Freezing meats is an alternative that can still result in a good product. You can freeze most meats for up to three months.

TIP

Rather than simply throwing the store-bought package straight into the freezer, we recommend opening the package, trimming extra skin or fat, and using zipper bags to prevent freezer burn. Zipper freezer bags are easy to use and come in different sizes, allowing you to divide meats into smaller or larger packages, depending on the number of people you'll be cooking for or the specifications of a given recipe. Be sure to label and date the bags before you place them in the freezer.

WARNING

To prevent bacterial contamination, don't thaw meats on the counter. Defrost meat, fish, or poultry in either the refrigerator or the microwave, using the defrost function. When defrosting in the refrigerator, be sure the meat is in a sealed bag or container and put it on a bottom shelf to minimize leaks and the chances of contaminating other foods.

FRESH POULTRY

Poultry pieces with the bones in and the skin on often cost less than their bone-less, skinless counterparts. Boning takes some skill and time, but removing the skin is an easy task. After you remove the skin, rinse the pieces under cold water, pat them dry, and freeze them in freezer bags. You can fit two portions in a quart-sized bag or four to six portions in a gallon-sized bag.

TIP

To facilitate removing one or two pieces at a time from the freezer, don't place pieces on top of one another when you freeze them, and try to leave a little space between the pieces.

You can cut large boneless chicken breasts into several smaller pieces. Some breasts are thick enough to cut in half lengthwise and then again crosswise, mak-ing thinner, smaller pieces. You can also cut boneless breast meat into strips for stir-fries or into chunks for chilis, stews, or salads. Thin pieces of boneless breast work well on the grill because they cook quickly and stay juicy.

FRESH PORK OR BEEF

REMEMBER

Lean is the key to healthy meats. Trim all visible fat from roasts or steaks before freezing. Use a large, lean cut, such as beef sirloin, to make strips for stir-fries. Freeze the strips in a single layer in quart-sized freezer bags.

Freeze individual steaks in a single layer in a freezer bag. You may purchase one large steak at the grocer, but keep in mind that your diet for hypertension requires you to limit the amount of beef and pork you eat. To that end, cut beef and pork steaks or chops into 4- to 6-ounce portions before you freeze them.

FISH AND SEAFOOD

You can freeze fillets whole or cut them into 6-ounce portions (about 2 to 3 inches apiece) before freezing. Use zipper freezer bags that are sized accordingly.

Easier yet, purchase pre-frozen fish fillets, shrimp, or scallops. You can find a variety of fish in the seafood freezer section of your grocery store. Fillets are flash-frozen so you can easily take them out of the bag one at a time. Look for weekly sales and stock up. Read the labels, though, because sometimes sodium is added.

Freezing fresh vegetables

When vegetables are in season or on sale, you may consider purchasing extras and freezing them for later. When you freeze fresh vegetables, you'll find that they're more flavorful than store-bought frozen veggies. You can even freeze leftover vegetables. For instance, if you steam a batch of fresh peas and have a little bit left over, place them in a zippered freezer bag and freeze them for use in another recipe. Fresh corn on the cob freezes well also. You can blanch it in boiling water for 3 minutes and then freeze it, or you can cut cooked corn off the cob and freeze it for another recipe in the future.

TIP

When freezing any vegetable, blanch it first. To blanch, bring a gallon of water to a boil. Wash and trim the fresh vegetables. You can either boil the vegetables in the water or steam them using a steaming basket. Place the vegetables into the steamer or pot and steam or boil them for 4 to 6 minutes (steaming usually takes a minute longer, and some veggies take less time). Plunge the vegetables into ice water immediately or place them in a colander and run cold water over them for a few minutes. Drain well and then pack them into zippered freezer bags. The nutrient quality of the frozen vegetables will be as good as the fresh ones.

Putting your slow cooker or Instant Pot to work

Nothing about a slow cooker will slow you down. This amazing, time-saving appliance can turn a few minutes of your morning into a flavor-packed dinner. If you have a slow cooker with a removable insert, you can assemble dinner before you go to bed, put it in the refrigerator, pull it out in the morning, place it into the slow cooker, and plug the slow cooker in. Voilà! A delicious dinner will be waiting for you when you arrive home at the end of the day.

Any recipe that requires long, slow, low heat is the perfect choice for a slow cooker. The following options all fit the bill:

>> Combine a pound of lean ground beef, chopped onion and jalapeño pepper, a 15-ounce can of no-added-salt tomato sauce drained and rinsed, 15-ounce cans of pinto and kidney beans, a tablespoon of chili powder, and a teaspoon of cumin in a 4- to 6-quart slow cooker and cook on low for 8 hours for a chillin' chili.

>> Try our Bold and Beefy Instant Pot Stew in Chapter 22.

>> Make the Hearty Southwest Slow-Cooker Soup in Chapter 22.

>> To make a rustic Italian vegetable soup in the Instant Pot, set the Instant Pot to Sauté and add olive oil and a chopped onion. Cook for 2 minutes. Then combine the following ingredients: 2 cups of low-sodium vegetable stock; a 15-ounce can of no-added-salt diced tomatoes; 2 cups of any of your favorite chopped veggies, such as carrots, celery and zucchini; a teaspoon of oregano, basil, and freshly ground black pepper; and 15-ounce cans of drained and

rinsed kidney and cannellini beans. Cover and set the pot on Manual/Pressure-Cook, High. Set the timer for 5 minutes. Cook until steam builds and the timer shuts off. Allow about 8 to 10 minutes for steam to release (or follow the manufacturer's instructions).

>> Asian mu shu pork wraps are a cinch in the slow cooker! Add a chopped onion and 2 pounds of pork tenderloin to a slow cooker and cook on low for 5 hours, or until the meat pulls apart easily with a fork. Shred the meat with a fork and add a cup of hoisin sauce, a tablespoon of agave nectar, and ¼ teaspoon ground ginger. Heat until the flavors blend and serve on a warm, whole-wheat tortilla with store-bought broccoli slaw.

TIP

Use a slow-cooker liner to make cleanup super-fast.

Cooking in batches

Batch cooking — cooking a lot of food in advance, and often freezing portions for later use — is handy for simplifying weeknight cooking, although it can make for a long cooking day. With batch cooking, you can cook up as much food as your freezer will hold or prepare scratch ingredients to use through the week (to prevent from having to purchase the processed equivalents, such as spaghetti sauce).

Preparing freezer meals involves totally prepping and cooking a full meal in advance and then freezing it for later use. The meal can be completely cooked and just thawed and reheated (such as a stew or lasagne), or assembled, frozen, and cooked at a later time.

TIP

Freezer meals are so handy when you absolutely have no time to prepare a meal at the last minute or if you need to take a meal to a friend who had surgery or just had a baby. It's like turning your freezer into a mini frozen food aisle at the grocery store but with healthier options! Obviously, you need the space to be able to do this method. A deep freezer is the perfect appliance for large-batch cooking.

You have a number of options to store food for freezing, such as foil casserole dishes, resealable plastic bags, vacuum sealers, and plastic storage containers in various sizes. You can plan a few weeks of menus, decide what recipes you want to use, and then buy all your ingredients in one trip. Then you devote an entire day to doing all the cooking. You may even dread that day, but when you're done cooking, you're all set with wonderful meals that you'll surely appreciate later!

A few recipes that work well as freezer meals (meaning they're less likely to dry out when reheated) are:

- » Lightened turkey tetrazzini (prepared with low-sodium chicken broth and low-fat dairy)

- » Louisiana Red Beans and Rice (Chapter 21)

- » Mini meatloaves

- » Most broth-based soups and stews

- » Stuffed shells, manicotti, and lasagne

TIP

After making a meal, keep the bacteria at bay by cooling it quickly. Let the baking container sit in a shallow container of ice water. Casserole-type dishes are easier to cut into portions when chilled. Dividing the dish into individual portions before freezing makes it easier to adhere to the appropriate servings and easier to reheat.

Making one-pot meals

A great way to get a quick dinner on the table on weeknights without breaking a sweat is to make one-pot meals. Every ingredient goes into the pot for cooking, and you can serve the meal right out of the pot. Try some of our favorites:

- » Caribbean Chicken Foil Pouches (Chapter 22)

- » Quick and Easy Shrimp Ancient Grain Bowl (Chapter 19)

- » Skillet scrambles such as Confetti Hash with Poached Eggs (Chapter 17)

- » Hearty Southwest Slow-Cooker Soup (Chapter 22)

TIP

Stir-fries are also one-pot meals, assuming you already have some rice made. Try our Stir-Fry Tofu with Mushrooms in Sichuan Sauce recipe in Chapter 21.

Livening up leftovers

You can always reheat your leftovers and eat them again. Some food actually tastes better the second day, like spaghetti sauce. On the other hand, some foods have a "warmed over" taste and unappealing texture when served a second time. Plus, it can get boring to eat the same few dishes all week. Welcome to the beauty of using your leftovers in creative ways that don't require a ton of effort! You can cook certain foods once and transform them into a totally new recipe. For example, you can take your roast chicken leftovers and make homemade chicken enchiladas, or mix your leftover grain with a rinsed can of beans and tuna the next day for a lunch salad.

REMEMBER

Leftovers can be the time-saving reward for cooking from scratch to begin with. Here are a few appealing ways to use leftovers that retain some of their original identity but are creative enough to get the family clamoring for more:

>> Reheat leftover salmon and serve it over a bed of fresh greens and a light balsamic dressing.

>> Mix leftover quinoa with rinsed, canned chickpeas, a chopped apple, and baby spinach.

>> Use leftover whole-wheat pasta in pasta salads or toss it into a homemade soup at the last minute.

>> Mix leftover cooked meat into enchiladas, quesadillas, casseroles, or even a stir-fry.

>> Use leftover roast or pork shoulder for burritos, tacos, stuffed peppers, lasagne, and sandwiches.

>> Use leftover roasted or grilled vegetables as a homemade pizza topping, mix them into fresh pasta sauce, make them into a wrap sandwich, or add them to a frittata.

>> Make dried whole-wheat bread into bread crumbs or croutons.

>> Wok-sear leftover brown rice and vegetables with a little oil and a scrambled egg.

IN THIS CHAPTER

» Thinking generally about heart-
healthy eating away from home

» Keeping DASH in mind at various
types of restaurants

» Staying on track when you travel

Chapter **15**

Dining Out and Traveling on DASH

You can't beat cooking and eating at home in terms of choosing the healthiest foods, but you may not always be able to get into the kitchen every day.
If you're like us, your schedule probably varies from day to day or month to
month. You also probably travel every so often, whether it's for business, to visit
relatives, or simply to get away from it all. This chapter aims to help you make
heart-healthy (or at least better) choices when cooking and dining at home isn't
an option.

REMEMBER

There may be times when you may not be able to meet every goal of the DASH diet
when dining out. That's okay. Just do your best and pick up where you left off at
the next meal. You may also not have too much control over sodium at times, so
keep this in mind, and reduce sodium at other meals and over the next day.

Dining Out with DASH, Generally Speaking

The DASH diet focuses on adding more fruits, vegetables, nuts, and seeds to your
diet. So when dining out, keep those food groups at the front of your mind. Look
for the vegetables on the menu and sneak in some milk or low-fat dairy foods
when you can.

TIP

DASH limits sodium, which is more difficult to control when dining out. Rather than worry too much about that, focus on what you can *include* with your choices. Consider these guidelines the next time you head out to eat:

» Rethink appetizers as possible entrees. Portions matter because the larger the portion, the higher the calorie content but also the higher the sodium content. Create a meal with an appetizer and add a side salad and baked potato.

» Look for vegetables. Be sure to add a side salad or a vegetable to your meal. To ensure you don't go overboard with the salad dressing, ask for it on the side. Watch out for crouton overload, as they can add 50 to 100 calories to your salad.

» Choose the side vegetable for your side dish. Choosing the green side veggie (such as asparagus, green beans, or a vegetable medley) adds antioxidants.

» Limit fried food; choose broiled, grilled, or baked instead.

» Going out to breakfast? Order the veggie omelet and ask for it to be made with two eggs rather than three. Once taboo, egg yolks are a great source of choline (essential for healthy metabolism and brain health), so it's fine to include them.

» Ask about changes to menu items. Often the cook or chef can skip the sauce, skip the salt, or lighten something up for you if you ask for it. Ask for sauces on the side.

» Rethink chicken. Chicken is known to be low in saturated fat, but restaurant chicken is often loaded with salt. Frozen chicken often has a salt solution added to it to retain moisture and extend its freezer life. Fresh beef or pork is often lower in sodium when dining out.

» Consider portion size. As we've said, the bigger the portion, the more sodium and fat. Choose 5-ounce steaks at the steakhouse, split an entree with someone, or eat half your meal and take half home.

» Skip the extra cheese. Though low-fat dairy is part of the DASH diet, chances are, the processed cheese used at most restaurants is full-fat and higher in sodium. Also, because most restaurant meals are generally higher in sodium, holding the cheese can help you reduce total sodium in that meal.

» Drink water with meals and monitor other beverages. Drinks high in sugar or alcohol can rack up calories and are not good for your blood pressure. If you enjoy them, limit alcoholic beverages to no more than one or two, and limit any sugary beverages to 8 ounces or less.

» Check out the nutrition information that chain and fast food restaurants offer on their websites.

TIP

Restaurant food is usually higher in sodium, so the next time you think about using the salt shaker on your food at the table, shake it into your hand. Just a few shakes can yield a quarter teaspoon (or about 600 milligrams of sodium).

Share and share alike

When dining out, sharing appetizers, meals, side dishes, or desserts is a great way to enjoy foods that you love. It's also a simple way to control your portion size. Considering the overly generous portions of food served up as entrees at restaurants these days, there's usually plenty on the plate for two (and your wallet will thank you as well).

Why worry about portions? Because bigger portions mean you get more of everything — good and bad. For the nutrients you want more of (like potassium, calcium, and vitamins A and C), be sure to have adequate portions from the food groups that provide them (fruits, vegetables, beans, nuts, seeds, and low-fat dairy). As for sodium, the larger the portion, the higher the sodium content. For high-sodium foods, this can really be a big deal. Half the portion means half the sodium too.

If you need a primer on proper portion sizes, check out Chapter 14.

Finding the Healthy Options at Various Types of Restaurants

Though sodium can be a major issue in a fine dining setting, you typically have plenty of choices to help you steer clear of high-sodium foods. In addition, you may have some bargaining power in the special request department, although it's often okay to make requests at fast food restaurants too. Ethnic restaurants can also have some healthy options, as long as you know what you're looking for.

Sit-down restaurants

Sit-down restaurants come in a few different flavors. At the lowest level are the casual chain restaurants. Next come the privately owned casual restaurants, followed by the more upscale restaurants (both chain and privately owned). In general, you have fewer choices at a chain restaurant than a privately owned establishment because most chains have set recipes and menus. Still, it doesn't hurt to ask your server if the kitchen can hold the salt or put the sauce on the side. You can also request the nutrition information from chains or check their websites or apps. Many now post the calories, at least, on the menu boards.

Following are our suggestions for finding the most DASH-friendly options when dining at sit-down restaurants:

>> Always add a side salad, preferably mixed field greens or added vegetables and nuts (look for healthy toppings such as roasted beets, almonds, or walnuts).

>> Choose the vegetable of the day for your side dish rather than fries or a potato, especially in steakhouses, where the potatoes are generally gigantic. (If you must have a steakhouse potato, just eat half.) You can also shake things up with a baked sweet potato once in a while.

>> If you're dining at a steakhouse, choose the smallest steak. Filet mignon is lowest in fat and is often offered as a 4-to-8-ounce portion.

>> For the sake of calorie control, it's best to skip dessert or to share dessert with a friend. "Better" choices: fruit crisp/cobblers, crème brûlée (milk and egg-based, often served with fresh berries), or sorbet.

Fast food places

Whether it's from a drive-through or a fast sit-down place, fast food gets a bad rap. No, it shouldn't be a daily (or even weekly) source of your food, but you can make informed choices when you get a fast food craving or if you're traveling and need a quick bite. Because you get a choice of portions (small, medium, large, humongous), you'll do best by sticking with the small or medium option (sometimes "medium" is the smallest choice). Value-type menus often have smaller-portion items, so they may be a safe bet too.

Saturated fat and sodium are two nutrients of concern on fast food menus, so be sure to take a look at them and choose the lower-sodium options. That smaller-portion rule works here (smaller portions mean less saturated fat and less sodium). Take a look at the simple math in Table 15-1 to see how you can reduce fat and sodium with smaller portion sizes at a typical chain steakhouse or a coffeehouse/bakery.

Other options that may surprise you are some typical café/bake-shop breakfast items, which we list in Table 15-2. Though the bagel is lowest in fat, it's still high in calories and sodium. The cheese in the egg sandwich adds about 450 milligrams of sodium (so if you just hold the cheese, you can reduce the sodium to 170 milligrams and the calories to around 550). As you can see from the numbers in Table 15-2, the parfait is a DASH diet winner! Keep balance in mind as you make choices as well. While Table 15-2 highlights fat and sodium, protein is important to satiety (helping you stay full longer and thus not take in more calories than you need through the day). Both the parfait and the egg sandwich offer you some protein as well. And, don't forget about the calories, sugar, and fat in fancy sweetened coffeehouse drinks. Ask for the breakdown if they aren't posted.

TABLE 15-1   Comparison of Various Portions of Similar Foods

Entree	Calories	Fat (g)	Sodium (mg)
4-oz cheeseburger	430	20	870
Small hamburger	230	8	490
Honey mustard chicken sandwich, whole	700	28	1,320
Honey mustard chicken sandwich, ½	350	14	660
Chicken and wild rice soup, 12 oz	300	17	1,450
Chicken and wild rice soup, 8 oz	200	12	970

TABLE 15-2   Calories, Fat, and Sodium in Typical Quick-Stop Breakfast Food

Food Item	Calories	Fat (g)	Sodium (mg)
Apple pastry	380	19	320
Cinnamon bagel	320	2	460
Egg and cheese breakfast sandwich	380	14	620
Strawberry granola yogurt parfait	310	12	100

Ethnic options

Just about every ethnicity offers beautiful traditional foods that are both healthy and not-so-healthy (but tasty no doubt). Saving those not-so-healthy options for special occasions and holidays is your best bet.

Table 15-3 focuses on the good choices you can make at various ethnic restaurants. Keep in mind, though, that sodium levels will still be higher than in food you cook at home (this is especially true with Chinese and Thai food, which can have more than 2,000 milligrams of sodium per serving). Skip fried choices. Ordering more vegetables is still a good addition to your diet. Ask for sauces on the side or ask for no MSG so you can better control the sodium.

TABLE 15-3   **Best Choices at Ethnic Restaurants**

Ethnicity	Best Choices
Mexican	Beans and rice, one crunchy taco, veggie burritos, fish tacos, a cup of black bean soup, Mexican salad of mixed greens and vegetables, guacamole, fajitas (shrimp, chicken, or beef with onions and bell peppers), salsa
Italian	Marinara sauces, baked or grilled fish with a side of pasta, ravioli, salads, Italian wedding soup, half portion of pasta with tomato sauce, pasta tossed in olive oil with vegetables, veal piccata with lemon butter and wine sauce
Chinese/Asian	Sushi, steamed brown/white rice, mixed vegetable stir-fry (garlic sauce or Szechuan), tofu with vegetables, chicken with broccoli, mixed vegetables, or snow peas
Middle Eastern	Falafel, tabbouleh, hummus, pita, fattoush, kebab, Greek salad
Indian	Curried vegetables, tandoori chicken or fish, steamed rice, lentil soup, chicken tikka masala, chicken vindaloo

Planning Ahead to Follow DASH on the Road

Planning ahead is the best strategy to ensure DASH-friendly eating, particularly when you're going to be traveling for any length of time. Vacations are often scheduled differently than your normal week, so when your environment changes, a little more planning can go a long way. A road trip may require different planning than going by air or boat, but it's all doable. Packing some snack items for the road helps eliminate choosing poor snack choices at convenience stops and saves money. Although you can't bring bottles of water through airport security, you can pack an apple and a bag of almonds and buy water or fill your reusable water bottle before you board.

Travel tips to help you stick to your goals

When you leave home for another destination, your routine is likely to change. You can go with the flow and still stick with your overall diet and exercise goals. Try not to get trapped into the mind-set of, "Well, I'm on vacation, so it's a free-for-all!" Instead, meet yourself halfway and think about how good you'll feel if you have some activity daily and eat well. You can still hold on to traditions and have that ice cream cone from that special ice cream parlor that you love, but you'll balance it out with healthy food and some exercise through the week.

Here's a simple game plan to think about the next time you leave town:

>> Pack a healthy snack to go.

>> Pack at least one set of exercise clothes and lightweight athletic shoes.

>> Plan some physical activity daily: walking, biking, kayaking, dancing.

>> Think about your meal plan at the beginning of the day.

>> Consider a larger lunch and a lighter dinner. You'll save money and have more time during the day to work it off!

>> Plan ahead if your hotel room has a kitchenette. If you pack a microwaveable egg cooker, you can make an egg sandwich in the morning on a whole-grain English muffin, or microwave a bowl of quick oats with fruit.

>> Do a grocery run if possible to pick up breakfast items and healthy snacks like eggs, quick-cooking oatmeal, fruit, carrot sticks, yogurt, cottage cheese, string cheese, whole-grain bread, nut butter, and nuts.

>> Don't skip breakfast because it's a chance to get important DASH foods in, such as low-fat dairy and fruit.

Simple portable snacks

Often when you're away from home, you may not have access to the same amount of space or conveniences. If you have a small refrigerator available, pack it with grab-and-go snacks. If you have a small kitchen available, plan to use it for breakfast each day. While we generally recommend you don't allow processed food to be a focus in your diet, some conveniences such as individually packaged nuts or snack bars can come in handy when traveling.

Consider these healthy convenience foods for the road:

>> Low-fat string cheese

>> Fruit cups, unsweetened or packed in their own juice (peaches, mixed fruit, applesauce)

>> Apples, bananas, pears (all are pretty hardy for travel bags compared to more delicate fruits)

>> Almonds, walnuts, or mixed nuts

>> Fruit and nut trail mix

>> Fruit and nut snack bars (look for brands that are comprised of mostly fruit and nuts — not chocolate-coated or sugary chewy types)

>> Yogurt cups (if you travel by car, a cooler is a great idea to have along)

>> Raw carrots, celery, or pepper strips

>> Whole-grain cereal (portion out snack bags to take along)

>> Water bottles

DASH EATING, AIRPORT STYLE

It may sound crazy, but you can make healthy choices in an airport (and you know you're not getting anything to eat on the plane, so plan ahead!). Most airports have both sit-down and counter-service options. If you're traveling by car and find yourself at a convenient mart, you can find good choices there as well. Look for foods that can serve as mini-meals:

- Yogurt or yogurt parfaits
- Small sandwiches (think two slices of whole-wheat bread, a wrap, or a small bun filled with turkey or ham, lettuce, and tomato)
- Fresh fruit; yes, there are apples, oranges, and bananas for sale
- Trail mix (nuts and dried fruit; compare sodium on labels and portion out small servings)
- Water, low-fat white or flavored milk
- Whole-grain cereal with fruit and low-fat milk
- Fresh fruit cups
- Small bags of baby carrots
- Small salads
- On a red-eye flight? Enjoy a nonfat latte.
- At a make-your-own sandwich place? Add lots of fresh veggies to your wrap or sandwich.

Chapter **16**

Adopting Everyday Lifestyle Changes

Sometimes life whizzes by so fast, you can't keep track of what you're supposed to be doing, and diet and lifestyle end up on the back burner. The irony of this problem is that a poor diet or lifestyle can exacerbate the stress that's making it so difficult to focus on diet and lifestyle! Prioritizing your diet and lifestyle goals is essential to feeling in control of your life and your health.

What do we mean by *lifestyle*? The term refers to what you do on a day-to-day basis. Do you have a sedentary job where you sit most of the day or does your job involve active labor? Do you try to eat right — fitting fruits and vegetables in daily, eating whole grains, and limiting fast food and fried foods? Do you dine out for lunch every day at work? Are you drinking enough water? Are you too rushed at meals? Do you do yardwork or housework and try to get some exercise every week? Do you smoke? What's your stress level like? These components of your life have a huge impact on your health and risk for disease.

Understanding the reasons behind the DASH diet and following it is one thing, but to be really successful for the long haul, you must develop a healthy lifestyle framework that includes managing stress, enlisting a support system, and tracking progress. This chapter helps you lay the groundwork for supporting your efforts to live a DASH-approved life.

Remembering That the Rat Race Isn't Really a Race

The alarm rings at 6 a.m. You get out of bed, make the coffee, jump in the shower, get to the kitchen, pour a travel mug, and out the door you go. Sound familiar? Life can get pretty busy, and often you may find yourself racing from one thing to the other, from 7 a.m. to 7 p.m., with no time in between to breathe — or eat properly! In the following sections, we help you figure out where you can slow things down a bit to buy yourself some breathing room.

REMEMBER

Don't forget the reason you're doing this: your health. Check out Chapters 2 and 3 whenever you're doubting yourself. Find motivation in the science behind DASH and how it can help.

Getting enough quality sleep

Sleeping well improves one's mood, reduces stress, helps with weight loss (and healthy weight maintenance), increases one's ability to stay focused and pay attention, and improves athletic performance. Good sleep is also your body's way of charging up for the next day, kind of like how you plug in your smartphone to charge it when the battery runs low. Getting enough sleep is even related to weight control.

The amount of sleep an adult needs to feel rested varies. The older you get, the less you may need. For example, school-age children need 10 to 11 hours a night, teens need 8.5 to 9.5 hours, and adults require 7 to 9 hours. It's up to you to decide how many hours you need — are you happy and do you feel good with 6 hours or do you really need 9 to feel right?

The quality of sleep matters too. If you're in bed for 9 hours but you're tossing and turning for most of them, you won't feel as well-rested as someone who got 6 hours of solid sleep.

WARNING

If you or a family member experiences daytime grogginess, snoring, gasping for breath, leg cramps, or difficulty breathing when sleeping, contact your primary physician right away because sleep apnea could be the culprit. It can impact your blood pressure. *Sleep apnea* is a sleep disorder that causes an individual to stop breathing momentarily, and repeatedly, while sleeping.

So how can you improve your odds of getting enough quality sleep? Follow our advice:

>> **Establish a consistent sleep-and-wake schedule.** Don't get too off-track on the weekends. In other words, go to bed around the same time each day, and wake up around the same time every day.

>> **Develop a relaxing bedtime routine.** A hot bath or shower, reading a book for pleasure, or listening to some soothing music all help get your body and mind ready for some good sleep.

>> **Create a sleep-inducing environment in your bedroom.** Try to keep your bedroom neat, dark, and comfortably cool. (Cooler temperatures are better for sleep.) Avoid watching TV or looking at any other type of screen in bed, especially if you're having issues with proper sleep, because research shows that bright screens relate to changes in the sleep hormone *melatonin*, making it more difficult to get to sleep.

>> **Avoid caffeine and alcohol close to bedtime.** Both can interfere with sleep, causing you to either have trouble falling asleep or have issues with waking up during sleep. One research study showed that caffeine six hours before bed reduced sleep time by one hour. Alcohol is associated with awakening in the second half of sleep and may cause night sweats or headache, both sleep disrupters.

>> **Exercise regularly.** A slightly tired physical body helps with the zzz's.

TECHNICAL STUFF

If your basal sleep needs and sleep debt are out of balance, you're going to feel it. *Basal sleep* is the amount of sleep your body requires on a regular basis for it to function optimally. *Sleep debt* is the accumulated sleep lost due to poor sleep habits, awakening, illness, or other causes. Think about times when you sleep great for three or four nights of the week but have two or three nights where you wake up in the middle of the night and can't fall back to sleep, or toss and turn. This sleep debt accumulates and can cause you to feel tired and less productive.

Savoring your food rather than scarfing it down

Science says that it takes about 20 minutes for your brain to register that your belly is full. This means that when you shovel down your lunch in 7 minutes flat, you may overeat and consequently find yourself left with an uncomfortable feeling of fullness a half-hour later.

Eating too quickly can easily become a bad habit, but you can work on breaking it. Here's how:

>> **Set a time to break for a meal.** Even if you only have a 30-minute lunch break (or no lunch break at all), do your best to allow yourself at least a 20-minute period to eat.

>> **Sit down.** Eating on the run, in your car, or standing up isn't a great habit. Sit down to eat so you can focus on not only the act of eating but also *what* you're eating.

>> **Enlist your eyes and nose.** Look at the food in front of you. Enjoy the colors and aromas.

>> **Slow your pace.** Sip on water and put your fork down between bites.

>> **Don't multi-task.** It may not seem like a big deal to watch TV or check email while you eat, but if you're not really focusing on your plate, you may eat too much. Treat yourself to an uninterrupted meal and break.

>> **Chew longer.** You may not even realize how quickly you chew and swallow your food. Not only is it easier on your digestive tract if you chew your food longer, but you may also absorb more nutrients that way.

Practicing mindfulness in your everyday life

Eating isn't the only activity you may do mindlessly. Do you ever find yourself driving along the highway and then suddenly wonder when you passed a landmark? After you park your car for work, do you find yourself sitting at your desk wondering, "What happened between there and here?"

Sometimes the chatter in your head is so loud and powerful that you can't turn it off, or maybe you don't even realize how continuous it is. Becoming more mindful in general can make your day-to-day life so much less stressful. Try these tactics to start living more mindfully:

>> **Take a deep breath.** Deep breathing is proven to lower stress. Sometimes just a few deep breaths can make a big difference. Sit quietly and close your eyes. Inhale to the count of 4 or 5. Exhale to the count of 4 or 5. Do this 3 to 5 times.

TIP

Taking 1 or 2 deep breaths before eating a meal (or any time of day really) can help you prepare for a more mindful experience.

>> **Be more compassionate.** Consideration of others and practicing gratitude can help you become more mindful. Work on becoming more self-compassionate as well. This involves becoming more aware of everything you do. Learn what's driving negative behaviors, as well as the situations that support positive

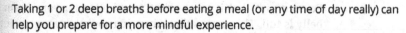

behaviors. Don't think of "me time" as selfish but as a vital way to maintain your overall health and well-being.

>> **Spend a few minutes at the beginning of each day planning out what you're going to accomplish.** You can also do this again at the end of the day or on Sunday, thinking about the week's to-do list.

>> **Focus on the positive.** Work on removing negative language from your vocabulary and thoughts. When it comes to your diet, focus on what you can eat, not what you can't.

The beauty of DASH is that you can eat plenty of food and enjoy a wide variety of fruits, vegetables, healthy fats, fiber, and low-fat dairy, as well as the occasional treat.

REMEMBER

TIP

Perhaps the most important trick to living mindfully is being grateful. Most people would say they're grateful for many things — their health, family, and home — but sometimes it's easy to ignore this gratitude or view things in a negative rather than positive way. For example, you may find yourself getting agitated as you sit in traffic when you're running late. Push those negative thoughts aside and use gratitude to change your attitude. Think: "I'm grateful I have a car, I'm grateful for the people who maintain these roads, and I'm grateful that I have somewhere to go." An attitude of gratitude wins the day!

Coping with Stress

You've probably heard somebody who's all stressed out complain that someone or something is "raising my blood pressure!" It doesn't quite work like that, but over time, stress plays a role in blood pressure and health in general.

Stress is a normal part of life, so it's important that you develop strategies to handle it. Finding ways to cope with daily stress can improve both your physical and mental health.

>> **Consider stress-reduction programs that may be offered through your workplace or health insurance plan.** You can't just wish stress away. There are techniques that you can use to gradually work at it, and a stress-management program helps you learn strategies to deal with life's stresses. Check with your local wellness center or medical center for local resources.

>> **Do a little deep breathing.** A few deep breaths work almost immediately to calm you down. The nearby sidebar walks you through how to do deep-breathing exercises.

>> **Plan some down time or a vacation.** There's nothing better than a few hours off to do something you really enjoy and forget about all the stressful things on your list. Even if you don't leave town, consider a "staycation" at home and plan some fun activities, take a morning walk, relax in the hammock with a good book, or take a nap!

The following sections take a deeper look at some of the best stress-busting strategies.

HOW TO DO DEEP BREATHING EXERCISES

Breathing is the only bodily function that is both voluntary and involuntary. It's your own yin-yang: inhale, exhale, expand, and contract. During emotional stress, the human nervous system stimulates a number of physical responses — your heart rate increases, you may perspire, your muscles tense, and your breathing becomes shallower. If you allow your body to operate this way for long periods of time, it can wreak havoc.

Take notice of how you breathe. Does your chest or abdomen expand when you take in a breath? Some people find that when they breathe in, they expand their chest and suck in their abdomen, which is inefficient. Rapid, shallow chest-breathing doesn't transfer as much oxygen to the blood. Abdominal breathing is more efficient. With a little practice, you can train yourself to breathe differently.

Abdominal breathing uses the *diaphragm* (a large muscle located between the chest and abdomen). Try this twice each day until it becomes habitual:

- Lie down in a comfortable, quiet spot. Place one hand on your chest and the other on your abdomen. Take a deep breath, focusing on raising the hand on your abdomen. The hand on your abdomen should rise higher than the hand on your chest. Practice this until you feel more comfortable with it.

- Exhale through your mouth. Try to do this for a count of 3, gradually increasing the count up to 7, or however long you can manage.

- Practice holding your breath. Breathe in deeply via your abdomen. Hold it for a count of 7 and then slowly exhale through your mouth for a count up to 7. Each time you exhale, think about breathing out all your worries.

- Repeat inhales and exhales up to 5 times, lengthening your exhale with each practice breath.

Breathing exercises are easy to do and very effective. After you're used to abdominal breathing, you won't have to think about it. You can do this anywhere, anytime — in your chair, on an airplane, waiting in line, and so on!

Exercising regularly

If you could simply walk away from your health problems, you would, right? It *can* be that easy. Virtually any type of exercise helps reduce stress. Activities such as walking, jogging, swimming, biking, dancing, yoga, weight lifting, rowing, housework, and gardening all count. In addition to stress reduction, exercise improves overall heart health, strength, and balance. Sit less and move more — it's that simple.

WARNING

Get your doctor's approval before beginning any type of exercise program. Immediately report any discomfort you experience to your doctor.

Exercise reduces stress over time in several ways:

>> Aerobic exercise has the ability to exhilarate you while also relaxing you. It also helps you sleep better, which reduces stress as well.

>> Exercise reduces the levels of the body's stress hormones (adrenaline and cortisol).

>> Exercise stimulates the production of endorphins, which elevate mood.

>> Exercise helps with weight control and builds muscle, giving you a sense of accomplishment.

REMEMBER

The better you feel, the easier it is to move about, and the less stress you'll have. Because weight control helps reduce blood pressure and lowers your risk for heart disease and diabetes, we can't overstate the important role physical activity plays in weight loss. Aerobic activity (along with calorie restriction) helps burn fat. Strength training builds muscle. The more muscle and the less fat you have, the faster and more efficient your metabolism is.

TIP

Most studies show that exercising 120 to 150 minutes weekly gives you the biggest benefit in terms of reducing your diabetes risk. You can even accomplish this in 10- or 15-minute increments. To ensure you stick to it, schedule an exercise plan into your calendar. If you have a smart watch, set it to cue you to stand up from sitting, and stick to a daily movement goal. Enlist a friend to join you to help you with compliance. Choose activities you enjoy and change up your routine from time to time to keep you interested and motivated.

Connecting the mind and body with yoga

Yoga is an ancient Hindu practice that aims to bring together the body and the mind. Yoga exercises, called poses or *asanas,* are designed to put mild pressure on the body's glandular systems. The beauty of yoga is that there's no one right way to do a pose. You just try the poses to the best of your ability and work on making improvements in flexibility, strength, and meditation. Breathing is an integral part of a yoga practice.

The best way to begin a yoga practice is to attend a class from a certified instructor. Different types of yoga exist, but hatha yoga is perhaps the most familiar. This practice combines various physical movements and postures with breathing.

Although the postures and breathing are important, yoga also encompasses a more mindful lifestyle, in which you make better choices about food, other types of exercise, and self-care. Yoga can help you with your dietary goals as you train yourself to become more mindful in all aspects of your life.

TIP

Although people often talk about multi-tasking, focusing on one thing at a time is actually healthier and more productive. Consider practicing "intentions." Each morning, think about your intention for the day. Perhaps you'll work on being more aware and focused on each little thing through the day. Start with your cup of coffee or tea. Avoid checking your smartphone or iPad while drinking your morning beverage. Just sit, breathe, and enjoy the warm beverage, and start your day with mindfulness.

To find out more about yoga, check out *Yoga For Dummies*, 3rd Edition, by Larry Payne and Georg Feuerstein (Wiley).

Meditating

Meditation has been shown to reduce anxiety, pain, and stress and help with insomnia, depression, and other emotional issues that may accompany a health diagnosis or disease (such as cancer or heart disease). As with yoga, meditation involves mindfulness. Think about what you'd like to achieve: Do you want to understand yourself better? Do you want to feel better? Do you want to learn to relax more? Do you want to learn how to enjoy "just being" instead of constantly "doing"?

You may view meditation as hocus-pocus, but we encourage you to have an open mind and give it a go. To begin trying meditation, do the following:

>> Choose a quiet, comfortable spot.

>> Don't try to meditate on an empty stomach, but you also don't want to be too full from a meal.

>> The lotus pose (cross-legged) is a good posture, but if this is uncomfortable, simply sit with your legs straight out, or sit up straight in a comfortable chair.

>> As you work on a proper posture (shoulders back, chin up slightly, back slightly arched), hold that posture, close your eyes, and begin taking mindful breaths.

>> Inhale and exhale until you've cleared all the thoughts from your mind and feel relaxed.

If you're having trouble meditating on your own, or if you just want a little guidance, check out apps like Headspace (www.headspace.com). For a low monthly fee, you can get a library of meditations for a variety of goals.

You may be wondering: How does meditation actually work? During periods of stress, the *sympathetic nervous system* mobilizes the body for action, causing blood vessels to constrict, your heart rate to increase, and your breathing to become more rapid. The *parasympathetic nervous system* does the opposite — it slows the heart rate, dilates the blood vessels, and increases the flow of digestive juices. It's thought that meditative practice helps increase the activity of the parasympathetic nervous system.

THE POWER OF POSITIVE THINKING

Positive thinking isn't about ignoring all the bad or unpleasant things life throws at you. Rather, it's about simply approaching them differently. "Self-talk" is the voice in your head — the endless stream of thoughts that go through your mind all day. You may feel constantly overwhelmed with your to-do list, for instance. Some self-talk may come from logic, but other self-talk may come from emotions or the misconceptions you create from a lack of knowledge or information.

Studies have shown that positive thinking can actually help your brain work better and reduce anxiety over time. Daily meditations can result in more positive emotions and a wide range of personal resources, such as more purpose in life, more mindfulness, and decreases in physical illness and symptoms. Because positive emotions tend to be more fleeting than negative ones (which are often more intense and attention-grabbing), finding ways to increase these positive thoughts is worth a try. In fact, some research shows that positive well-being was associated with nearly a one-third reduction in heart disease in a high-risk population that had a family history. Smile, that's pretty powerful!

Calling on Your Support System

Lifestyle changes are an everyday proposition, 365 days a year. Although you may not exercise every single day (nor do you have to), you will eat, sleep, and deal with stress daily. A support system can only help you in the long run. If you don't already have a support system in place, start building one. Turn to your friends and family first, but don't forget about your doctor, and maybe even your coworkers. All these people will help you create a positive environment of support. Your doctor in particular can be an excellent resource if you've been newly diagnosed with hypertension or heart disease and want help understanding your condition.

REMEMBER

When it comes to the medical stuff, don't be afraid to ask questions. Ask for specific advice at the doctor's office. Ask the nurse about smoking cessation, and ask the dietitian about your diet and nutrition status (if you don't have a dietitian, ask your doctor to refer you to one). Ask them to provide you with a good resource list (including this book!). Your doctor can only help you as much as you can help yourself. Listen to your body and keep track of changes, and then communicate the information to your doctor at your next visit (consider self-monitoring your blood pressure, as discussed in Chapter 6).

TIP

If you're really struggling to make the lifestyle changes you need to make for better heart health and wellness, consider speaking with a behavior therapist or psychologist.

Figuring out how family and friends can help

Family and friends can help you stay well or get well and be role models for good behaviors. They can also help you stay accountable to your goals. Consider enlisting your family members and friends to help you

>> Add more fruit to your diet by preparing breakfast in the morning together.

>> Grocery shop together or sit down once a week to create your shopping list (use the guidelines in Chapter 12).

>> Like competition? Try pairing up with a pal and counting your daily steps using a pedometer or join a social media fitness support group. Or consider purchasing a digital fitness device that connects via an app to social media and reports your progress.

>> Schedule an active family night once a week. Get out for a bike ride together on the bike path or take a hike through the woods.

>> Unplug as a family. Electronics have their benefits, but sometimes you need to step away. Encourage everyone to put all the electronic devices to sleep for one evening a week. This automatically redirects you, possibly into more mindful or interactive activities.

TIP

Choose different people to help you in different areas. For instance, go grocery shopping with your spouse and go for nightly walks with your son or daughter. Or take a friend up on her offer to help you quit smoking. The important thing is having someone else help you with your accountability.

Enlisting an exercise partner

Exercise is as important as the other dietary and lifestyle changes involved in heart health. The most important thing about exercise is consistency. Finding an exercise buddy helps improve your accountability because when people make an appointment with someone, they generally want to keep it. Exercising with a friend also makes the time pass more quickly. Before you know it, your workout is over. It can even help you push your fitness levels up by providing a little friendly competition.

When exercising with a partner, start small and make sure you're on the same page. Your workout buddy should be at about the same fitness level as you for the experience to be enjoyable for both of you. If you're just starting out with an exercise program and your exercise partner is pretty advanced, your joint-workout days will likely be numbered even before you get started.

Here are a couple ideas for working out with a friend:

>> Schedule two gym days a week to meet a friend for a workout or game of racquetball.

>> Join a tennis or golf league for companionship and a built-in schedule.

>> Look for a Masters swim group or a local cycling group that meets weekly.

>> Schedule three days a week to meet an exercise partner for some aerobic exercise, such as walking, jogging, weight lifting, yoga, cycling, or swimming.

>> Consider splitting the cost of a personal trainer with a friend.

Sticking to the DASH Plan

Making lifestyle changes isn't easy, even when you're adopting a way of life that's as flexible and easy to follow as DASH. Allow yourself the time necessary to see results and make your new, healthier behaviors feel like old habits. Setting realistic goals, tracking your progress toward those goals, and knowing how to handle setbacks and slip-ups helps you in your journey toward a truly DASHing lifestyle.

Building strategies toward lasting success

To fully adopt a new lifestyle or make a change, you need to continually develop small strategies to maintain the change, and be happy with it. Realistic goal-setting is so critical to making successful lifestyle changes — such as adopting the DASH way of life — that even though we walk you through how to set SMART goals in Chapter 4, we had to touch on goal-setting again here. You should have long-term goals, but you should also keep short-term ones in the front of your mind. For instance, if you eat out for dinner four times a week, you know you'd have more control over sodium and be able to add more veggies if you swapped out two of those nights for eating at home. You have to create a goal and have a strategy for making this happen. Because life is ever-changing, new strategies are required to maintain your long-term goals.

Be patient. Your goals should always be realistic, but they should also challenge you a little. For example, if you have trouble drinking enough water daily, why not tell yourself that tomorrow morning you're going to fill a large water bottle in the morning, keep track of how much water you drink, and really work on it?

REMEMBER

Don't focus on only one set of goals. If weight loss is one of your goals, consider other health parameters too — lowering cholesterol, improving blood pressure readings, reducing medications. These are all very important and may occur even when you fall short of your weight-loss goal. Also, don't try to accomplish all your goals at once. Choose one to three behaviors to work on every week. After they become habitual, move on to the next set.

TIP

Track your weight loss monthly, not daily. Don't overuse the scale. Getting on the scale every day can be very discouraging. Stick with your meal plan and exercise schedule, and the weight will drop.

Keeping track of where you're at with a journal or app

Research has shown that writing down what you eat helps you eat less and makes you more aware of your hunger patterns and eating habits. So it's definitely worth a try, especially if you've hit a rut.

Lots of diet and fitness apps exist that can help you stay on track (some examples include Lose It!, MyFitnessPal, and Noom). Many of them allow you to enter your food or calorie intake and then do the math for you, letting you know how many calories you have left that day. Or you can go the old-school route and use a paper tracker. Because the goals of DASH are so specific, you may want to consider writing up a custom food record for yourself.

TIP

When you're tracking, focus on all your results. If you want to lose weight and the pounds are coming off very slowly but your blood pressure is better, then focus on the positive. Accept the slow weight loss in exchange for better blood pressure and perhaps lower cholesterol levels. Also be aware that accomplishing goals such as increasing your fruit and vegetable intake or decreasing processed foods is a success in itself that, over time, will yield positive health outcomes.

An added bonus of tracking is that you can reward yourself after you've accomplished a few goals and stuck to them for a few weeks. Go to the movies or buy yourself a new outfit or new set of workout clothes.

Dealing with falling off the wagon

Despite what some appearances may suggest, nobody can eat and exercise perfectly 365 days of the year. Sometimes you may fall off the health wagon. In those cases, the best strategy is to get back on track as soon as possible.

REMEMBER

The key to dealing with setbacks in making lifestyle changes is not to give up on the whole day if you make one mistake. If you splurge on a meal or miss a workout, don't decide that the day's a wash and that you'll start over tomorrow. Instead, plan to make more DASH-friendly choices at the very next meal or snack. Plan and portion out snacks. It's not that you can't snack — it's the amount that matters. Portion out 6 olives, a quarter cup of nuts, and so on. Work on ways to move more, too. Plan to take the stairs the rest of the day rather than the elevator. Also, take a moment to think about what situation may have triggered your setback or overindulgence. Simply recognize it and consider how you can eliminate the trigger, if possible; then let it go and move forward. The DASH diet isn't about becoming a supermodel; it's about improving your overall health. So keep your body's health in the front of your mind as you make choices.

TIP

If you mindlessly just ate nearly an entire jar of dry-roasted peanuts, put them away and take a walk to clear your head. Sometimes overeating is a cue that something's bothering you. Some fresh air or exercise can do you good and empower you to get back on track for the rest of your day.

Look at slip-ups as an opportunity to learn from your mistakes. If you went to a party too hungry and couldn't control overeating, think about how to deal with the situation in the future. Also, remember that life isn't stagnant. Things change. What works for you today in terms of meal planning and exercise may not be a good fit at all one year from now, one month from now, or even one week from now. Take the time to realize this and either create a new plan or get some support from a registered dietitian nutritionist to help get you on a new track.

WARNING

A special note on vacations: Considering a vacation a free pass can sabotage you. If you take two or more weeks of vacation a year, it's important to learn how to continue managing your eating and activity during that time. You don't want to lose all your gains. This doesn't mean you can't have any fun! You should enjoy vacation time, but if it involves too much overeating or alcohol overindulgence, you'll end up feeling not-so-rested. Enjoy special foods on vacation but in small portions (share an appetizer or entree or split desserts). Look for ways to add activity. Walk wherever you can, rent a bike to tour the area, go golfing, or find a beach yoga class. Fit some movement in every day.

4

Smashing DASH Recipes

Find out how to incorporate multiple food groups in your morning meal to help keep your appetite level low and your energy level high.

Serve up salads, sandwiches, and soups to satisfy midday hunger pangs. (With a little strategizing and prepping ahead of time, you can even take these meals to work — a surefire way to say "no" to the drive-through.)

Incorporate lean protein from beef, chicken, fish, lamb, pork, and shellfish into your entrees using proper portions. A 3-ounce serving is all you need to get the health benefits without excess calories or fat.

Get adventurous with new ways to make vegetables dishes crave-worthy while upping your fiber intake with creative grain dishes.

Pair vegetables and whole grains to create tasty and satisfying meatless main dish options. It's all about changing your expectations of how vegetables "have" to be prepared and experimenting with delicious new combinations and techniques.

Whip up DASH-approved meals with minimal kitchen mess by embracing one-dish meals. Your dishwasher will thank you!

Discover how you can include dessert in your meal plan while also creating treats that incorporate part of your fruit servings into your day.

IN THIS CHAPTER

» Discovering how to include more food groups in your morning meal

» Making a variety of easy and healthy breakfast recipes

Chapter 17

Delicious Breakfasts and Brunches

R ise and shine! Rise and dine! What a perfect way to start the day divine. Breakfast can boost metabolism and wake up the brain for better mental acuity and cognitive function. It's also the perfect time to boost your diet with the fiber, calcium, and delicious, incredible protein found in eggs. Simplicity and freshness are key.

Then there's brunch — the new happy hour — a fun way to reconnect with family and friends on a lazy weekend morning. Brunch is a flexible meal that can top off a round of golf or celebrate a festive occasion such as Easter or Mother's Day. Brunch can be a hybrid of breakfast and lunch dishes, with an exciting balance of savory and sweet, rich and low-calorie options.

Unscrambling Breakfast, the Most Important Meal of the Day

Breakfast is an opportunity to break your fast after a good night's rest. You may eat less breakfast some days than others, and that's okay because you can make up the difference at lunch or dinner. The goal is to make improvements — not try to be perfect.

TIP

If you're adding breakfast for the first time when you normally omit that meal, start small, go easy on yourself, and choose meal ideas that are realistic and enjoyable. Have a simple hard-cooked egg with a piece of fruit or a slice of good, grainy bread spread with nut butter.

There are no hard and fast rules about what specific foods to include at breakfast or brunch. As with any healthy eating plan, it's important to focus on choosing a variety of different foods and spacing your meals throughout the day.

Getting Creative with the Food Groups

Breads, cereal, and fruit typically come to mind when people think of breakfast, but don't let those common options limit you in your breakfast choices. Why not incorporate more food groups into your morning? Combining foods from the major food groups helps you build a better meal, whether it's usual breakfast food or not. A multi-food-group breakfast should

>> Include protein, whole grains, and some fat to satisfy hunger and taste.

>> Help you maintain proper blood sugar levels, keeping appetite low and energy levels high.

>> Incorporate a variety of foods to maximize the most nutrients.

Try some new recipes (like the ones in this chapter!) and round out your meal with a serving of low-fat milk or yogurt, hearty whole-grain bread, or an additional fruit or vegetable. You can even add in a vegetable for a real nutritional bonus that doesn't add many calories. Mix and match selections from the different food groups and remember to limit the amount of extra sugar and fat in all your meals.

TIP

Here are some tasty combos you can make using some of the recipes in this chapter:

>> Crave-Worthy Toast and ½ cup of fruit salad with a dollop of low-fat lemon-flavored Greek yogurt

>> A serving of Easy Shakshuka with a slice of hearty whole-grain naan bread

>> A cup of low-fat vanilla-flavored Greek yogurt topped with blueberries and 2 tablespoons of granola with nuts

Easy Shakshuka

PREP TIME: 10 MIN | COOK TIME: 40 MIN | YIELD: 4 SERVINGS

INGREDIENTS

1 tablespoon extra-virgin olive oil

½ small sweet onion, chopped

1 small red bell pepper, seeded and diced

2 large garlic cloves, minced

½ teaspoon smoked paprika

¼ to ½ teaspoon cumin

One 28-ounce jar low-sodium marinara sauce

1 cup fresh baby spinach, chopped

8 large eggs

1 small avocado, sliced

¼ cup crumbled reduced-fat feta cheese

Fresh parsley, chopped, for garnish

2 pieces naan bread, toasted and cut into 8 pieces

DIRECTIONS

1 In a 10-inch deep skillet, heat the oil over medium-high heat. Add the onion, red bell pepper, and garlic; sauté until the onion is translucent, about 5 to 6 minutes.

2 Add the paprika and cumin and cook for 1 minute. Add the marinara sauce and simmer on low heat for 20 to 22 minutes, until the sauce has thickened and the flavors have blended. Add the spinach and stir until wilted.

3 Using a spoon, make four wells in the sauce. Crack each egg and gently lay the eggs on top of the tomato mixture in the wells. Cover and continuing cooking 6 to 8 minutes, or until the whites are set and the yolks are done to your desired consistency.

4 Scoop each egg from the pan, bringing the sauce with it, and transfer to a dish. Sprinkle with feta and garnish with parsley. Serve with a few slices of avocado and the toasted naan.

PER SERVING: *Calories 454 (From Fat 206); Fat 23g (Saturated 6g); Cholesterol 21mg; Sodium 604mg; Carbohydrate 45g (Dietary Fiber 6g); Protein 18g.*

TIP: For a lower-sodium sauce, cut 6 to 8 fresh, ripe, whole tomatoes and 1 red bell pepper, into chunks instead of using store-bought sauce or canned tomatoes. Follow the recipe through step 2. Instead of adding the sauce, add the tomatoes and bell pepper and simmer and stir until they're softened. It takes a little longer to make the sauce using the fresh vegetables, but it's worth it!

NOTE: Naan bread can be found in most grocery stores. Place in the toaster to warm the bread. You can also use whole-wheat pita bread or crusty white bread instead of naan.

VARY IT! If you prefer a spicy option, add minced jalapeño peppers and a dash or two of cayenne pepper when cooking the sauce. Instead of feta cheese, try Cotija. For garnish, use cilantro instead of parsley.

NOTE: This dish is finally making a name for itself as a healthy breakfast, brunch, or even dinner option, but has been around in Mediterranean cultures for centuries.

Open-Faced Egg Sandwich

PREP TIME: 10 MIN | YIELD: 4 SERVINGS

INGREDIENTS

4 tablespoons plain Greek yogurt

1 teaspoon spicy mustard

1 teaspoon non-pareil capers

4 whole-wheat English muffins, split in half

1 cup fresh baby spinach

8 tomato slices

4 hard-cooked eggs, sliced

½ teaspoon oregano

Freshly ground black pepper

DIRECTIONS

1 In a small bowl, combine the yogurt, mustard, and capers.

2 Toast the English-muffin halves and place them on a serving plate. Spread each half with the yogurt-mustard mixture, a small amount of spinach, a tomato slice, and hard-cooked egg slices (½ egg each).

3 Sprinkle each sandwich with oregano and pepper before serving.

PER SERVING: *Calories 247 (From Fat 63); Fat 7g (Saturated 2g); Cholesterol 187mg; Sodium 380mg; Carbohydrate 32g (Dietary Fiber 7g); Protein 14g.*

NOTE: Eggs are popular with our authors. Rosanne even has eggs in the backyard gathered fresh every day. One egg white provides only 16 of the 70 calories in a whole egg and about half the protein, 3 of the 6 grams. The egg yolk provides the other 54 calories, 3 grams of protein, and all the cholesterol (about 185 milligrams). You can use two whites for every one whole egg listed in a recipe to lower the cholesterol content. Eggs are an egg-ceptional source of protein for a meal or snack any time of day!

TIP: Purchase already hard-cooked, peeled eggs in your grocer's dairy aisle for a versatile, nutritious option that has a long shelf life. Also consider prepping your ingredients the night before and storing them in small plastic containers for easy assembly in the morning when you're in a time crunch.

VARY IT! Chop the eggs and combine with the yogurt-mustard mixture; scoop equal amounts on each English muffin; top with spinach, tomato, and grated part-skim mozzarella cheese; and broil until the cheese melts — about 4 minutes.

Breakfast Smoothie Bowl

PREP TIME: 5 MIN	YIELD: 1 SERVING

INGREDIENTS

1 cup frozen mixed berries

1 banana, frozen

1½ tablespoons almond butter or preferred nut butter

½ cup packed baby spinach

1 tablespoon granola (optional)

1 tablespoon unsweetened flaked coconut (optional)

1 tablespoon fresh blueberries (optional)

1 tablespoon fresh strawberries (optional)

1 sliced kiwi (optional)

1 teaspoon chia seeds (optional)

1 tablespoon pomegranate arils (optional)

2 teaspoons pumpkin seeds (optional)

DIRECTIONS

1 In a high-tech blender (such as a Vitamix), place the berries, banana, nut butter, and spinach. Process until the mixture is thick and creamy, scraping down the sides as needed.

2 Scoop into a bowl and garnish with 4 or 5 different toppings of your choice.

PER SERVING: Calories 232 (From Fat 49); Fat 5g (Saturated 1g); Cholesterol 0mg; Sodium 53mg; Carbohydrate 48g (Dietary Fiber 8g); Protein 4g.

TIP: This recipe tastes best fresh, but you can double it or make it ahead of time if you like. Leftovers can be frozen for a week. Thaw before serving by bringing to room temperature for 15 minutes or microwave for 20 to 30 seconds.

TIP: A conventional blender can do the job but the results won't be as smooth and spoon-thick! If you love smoothies and smoothie bowls, look for a blender that has a powerful and long-lasting reliable motor.

NOTE: You can assemble make-ahead smoothie bags for the freezer, adding 1 cup of fruit to each bag. You can also freeze your favorite Greek yogurt in ice cube trays and add a few cubes to each bag for added calcium and protein. When ready to serve, blend the fruit with the Greek yogurt.

VARY IT! Get creative — the variations are endless! Some flavorful combinations are kiwi, apple, banana, and spinach; blackberry, raspberry, strawberry, and beets; and mango, pineapple, banana, and kale. Making the fruit bags ahead of time is one less thing to think about on hectic mornings!

Banana Nut Hot Oatmeal

PREP TIME: 5 MIN	COOK TIME: 5 MIN	YIELD: 2 SERVINGS

INGREDIENTS

1 cup skim milk

1 cup old-fashioned rolled oats

1 tablespoon chia seeds or ground flaxseeds

1 small ripe banana, mashed

¼ cup honey-flavored Greek yogurt

½ banana, sliced

2 tablespoons chopped pecans, toasted

2 teaspoons honey

DIRECTIONS

1 In a small saucepan, bring the milk to boil over medium–high heat.

2 Stir in the oats and seeds and cook over medium heat, while stirring, approximately 5 minutes. Remove from the heat and stir in the banana and yogurt.

3 Divide the oatmeal between 2 bowls. Top with banana, pecans, and honey.

PER SERVING: *Calories 342 (From Fat 61); Fat 7g (Saturated 1g); Cholesterol 2mg; Sodium 67mg; Carbohydrate 60g (Dietary Fiber 7g); Protein 14g.*

NOTE: If you don't have old-fashioned rolled oats, you can use plain instant oatmeal instead. It provides the same nutritional benefits; it just has less protein. Many instant oatmeal packets are high in sugar, so be sure to choose the plain version.

VARY IT! Add your favorite fruit to your cereal to up the sweetness, fiber, and potassium without added sugar. Add your favorite nuts to increase the protein and fiber. Vary your toppings based on the seasons — apples in fall, citrus in winter, berries in spring, and peaches in summer!

Crave-Worthy Toast

PREP TIME: 5 MIN	YIELD: 2 SERVINGS

INGREDIENTS

1 small ripe avocado, washed, cut in half, and pitted

Squeeze of fresh lime

1 green onion, chopped

Chopped cilantro to taste

2 thickly sliced pumpernickel bread slices, well toasted

1 ounce thinly sliced smoked salmon

1 tablespoon crème fraîche

2 sprigs dill

DIRECTIONS

1 Scoop the avocado out of the skin, place it in a bowl, and mash it to your desired texture. Add the lime juice, green onion, and cilantro, and mix together.

2 Divide the mixture between the two pieces of toast. Top each piece of toast with salmon, a dollop of crème fraîche, and dill.

PER SERVING: *Calories 234 (From Fat 131); Fat 15g (Saturated 4g); Cholesterol12 mg; Sodium 342mg; Carbohydrate 21g (Dietary Fiber 7g); Protein 7g.*

NOTE: Avocados are nature's butter! Choose an avocado that yields a bit to a gentle squeeze. Avocados are a wonderful source of monounsaturated fat, but be aware: Like other fats, they're high in calories.

VARY IT! Move over avocado toast, there are more toppings to love! Just use your creativity and choose good-quality ingredients like delicious and rustic whole-grain bread from the bakery — well-toasted, thick, sturdy bread is a wonderful foundation for the delicious and creamy toppings. Try heirloom tomatoes, Burrata cheese, and fresh basil; mashed avocado and diced mangoes with a drizzle of lime juice; ricotta, fresh berries, mint, and a drizzle of honey; goat cheese, strawberries, and basil leaves; or a drizzle of balsamic glaze, tahini, fresh or dried figs, and drizzle of maple syrup. Get the whole family involved and make a competition out of it!

Confetti Hash with Poached Eggs

PREP TIME: 15 MIN	COOK TIME: 20 MIN	YIELD: 6 SERVINGS

INGREDIENTS

2 tablespoons extra-virgin olive oil

1 tablespoon unsalted butter

1 medium shallot, chopped

½ teaspoon ground nutmeg

1 pound Brussels sprouts, shredded or thinly sliced

Freshly ground pepper to taste

5 cups shredded hash browns, refrigerated or frozen

¼ cup chopped pecans, toasted

¼ cup dried cranberries

6 large eggs

DIRECTIONS

1 Heat the oil and butter in a large skillet. Add the shallot, nutmeg, and Brussels sprouts. Add some ground black pepper to taste. Cook 2 minutes, or until the Brussels sprouts are bright green. Add the hash browns and cook undisturbed (to allow browning) for about 3 to 4 minutes. Stir the hash browns, turn them, and cook 3 to 4 minutes longer, or until the potatoes are tender, golden-brown, and crispy.

2 Add the pecans and cranberries. Divide the hash among four plates and keep warm.

3 Bring 2 inches of water to a boil in a large saucepan or skillet (a 12-inch skillet works well). Reduce to a simmer. Break an egg into a small bowl and gently slide the egg into the water. Repeat with the remaining 5 eggs. Cook for 5 minutes for a medium-set egg. Gently remove the eggs with a slotted spoon and serve over the confetti hash (cook in two batches of 3 eggs at a time, if using a smaller skillet).

PER SERVING: *Calories 328 (From Fat 135); Fat 15g (Saturated 4g); Cholesterol 191mg; Sodium 182mg; Carbohydrate 39g (Dietary Fiber 5g); Protein 11g.*

NOTE: Cook the eggs in two batches of 3 if you're using a smaller skillet.

TIP: Shredded potatoes can be found in your grocer's dairy aisle. You can also use frozen shredded potatoes and cook them according to the package directions.

VARY IT! You can easily turn this dish into a skillet meal: After the potatoes, shallot, and Brussels sprouts are cooked, beat together the eggs. Next, add the eggs to the skillet and cook until the eggs are set, stirring frequently.

Chapter **18**

Quick and Healthy Lunches

M aking time for a midday meal refuels and reenergizes you so you can be more productive. Lunch can also fuel your motivation to work to the end of the day. Not only that, but skipping — or skimping on — lunch may cause you to snack poorly in the afternoon or overeat at dinner, making nutritionally unbalanced food choices.

Lunch should make up one-third of your nutrient requirements for the day. Fortunately, surviving the lunch crunch can be as easy as heating up some leftovers or nibbling on simple, delicious ingredients from the fridge. Or you can whip up out-of-the-box sandwiches, sassy salads, and savory soups by following the recipes in this chapter. They're a cinch to make and comforting too.

Preparing the Big Three: Sandwiches, Salads, and Soups

Whether you're home during the day or at the office, have a plan in place for lunchtime. Menu planning for lunch is an important strategy to improve overall health and establish good eating habits. Make every meal count! With some planning, you can choose foods and recipes that align with the goals of DASH, utilize leftovers, and also save time and money. Sandwiches, salads, and soups are also easy to prepare ahead of time and use for lunch the next day.

» You can make sandwiches open-faced to limit calories from the extra serving of bread, such as our Open-Faced Roast Beef Sandwich with Horseradish Sauce (see the first recipe in this chapter). Always take opportunities to add more vegetables such as sliced tomatoes, roasted red bell peppers, spinach, chile peppers, sliced cucumbers, and green bell peppers in place of cheese or a large portion of animal protein. Key ingredients can add a great deal of flavor and make lunchtime exciting and healthy. Mashed avocado in place of mayo-type spreads adds monounsaturated fat in place of unhealthy saturated fat. Pesto — traditionally made from olive oil, basil, garlic, and pine nuts (you can also use omega-3-rich walnuts in place of pine nuts) — is high in calories, but a little goes a long way with flavor. Adding a teaspoon of prepared horseradish, a dash of wasabi powder, or any number of hot sauces to light mayo can add a pop of flavor.

» Salads can be a quick and easy lunchtime meal incorporating leftovers and seasonal ingredients that are full of exceptional flavor. Put lots of colorful vegetables into your salad to meet your four to five servings per day. Try some new creative combinations. Start with a foundation of various types of greens or use quinoa or farro. Add plenty of veggies for crunch, flavor, and disease-fighting nutrients. Tofu, beans, cottage cheese, tuna, or grilled salmon can be a delicious added protein for a main dish. For a bit of extra flavor, add sunflower seeds, sun-dried tomatoes, or even fresh ginger. A few olives and capers add a punch of salty flavor and only provide a small amount of sodium (they also provide healthy fats!). A splash of extra-virgin olive oil and a flavored vinegar such as fig, champagne, or chipotle balsamic piques your taste buds.

>> Soups are a meal in a bowl and are nutritionally complete with vitamins, minerals, and fiber. Whether you make them from scratch or use leftovers such as roasted chicken, soups and stews are sure to be a winner. They can be broth-based and light or thickened with pureed vegetables to provide some depth, such as our Velvety Vegetable Soup with Tarragon Cream (see the recipe in this chapter). Some studies show that eating soup (and salad) can give you the feeling of fullness and help provide the willpower to resist heavy entrees.

TIP

If lunch gets too repetitive, you won't be inspired to eat it. The result: wasted time and wasted food, which fuels the desire to buy the quick lunch you may regret. So don't let yourself get into a rut.

WARNING

When planning to eat out for lunch, prevent temptations by preplanning what you may order before walking into a restaurant. Be sure to review the nutritional information. The huge, sodium-heavy, and saturated-fat-laden portions at many fast food establishments won't do much good for your blood pressure, nor your waistline. Balance a fast food meal with a nutritious breakfast and dinner that includes less fat calories and more vegetables, fruit, and lower-fat dairy. If you must buy from vending machines and gas stations, choose a hard-boiled egg, cheese sticks, a snack-size veggie pouch, a turkey sandwich, whole fruit, or a fruit cup. By making even a minimal effort to plan and prep your lunches, you'll have a great meal to look forward to that's delicious *and* nutritious.

Open-Faced Roast Beef Sandwich with Horseradish Sauce

| PREP TIME: 10 MIN | YIELD: 4 SERVINGS |

INGREDIENTS

2 ounces Neufchâtel cream cheese, softened

¼ cup plain Greek yogurt

1 tablespoon Dijon mustard

1 tablespoon prepared horseradish

¼ teaspoon garlic powder

Freshly ground pepper to taste

12 ounces low-sodium deli roast beef, thinly sliced and divided into 4 equal portions

2 crusty ciabatta rolls or crusty whole-wheat rolls, cut in half

½ tablespoon extra-virgin olive oil

1 tablespoon white-wine vinegar

2 cups mixed baby greens

DIRECTIONS

1 To make the sauce, combine the softened cream cheese, yogurt, mustard, horseradish, garlic powder, and pepper to taste in a small bowl. Mix until well blended.

2 Place the roast beef on top of each of the four roll halves. Spoon the sauce on top of the roast beef.

3 Just before serving, combine the olive oil and vinegar and toss with the mixed greens. Place the mixed greens on top of the sauce and serve.

PER SERVING: *Calories 251 (From Fat 90); Fat 10g (Saturated 5g); Cholesterol 63mg; Sodium 396mg; Carbohydrate 13g (Dietary Fiber 1g); Protein 26g.*

NOTE: Low-sodium, oven-roasted roast beef is a nice change from turkey or ham. If you purchase higher-end brands, the sodium content is lower because the companies use quality ingredients, making it unnecessary to overuse salt as a flavor enhancer.

TIP: If you have leftover whole-grain baguettes, slice them into ½-inch-thick pieces, brush both sides with olive oil, and bake them in a preheated oven for 10 minutes. This is a great way to utilize bread when it's slightly stale instead of buying special rolls.

VARY IT! Use a commercially prepared horseradish sauce, which may be slightly higher in sodium, or replace the tablespoon of horseradish sauce with a tablespoon of spicy brown mustard. You can also use less horseradish, as little as ½ tablespoon, if you prefer less spice.

Chicken Wrap with Spicy Peanut Sauce

PREP TIME: 15 MIN	YIELD: 4 SERVINGS

INGREDIENTS

2 cups cooked chicken breasts, chopped

¼ cucumber, peeled, seeded, and thinly sliced (see Figure 18-1)

¼ cup shredded carrots

2 green onions, diagonally sliced

¼ cup shredded Chinese cabbage

1 teaspoon toasted sesame seeds

2 tablespoons chopped fresh cilantro leaves

4 multi-grain flatbreads with flax

⅓ cup store-bought spicy peanut sauce (optional)

DIRECTIONS

1 In a medium bowl, toss together all the ingredients except the flatbread and optional sauce until well blended.

2 Divide the mixture among the four flatbreads and tightly roll up the wraps.

3 Serve with spicy peanut sauce, if desired.

PER SERVING: *Calories 228 (From Fat 45); Fat 5g (Saturated 1g); Cholesterol 60mg; Sodium 368mg; Carbohydrate 19g (Dietary Fiber 9g); Protein 31g.*

TIP: If you prefer to make your own spicy peanut sauce, soften 2 tablespoons low-sodium peanut butter in the microwave and stir in 2 tablespoons low-sodium soy sauce, 2 tablespoons low-sodium chicken stock, 1 tablespoon brown sugar, ⅛ teaspoon ground ginger, 1 minced garlic clove, and ⅛ to ¼ teaspoon cayenne pepper and mix well.

VARY IT! In place of the spicy peanut sauce, combine ½ cup Greek yogurt, 2 tablespoons light mayonnaise, and 2 tablespoons Dijon mustard for the dressing. Mix together your favorite pantry ingredients with the chopped chicken, such as toasted walnuts, dried cranberries, a dash of dried tarragon, diced celery, and rinsed and chopped water chestnuts.

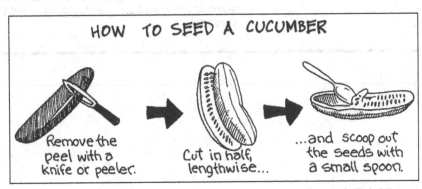

FIGURE 18-1: How to seed a cucumber.

HOW TO SEED A CUCUMBER

Remove the peel with a knife or peeler.

Cut in half, lengthwise...

...and scoop out the seeds with a small spoon.

Illustration by Elizabeth Kurtzman

Confetti Quesadillas

PREP TIME: 10 MIN	COOK TIME: 10 MIN	YIELD: 8 SERVINGS

INGREDIENTS

Eight 8-inch corn tortillas or fat-free flour tortillas

1 cup shredded Mexi-blend cheese

1 cup frozen corn, thawed

½ cup minced red bell pepper

½ cup minced green bell pepper

½ cup fresh salsa

DIRECTIONS

1 Heat a griddle on medium heat. Spritz nonstick cooking spray lightly over a tortilla. Place the tortilla sprayed side down in the hot skillet.

2 Top the tortilla with ⅛ of the cheese, corn, and peppers and heat for 30 seconds. Fold over the tortilla, gently press it down with a spatula, and continue to heat until golden-brown. Flip over and heat the other side until it's golden and the cheese is melted.

3 Repeat the process with the remaining tortillas.

4 Cut each folded tortilla into four equal pieces and serve with your favorite salsa.

PER SERVING: *Calories 203 (From Fat 54); Fat 6g (Saturated 3g); Cholesterol 15mg; Sodium 158mg; Carbohydrate 31g (Dietary Fiber 3g); Protein 6g; Potassium 93mg.*

NOTE: Quesadillas are the new grilled cheese sandwich. Using a griddle instead of a skillet to cook the quesadillas allows you to make four at the same time.

TIP: Quesadillas are the perfect way to use up leftovers — veggies, meat, seafood, and even fruit — and nothing is better than grilled apple and cheddar.

Lemon Pepper Tuna and White Bean Salad

PREP TIME: 10 MIN | **YIELD: 2 SERVINGS**

INGREDIENTS

1½ teaspoons lemon juice

1 tablespoon extra-virgin olive oil

1 small garlic clove, minced

1 cup low-sodium cannellini beans, rinsed and drained

¼ cup chopped red bell pepper

2 tablespoons minced red onion

One 2.6-ounce lemon-pepper-flavored tuna pouch

Freshly ground pepper to taste

2 cups arugula

DIRECTIONS

1 In a small bowl, combine the lemon juice, olive oil, and garlic; set aside.

2 In a medium bowl, combine the beans, red bell pepper, onion, and tuna.

3 Add the dressing to the bowl with the tuna, and gently stir until the ingredients are combined.

4 Divide the arugula between 2 plates. Spoon the salad on top of the arugula.

PER SERVING: *Calories 229 (From Fat 65); Fat 7g (Saturated 1g); Cholesterol 17mg; Sodium 267mg; Carbohydrate 25g (Dietary Fiber 9g); Protein 17g.*

TIP: Mash any leftover beans and spoon on top of your fancy toast in the morning; toss the beans in a salad at lunch; or blend the bean in a food processor with olive oil and make a hummus-type dip.

TIP: Rinsing canned beans can reduce the sodium by up to 40 percent!

NOTE: Light tuna is the best choice for omega-3 fatty acids. Incorporating more than 2 servings of fatty fish per week may reduce the risk of coronary heart disease. Canned tuna packed in oil is flavorful, and you can use the oil as part of the dressing!

VARY IT! If you prefer, you can substitute leftover cooked or canned salmon for the tuna or change up the type of beans, such as Great Northern. The tuna pouches also come in a variety of flavors such as sweet 'n' spicy, hickory smoked, and more. Mix in a smidge of mayonnaise, Greek yogurt, or avocado, and spread on a whole-grain tortilla for a roll-up!

Fruit and Nut Chicken Salad Lettuce Wraps

PREP TIME: 20 MIN	YIELD: 8 SERVINGS

INGREDIENTS

¼ cup plain Greek yogurt

¼ cup mayonnaise

1 tablespoon lemon juice

1 teaspoon sugar

Freshly ground pepper to taste

2 stalks celery, chopped

1 medium crisp red apple, chopped

1 cup seedless red grapes, cut in half

2 cups shredded chicken from a purchased rotisserie chicken

¾ cup toasted walnuts, roughly chopped

2 heads butter lettuce, washed and leaves separated

DIRECTIONS

1 In a medium bowl, whisk together the yogurt, mayonnaise, lemon juice, sugar, and pepper.

2 Stir in the celery, apple, grapes, chicken, and walnuts.

3 Spoon the salad mixture into the lettuce leaves and serve.

PER SERVING: *Calories 183 (From Fat 90); Fat 10g (Saturated 1g); Cholesterol 32mg; Sodium 93mg; Carbohydrate 10g (Dietary Fiber 2g); Protein 14g.*

TIP: Store-bought rotisserie chickens are a timesaver! Tear it apart, discarding the skin and bones and shred the meat with your fingers. Any leftovers can be reserved for a midday snack or frozen for future use. If you're following a very low-sodium restriction, you can poach chicken breasts by covering them with water and adding a bay leaf, smashed garlic clove, or any herb. Bring to boil and simmer until the chicken is cooked through, 10 to 14 minutes. The low temperature prevents the chicken from becoming tough. To be sure they're cooked, use an instant-read thermometer and make sure the internal temperature is at least 165 degrees.

TIP: You can purchase already toasted walnuts or toast them yourself in the oven. Preheat the oven to 350 degrees. Place the nut halves in a single layer on a baking sheet and bake about 5 minutes or until golden brown. Stir during toasting for even browning. They continue to brown after removing from the oven. Cool for a few minutes and then chop to the desired consistency.

VARY IT! Substitute your favorite apple, grapes, or nuts! Can't find butter lettuce? Try romaine gems or serve over a bed of shredded lettuce. You can also use leftover pork tenderloin from a previous dinner if you don't have chicken on hand.

Grilled Shrimp Salad with Creamy Mango-Lime Dressing

PREP TIME: 20–30 MIN | COOK TIME: 16–18 MIN | YIELD: 4 SERVINGS

INGREDIENTS

2 large, fresh, ripe mangoes, peeled and cut into cubes

Juice of 1 small lime or 2 tablespoons lime juice

½ cup light mayonnaise

1 tablespoon extra-virgin olive oil

½ teaspoon crushed garlic

1 teaspoon sugar

1 tablespoon orange juice to thin (optional)

1 pound large shrimp, peeled and deveined

2 tablespoons zesty Italian dressing

⅓ cup pine nuts, toasted

1½ cups sliced asparagus, blanched

8 cups torn or cut mixed salad greens

2 celery ribs, sliced

¼ small red onion, thinly sliced

1 to 2 tablespoons chopped fresh cilantro

DIRECTIONS

1 To make the salad dressing, place ¼ cup of the mango cubes, lime juice, mayonnaise, olive oil, garlic, and sugar in a mini food processor. Add the orange juice, if desired, to thin the dressing. Blend well and set aside.

2 Place shrimp in a shallow container. Add the Italian dressing to coat the shrimp evenly. Cover and marinate on the counter for 10 minutes.

3 Roast the pine nuts in a dry skillet over medium-low heat. Watch closely; they brown quickly. Shake the skillet for even browning. When the pine nuts are golden in color, remove them from the heat.

4 Blanch the asparagus in boiling water for 2 minutes, drain, and refresh in cold water. Drain again and set aside.

5 Divide the mixed salad greens among four dinner plates and top with the asparagus, remaining cubed mango, celery, red onion, and pine nuts.

6 Spray a grill with nonstick cooking spray and heat it to medium. Remove the shrimp from the marinade and place it over direct heat, cooking for 1 to 2 minutes on one side and 30 seconds to 1 minute on the other side. The shrimp is done when the inside is opaque.

7 Arrange the grilled shrimp on top of the mixed greens and sprinkle with cilantro to garnish. Drizzle the mango-lime dressing over the salad and serve.

PER SERVING: Calories 458 (From Fat 234); Fat 26g (Saturated 3g); Cholesterol 182mg; Sodium 593mg; Carbohydrate 33g (Dietary Fiber 6g); Protein 27g; Potassium 572mg.

Shrimp Avocado Ceviche

PREP TIME: 1 HR 15 MIN YIELD: 4 SERVINGS

INGREDIENTS

¾ pound small cooked salad shrimp, tails removed

Juice of 1 small lemon

Juice of 1 small lime

Juice of 1 small orange

1 cup peeled cucumber, ¼-inch dice

½ cup red onion, minced

1 small jalapeño pepper, seeded and minced

1 small tomato, diced

1 small avocado, peeled and chopped

1 tablespoon chopped cilantro

Butter lettuce leaves (optional)

Whole-wheat tortilla or pita chips (optional)

DIRECTIONS

1 In a glass bowl, combine the shrimp, lemon juice, lime juice, and orange juice. Stir in the cucumber, onion, and jalapeño. Refrigerate at least 1 hour to allow the flavors to blend.

2 Add the tomato, avocado, and cilantro to the shrimp mixture and combine. Garnish with cilantro sprigs, and serve in lettuce leaves or with whole-wheat tortilla or pita chips.

PER SERVING: *Calories 174 (From Fat 59); Fat 7g (Saturated 1g); Cholesterol 129mg; Sodium 133mg; Carbohydrate 11g (Dietary Fiber 3g); Protein 19g.*

TIP: If you can't find salad shrimp, buy medium-size shrimp and chop to the desired size.

NOTE: Traditionally ceviche uses citrus to "cook" raw seafood. In this recipe the citrus is used to flavor the seafood that's already cooked.

VARY IT! Adjust the amount of jalapeños to your spice tolerance. If you have leftover cooked fish, such as mahi-mahi or halibut, you can toss it together with the shrimp for a delightful variation. Fresh chopped mango is delicious with halibut and mahi-mahi, too!

Velvety Vegetable Soup with Tarragon Cream

PREP TIME: 15 MIN	COOK TIME: 60 MIN	YIELD: 7 SERVINGS

INGREDIENTS

1 yellow onion, peeled and chopped

4 celery ribs, chopped

4 medium carrots, chopped

2 medium leeks, chopped

1 rutabaga, peeled and chopped

3 large parsnips, peeled and chopped

6 cups unsalted vegetable stock

1 teaspoon dried thyme

3 bay leaves

Freshly ground pepper to taste

3 tablespoons fresh tarragon, chopped

¾ cup fat-free, plain Greek yogurt

DIRECTIONS

1 Place all the chopped vegetables in a Dutch oven.

2 Pour the vegetable stock over the vegetables and add the thyme and bay leaves. Bring to a boil over high heat. Reduce to simmer for about 45 to 60 minutes, or until all the vegetables are tender.

3 Remove the bay leaves and purée the soup in a blender in small batches until smooth. (Alternatively, remove the pot from the stove and use an immersion blender to blend until smooth.)

4 Return the soup to the Dutch oven and add pepper to taste. Place the soup over low heat to keep it warm.

5 Just before serving, make the tarragon cream by stirring the tarragon into the Greek yogurt. Place ½ tablespoon of the tarragon cream on top of each bowl of soup.

6 Sprinkle with extra chopped tarragon as a garnish.

PER SERVING: *Calories 150 (From Fat 18); Fat 2g (Saturated 0.5g); Cholesterol 0mg; Sodium 107mg; Carbohydrate 28g (Dietary Fiber 7g); Protein 9g; Potassium 657mg.*

NOTE: Often overlooked and underappreciated, root veggies such as rutabaga and parsnips are at their peak in the winter months, when their robust flavors come alive. These nutritional powerhouses are versatile and inexpensive. Roots taste delightful roasted and caramelized for an easy side dish in the winter months, and roasting may be the trick that gets your kids to eat their veggies (it worked for coauthor Cindy!).

TIP: When purchasing root veggies, choose those that have a more regular shape to make peeling easier. Store the veggies in a cool, dry place.

Crab Louis Mason Jar Salad

PREP TIME: 25 MIN	YIELD: 2 SERVINGS

INGREDIENTS

2 tablespoons mayonnaise

2 tablespoons chili sauce

½ tablespoon Dijon mustard

¼ teaspoon prepared horseradish

¼ pound fresh crabmeat

¼ pound cooked, small shrimp, peeled and tails removed

3 green onions, sliced

½ cup cherub tomatoes, cut in half

1 ripe avocado, seeded, peeled, and cut into slices

2 cups chopped Romaine lettuce

¼ cup slivered almonds, toasted

DIRECTIONS

1 In a medium bowl, combine the mayonnaise, chili sauce, mustard, and horseradish; mix well.

2 In a separate bowl, toss together the crabmeat and shrimp.

3 Divide the dressing from Step 1 between two 1-quart mason jars. Then divide the crab and shrimp mixture between the mason jars, on top of the dressing. Place the onions, tomato, and avocado on top of the crab and shrimp mixture, followed by the lettuce. Refrigerate at least an hour, or until ready to serve.

4 Store the nuts separately in a resealable plastic bag to keep them crunchy.

5 Serve by shaking the mixture into a large bowl or plate and toss the ingredients so that the dressing gets distributed over the salad. Sprinkle with the toasted almonds.

PER SERVING: Calories 349 (From Fat 191); Fat 21g (Saturated 2g); Cholesterol 147mg; Sodium 394mg; Carbohydrate 17g (Dietary Fiber 7g); Protein 26g.

TIP: You can make this recipe ahead and store in the refrigerator 2 to 3 days.

TIP: You can purchase almonds already toasted or toast small amounts on the stove in a skillet. Place them in a dry skillet and heat over medium heat for about 4 to 5 minutes, or until golden brown. It'll take more time if you're using whole almonds or less time if you're using almond slices.

VARY IT! There are so many variations of this recipe — think about what you like best! For example, if a chef's salad is your favorite, add lean turkey and low-sodium ham with hard-boiled egg slices, strips of cheddar cheese, cherry tomatoes, red onions, red wine vinegar, and extra-virgin olive oil.

Chapter **19**

Mouth-Watering Entrees

Protein-rich foods, such as fresh seafood, poultry, pork, beef, and lamb, are a natural entree choice. They're lower in sodium than processed and cured meats such as bacon, ham, sausage, and many deli meats, which means they fit into a DASH eating plan pretty much perfectly. In this chapter, we provide you with a collection of recipes that gives you a wide variety of choices to take your entree options from ho-hum to yum!

Keeping Protein Portions in Perspective

Traditionally, the entree has been the centerpiece on the plate, but this isn't a good idea from a heart-healthy nutritional standpoint. As you transform your lifestyle to DASH, your protein portion will only take up one-fourth of the plate and will be accompanied by whole-grain side dishes and a variety of colorful and seasonal vegetables. The size of that protein portion is key. A 3-ounce serving of fresh meat, poultry, or seafood has just 30 to

90 milligrams of sodium, but obviously that fairly low sodium count can rise quickly when you start bumping up the portion size. Table 19-1 shows how 3-ounce servings of various types of chicken, pork, beef, and fish match up in terms of calories, fat, and saturated fat, according to data from the USDA Nutrient Database for Standard Reference.

TABLE 19-1   ## Comparing Chicken, Pork, Beef, and Fish

Per 3-Ounce Serving of . . .	Calories	Fat (in Grams)	Saturated Fat (in Grams)
Skinless chicken breast	123	3.0	1.0
Skinless chicken thigh	193	9.6	2.7
Pork tenderloin	122	3.0	1.0
Pork, boneless top loin chop	167	7.7	2.6
Pork, top loin roast	147	5.3	1.6
Beef, top round	172	6.2	2.2
Beef, top sirloin	180	8.2	3.2
Beef tenderloin	179	7.6	3.0
Cod	84	0.25	0.5
Salmon	155	6.9	1.06

When picking cuts of pork or beef, opt for lean cuts, which generally have the word *loin* in the description, such as pork tenderloin or beef tenderloin. Also, purchase choice grades of meat when you can because the quality is good and the meat has less marbling.

TIP

Research suggests that consuming about 8 ounces per week of a variety of seafood is associated with reduced cardiac deaths among individuals with and without preexisting heart disease. Seafood contributes healthy fats, including omega-3 fatty acids, eicosatetraenoic acid (EPA), and docosahexaenoic acid (DHA). Table 19-2 shows you how much EPA and DHA exist in 3-ounce cooked servings of various seafood (fish and shellfish), according to the USDA Data for High Omega-3 Fish Analysis. The recipes in this chapter include some mouth-watering seafood favorites that your family is sure to enjoy — even those who generally turn up their noses. The good news is that fish is a timesaver. These dishes take no time at all to prepare.

TABLE 19-2 **EPA and DHA Content in Various Types of Seafood**

Type of Seafood (Cooked)	Milligrams of EPA and DHA per 3 Ounces
Salmon	1,825
Mackerel, Atlantic and Pacific (not King)	1,023
Bluefin and albacore tuna	1,278
Halibut	395
Rainbow trout, wild	840
Canned albacore tuna	733
Yellowfin tuna	237
Red snapper	273
Shrimp	268

*Source: FoodData Central (*https://fdc.nal.usda.gov*)*

REMEMBER

Whichever form of protein you choose for your entree, stick to a 2- to 3-ounce serving per meal to keep within the goal of the DASH diet (consume about 6 ounces of protein total per day, depending on calorie level; see Chapter 5 for more DASH nutrition basics).

Building Flavor with Techniques and Seasonings

If you think DASH eating means giving up feeling satisfied, think again. These hearty, flavor-packed dishes are proof that less can really be more and that these cooking methods can add flavor without the addition of sodium.

Using the right cooking method for each type of protein guarantees more flavorful and tender results. The recipes we include in this chapter use searing and grilling to bring out the natural flavor of the featured protein source. Both techniques use high heat to provide color and a distinctive flavor that you can accomplish on a charcoal or gas grill or by using a cast-iron, stove-top grill over high heat. For convenience, we use a gas grill, but charcoal grilling can add a smoky flavor.

To create more complex taste sensations, you can turn to simple herb and spice mixtures and marinades. The combinations can lock in moisture, producing a juicy and tasty end product. Garnishes such as a fruit salsa (such as the Jamaican Jerk Chicken with Cha-Cha Salsa in this chapter) or grilled lemon can also serve as a special bonus of visual appeal and added antioxidants. You can sprinkle on spices as a dry rub or make them into a wet rub with the addition of heart-healthy oil, crushed garlic and mustard, or acidic ingredients such as vinegar or fruit juice to tenderize and flavor meat. The biggest bonus is, there's no need to add salt!

Seared Scallops with Pistachio Sauce

PREP TIME: 10 MIN	COOK TIME: 8 MIN	YIELD: 4 SERVINGS

INGREDIENTS

1½ pounds large sea scallops

1 tablespoon extra-virgin olive oil, divided

Freshly ground black pepper to taste

¼ cup chopped unsalted pistachios

1 tablespoon unsalted butter

DIRECTIONS

1 Dry the scallops well with paper towels, removing as much water as possible. Heat ½ tablespoon of the olive oil on high in a large, nonstick skillet. Season the scallops with the freshly ground pepper.

2 Place half of the scallops onto the hot pan and sear them without turning them until they're well browned, about 2 minutes. Turn the scallops and cook until the sides are firm and the centers are opaque, about 2 to 3 minutes.

3 Transfer the scallops to a serving plate and loosely tent them with foil (fold a piece of aluminum foil in half and loosely cover the plate). Repeat with the remaining oil and scallops and transfer them to the plate.

4 Add the chopped pistachios and butter to the skillet and cook until the butter is lightly browned, about 3 minutes. Pour the sauce over the scallops and serve.

PER SERVING: *Calories 289 (From Fat 108); Fat 12g (Saturated 3g); Cholesterol 98mg; Sodium 451mg; Carbohydrate 2g (Dietary Fiber 1g); Protein 41g; Potassium 889mg.*

TIP: Don't crowd the pan with too many scallops at once. The scallops should sizzle when they hit the pan.

TIP: Always buy "dry" scallops, which haven't been treated with a sodium solution that acts as a preservative and keeps them plump and white. They should be consistent in color, smell briny, and not have an iodine odor. Fresh scallops are more translucent and firm. If you buy frozen, keep them frozen. If you buy previously frozen, thaw them and don't refreeze them. Ask for a bag of ice at the grocery store to keep your seafood cold for the ride home. Store scallops in the coldest part of your refrigerator.

Curry-Crusted Roasted Salmon

PREP TIME: 5 MIN | COOK TIME: 12 MIN | YIELD: 2 SERVINGS

INGREDIENTS

Two 4-ounce salmon fillets, with skin

2 teaspoons mayonnaise

1½ teaspoons curry powder

¼ cup panko breadcrumbs

2 teaspoons extra-virgin olive oil

1 green onion, sliced

DIRECTIONS

1 Preheat the oven to 450 degrees. Dry the fish with paper towel. Place the fish on a baking sheet lined with parchment paper or a silicone baking mat.

2 In a small cup, combine the mayonnaise and the curry powder. Spread the mayonnaise mixture over the salmon. Top with the breadcrumbs and press gently so that the crumbs adhere to the fish. Lightly drizzle with the olive oil.

3 Place the pan in the oven and roast 10 to 12 minutes or until browned and cooked through. Remove from the oven and garnish with onions.

PER SERVING: *Calories 217 (From Fat 81); Fat 9g (Saturated 2g); Cholesterol 48mg; Sodium 175mg; Carbohydrate 11g (Dietary Fiber 1g); Protein 22g.*

TIP: Salmon is one of the best sources of omega-3 fatty acids, which are essential for heart health. Eating fatty fish at least twice a week will give you the amount you need.

NOTE: The cook time for the fish will depend on the thickness. A general rule is 10 to 12 minutes per inch of thickness. For a more accurate method of testing doneness, cook until an instant-read thermometer registers 145 degrees.

NOTE: Roasted and grilled fish with the skin on keeps the integrity of the fish while cooking. It's also edible!

VARY IT! Don't like the flavor of curry? Skip the curry powder and use smoked paprika or jerk seasoning instead.

Quick and Easy Shrimp Ancient Grain Bowl

PREP TIME: 15 MIN	COOK TIME: 5 MIN	YIELD: 2 SERVINGS

INGREDIENTS

4 ounces medium-size raw shrimp, peeled and deveined

3 tablespoons sesame-ginger salad dressing, divided

One 11-ounce can mandarin oranges, in juice, drained

2 cups pre-shredded coleslaw mix

3 tablespoons slivered almonds, toasted

2 green onions, sliced diagonally

½ cup snap peas, blanched

½ cup cooked tri-color quinoa

DIRECTIONS

1 In a large bowl, marinate the shrimp in 1 tablespoon of the salad dressing for 15 minutes.

2 To assemble, divide between 2 shallow bowls the oranges, coleslaw mix, almonds, onions, snap peas, and quinoa in little mounds.

3 Heat a nonstick skillet on high and cook the shrimp until they turn pink, about 4 to 5 minutes.

4 Divide the shrimp between the two bowls. Drizzle an additional 1 tablespoon of dressing over each bowl before serving.

PER SERVING: *Calories 269 (From Fat 105); Fat 12g (Saturated 2g); Cholesterol 65mg; Sodium 351mg; Carbohydrate 29g (Dietary Fiber 6g); Protein 14g.*

TIP: This one-dish wonder makes for an incredibly satisfying meal. The best approach is to utilize leftovers from previous meals. All the ingredients can be made ahead and refrigerated in separate airtight containers.

NOTE: When deciding on your favorite combinations, think about adding a grain, a green, and a protein. Add a quality dressing or pesto, if desired, to round out the flavor, and enjoy!

TIP: You can use any dressing to get your desired flavor. Try a store-bought spicy Thai dressing or Mediterranean dressing with feta cheese for a different twist.

TIP: You can purchase toasted almonds or toast them at home. Preheat the oven to 350 degrees. Spread the slivered almond on a baking sheet in an even layer and bake for 5 minutes. Remove from the oven and stir to help them roast evenly. Return to the oven for 3 more minutes. Watch closely — they burn quickly. Let them cool before serving.

TIP: The best way to blanch snap peas is to bring 4 cups of water to boil, add the peas, and cook until they're tender-crisp, about 1 to 2 minutes. Using a slotted spoon, transfer the peas to an ice-water bath; drain and pat dry. This softens the peas and brightens their color.

Jamaican Jerk Chicken with Cha-Cha Salsa

PREP TIME: 20 MIN, PLUS MARINATING TIME	COOK TIME: 10 MIN	YIELD: 6 SERVINGS

INGREDIENTS

3 tablespoons salt-free Jamaican jerk seasoning

3 tablespoons canola oil

2 tablespoons reduced-sodium soy sauce

1 tablespoon cider vinegar

6 boneless skinless chicken breasts

Nonstick cooking spray

1 ripe mango, peeled, seeded, and diced

½ small cucumber, scrubbed, seeded, and diced

¼ small red onion, diced

1 cup chopped fresh cilantro

1 small jalapeño pepper, seeded and minced

1 tablespoon fresh lime juice

DIRECTIONS

1   Combine the jerk seasoning, oil, soy sauce, and cider vinegar and pour the mixture over the chicken breasts. Refrigerate for at least 30 minutes or up to 8 hours.

2   Preheat your grill on high for 15 to 20 minutes to ensure maximum heat is achieved. Coat the grill rack with cooking spray and place the marinated chicken on the rack. Grill 4 to 6 minutes on each side, or until cooked thoroughly. Do not overcook.

3   While the chicken grills, prepare the salsa. Combine the mango, cucumber, onion, cilantro, jalapeño pepper, and lime juice in a small bowl. Serve with the grilled chicken.

PER SERVING: *Calories 419 (From Fat 135); Fat 15g (Saturated 3g); Cholesterol 157mg; Sodium 372mg; Carbohydrate 9g (Dietary Fiber 1g); Protein 59g; Potassium 596mg.*

NOTE: If it's the dead of winter or you just want to keep things simple, an alternate method of cooking is an indoor electric grill. The cooking is fast and the cleanup is even quicker.

TIP: The salsa tastes best when it's served within a few hours of preparation.

VARY IT! Combine the jerk seasoning and canola oil and use it as a dry rub instead of adding soy and cider vinegar. It works well on all types of meat and seafood and saves a few milligrams of sodium too!

Herbed Baked Chicken with Artichokes

PREP TIME: 10 MIN	COOK TIME: 50 MIN	YIELD: 6 SERVINGS

INGREDIENTS

1½ pounds boneless, skinless chicken breasts, split

Two 15-ounce cans small artichoke hearts, in water, drained, and rinsed well

6–8 garlic cloves, crushed

Freshly ground black pepper to taste

1 tablespoon fresh rosemary, chopped

1 tablespoon fresh thyme, chopped

1 tablespoon fresh mint, chopped

1 tablespoon chopped sage

1 teaspoon fresh chopped marjoram

2 bay leaves, cut in half

2 tablespoons extra-virgin olive oil

DIRECTIONS

1 Preheat the oven to 375 degrees. Cut the chicken breasts into six equal-sized pieces. Place the chicken and artichoke hearts in a large Dutch oven.

2 Combine the garlic, pepper, herbs, and oil and pour the mixture over the chicken and artichoke hearts.

3 Cover the Dutch oven and place it over high heat on top of the stove. When the oil begins to sizzle and the chicken begins to brown, place the Dutch oven in the oven and bake for 25 to 35 minutes. Check after 20 minutes and add up to a cup of water if needed.

4 Just before serving, remove the bay leaves. Serve the chicken with equal amounts of artichokes and sauce.

PER SERVING: *Calories 309 (From Fat 18); Fat 9g (Saturated 2g); Cholesterol 96mg; Sodium 170mg; Carbohydrate 19g (Dietary Fiber 13g); Protein 40g.*

TIP: Organic chicken breasts are typically smaller and more tender.

TIP: Serve this recipe with your favorite whole-grain side dish.

VARY IT! Along with the chicken, add shallots, Roma tomatoes, baby carrots, and haricot verts (thin green beans) to the Dutch oven and cook as directed. You can also add up to 1 cup of your favorite dry white wine during baking for additional flavor.

Grilled Pork Tenderloin Medallions

PREP TIME: 10 MIN, PLUS MARINATING TIME	COOK TIME: 5 MIN	YIELD: 4 SERVINGS

INGREDIENTS

One 1-pound pork tenderloin

2 tablespoons canola oil

1 tablespoon lemon juice

2 cloves garlic, minced (see Figure 19-1)

1 teaspoon dried basil

1 teaspoon dried rosemary

1 teaspoon dried thyme

1 teaspoon Dijon mustard

Freshly ground pepper to taste

DIRECTIONS

1 Slice the tenderloin crosswise into eight ¾-inch-thick slices, called *medallions*.

2 Combine the remaining ingredients. Place the pork in a baking dish. Pour the marinade over the pork and marinate 3 to 4 hours.

3 When you're ready to cook, preheat your gas grill on high and grill the medallions for 2 to 3 minutes on each side, until done. Do not overcook.

PER SERVING: *Calories 190 (From Fat 90); Fat 10g (Saturated 2g); Cholesterol 56mg; Sodium 72mg; Carbohydrate 1g (Dietary Fiber 0.5g); Protein 23g; Potassium 617mg.*

NOTE: Cutting the tenderloin into small medallions allows it to cook faster and makes a great hearty appetizer or finger food for a party. Serve it plain or with your favorite sauce.

TIP: Feel free to keep a tinge of pink when cooking pork. It will be more tender and succulent than if you cook it to death. The dreaded risk of trichinosis is virtually nonexistent. Here's a temperature guide for cooking pork: 130–140 degrees for medium, 140–150 degrees for medium-well, and 150–155 degrees for well done.

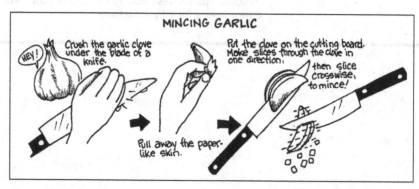

FIGURE 19-1: How to mince garlic.

Illustration by Elizabeth Kurtzman

Black-Tie Flat-Iron Steak

PREP TIME: 5 MIN, PLUS MARINATING TIME	COOK TIME: 15 MIN	YIELD: 4 SERVINGS

INGREDIENTS

1 clove garlic, minced

1 tablespoon extra-virgin olive oil, plus 2 teaspoons

¼ cup red wine vinegar

2 tablespoons low-sodium ketchup

1½ teaspoons Worcestershire sauce

1 teaspoon sugar

1 teaspoon dried basil

One 1½ – 2 pounds flat-iron steak

8 ounces fresh button mushrooms, sliced

¼ cup green onions, sliced into ¼-inch pieces

DIRECTIONS

1 In a small saucepan, cook the garlic in the olive oil until it's fragrant and begins to brown slightly. Remove from heat. Stir in the red wine vinegar, ketchup, Worcestershire sauce, sugar, and basil.

2 Place the steak in a resealable plastic bag and pour the marinade over the meat. Close the bag, place it in a shallow pan, and refrigerate for 6 hours or overnight.

3 When you're ready to cook, bring the meat to room temperature in the bag. Drain the meat but reserve the marinade. Preheat the grill to medium-high heat. Grill the steak over moderately high heat until it's well-browned and medium-rare, about 3 to 4 minutes per side.

4 In a small nonstick saucepan, heat 2 teaspoons of olive oil and add the mushrooms and onions. Cook until the mushrooms are soft, about 3 minutes. Pour the reserved marinade into another saucepan and bring to a boil. Cook for at least 3 minutes to kill any germs that may have been transferred from the food. Add the cooked mushrooms and onions, and simmer for 2 minutes.

5 Transfer the steak to a carving board and let it rest for 5 to 8 minutes. Carve the meat across the grain in thin slices. Serve with the mushroom sauce.

PER SERVING: Calories 421 (From Fat 180); Fat 20g (Saturated 6g); Cholesterol 155mg; Sodium 142mg; Carbohydrate 4g (Dietary Fiber 0g); Protein 52g.

NOTE: The flat-iron steak is also known as *top blade steak* (from the shoulder of the cow). It's nearly perfect for marinating and grilling — it's flavorful, tender, and really lean. It's best grilled over medium-high heat and cooked rare to medium.

VARY IT! After grilling, serve the steak with chimichurri sauce made by pureeing the following ingredients in a food processor in this order: ½ cup cilantro leaves, ½ cup flat leaf parsley, 2 tablespoons minced garlic, 3 tablespoons lemon juice, 2 teaspoons red wine vinegar, ½ teaspoon cayenne pepper, and ½ cup olive oil.

Herbs de Provence Lamb Chops

PREP TIME: 5 MIN	COOK TIME: 6 MIN	YIELD: 4 SERVINGS

INGREDIENTS

Four 4-ounce lamb loin chops

½ teaspoon freshly ground pepper

3 tablespoons Herbs de Provence

1 tablespoon extra-virgin olive oil

DIRECTIONS

1 Trim any visible fat from around the edges of the lamb chops and sprinkle them with fresh pepper.

2 Combine the Herbs de Provence with olive oil and brush on both sides of the lamb chops.

3 Preheat the grill on high. Add the chops and sear for about 2 minutes. Turn the chops and cook another 3 minutes for medium-rare or 3½ minutes for medium.

PER SERVING: *Calories 274 (From Fat 180); Fat 20g (Saturated 8g); Cholesterol 75mg; Sodium 68mg; Carbohydrate 2g (Dietary Fiber 1g); Protein 21g.*

TIP: Most cuts of lamb are fairly tender and lend themselves to quick cooking methods like grilling or pan-frying. Lamb chops develop a gamey flavor when well done or overcooked. Here's a temperature guide for cooking lamb: 125–130 degrees for medium-rare, 130–135 degrees for medium, and 135–140 degrees for well done.

TIP: When purchasing lamb, look for lamb that is raised on pasture and grass-fed, and be sure the fat is a light, creamy fat and isn't yellow or dark, which indicates an older, mature sheep.

VARY IT! Make a quick rub to marinate the lamb. Add a few cloves of garlic, 2 tablespoons fresh rosemary, 1 teaspoon thyme, a pinch of cayenne pepper, and 2 tablespoons olive oil in the bowl of a food processor and pulse into a paste. Rub the paste on both sides of the lamb and marinate an hour before grilling. Another alternative is to use your favorite balsamic vinegar dressing to marinate the lamb before grilling.

Dressed-Up Butternut Squash Ravioli

PREP TIME: 10 MIN	COOK TIME: 10 MIN	YIELD: 6 SERVINGS

INGREDIENTS

Two 10-ounce packages butternut squash ravioli

2 teaspoons extra-virgin olive oil

6 ounces (2½ cups) fresh kale, washed and ribs removed and chopped

One 25-ounce jar butternut squash sauce

2 cups shredded chicken from store-bought Rotisserie chicken

4 tablespoons unsalted roasted pumpkin seeds, for garnish

DIRECTIONS

1 Add the butternut squash ravioli to 6 quarts of water and cook on high for 4 minutes. Drain, reserving ¼ cup of the cooking liquid.

2 In the meantime, heat the olive oil in a skillet and sauté the kale for 1 minute. Add the butternut squash sauce, chicken, and some of the pasta cooking liquid to get your desired consistency. Continue cooking for 3 to 5 minutes, just until the kale is tender.

3 Mix the cooked ravioli with the butternut squash mixture and garnish with the pumpkin seeds.

PER SERVING: Calories 429 (From Fat 114); Fat 13g (Saturated 6g); Cholesterol 90mg; Sodium 589mg; Carbohydrate 58g (Dietary Fiber 8g); Protein 24g.

TIP: For a quick and easy meal, buy fresh pasta and a jar of high-quality sauce. Your meal is ready in a flash! Embellish it with a nutrient-dense vegetable and add a protein. This is a great way to break the take-out routine.

NOTE: If you can't find butternut squash ravioli, substitute fresh cheese or spinach ravioli from the refrigerator case in the grocery story deli area. This recipe is an example of how you can elevate fresh pasta from your grocer's refrigerated aisle into a special dish with the addition of more vegetables and a variety of sauces.

VARY IT! Can't find butternut squash sauce? Use your favorite low-sodium marinara sauce instead. It's still delish! Don't like kale? Use baby spinach or arugula instead. Feeling like seafood? Add cooked shrimp.

Sesame-Infused Steamed Haddock

PREP TIME: 5 MIN | COOK TIME: 10MIN | YIELD: 4 SERVINGS

INGREDIENTS

2 tablespoons chili paste

2 tablespoons rice wine

1 tablespoon sesame oil

Four 4-ounce haddock fillets, with skin

1 green onion cut in long diagonal slices

2 tablespoons black sesame seeds, for garnish

DIRECTIONS

1 In a small bowl, combine the chili paste, rice wine, and sesame oil. Set aside.

2 In a large, deep pan, add 2 inches of water. Place a vegetable steamer in the pan and bring the water to a boil. Place the fish fillets in the steamer, making sure the rack is elevated above the water. Cover the pan loosely and steam the fish 8 to 10 minutes. Cook just until the entire piece of fish goes from shiny and translucent to opaque and easily flakes when tested with a fork.

3 Brush the sesame oil mixture onto the fish fillets and top with green onions. Garnish with sesame seeds.

PER SERVING: *Calories 135 (From Fat 56); Fat 6g (Saturated 1g); Cholesterol 48mg; Sodium 208mg; Carbohydrate 1g (Dietary Fiber 1g); Protein 17g.*

TIP: A bamboo steamer is also a good choice to steam the fish. Line the steamer with kale or spinach for easy cleanup!

NOTE: Use an instant-read thermometer to test the fish for doneness. It should register 145 degrees.

VARY IT! Other types of fish to steam are cod, grouper, snapper, tilapia, sea bass, and salmon. Haddock and cod are used almost interchangeably — both are great sustainable choices, delicious and versatile.

Chapter 20

Savory Side Dishes

Move over, white rice and potatoes. The recipes in this chapter kick those old standbys to the curb in favor of whole grains and a variety of vegetables that contain the antioxidants and phytochemicals that are beneficial in the DASH diet. Even if vegetables aren't on your list of favorites, try to have an open mind about some of our sneaky healthy-eating suggestions and give vegetables and whole grains another chance. Go ahead and break out of your same-old-same-old side dish rut — we dare you!

Embracing the Complexity and Tastiness of Whole Grains and Vegetables

Starchy carbohydrates have gotten a bad rap over the years, but we assert that the popular notion that "carbs make you fat" is unfounded, because not all carbs are alike. Wholesome complex carbohydrates supplied by grains, fruits, and vegetables provide the main source of energy in your diet. You read that right. Your muscles prefer complex carbs to protein as an energy source. Complex carbs also supply specific nutrients and fiber, important to the blood-pressure-regulating role of the DASH diet. You'd be hard-pressed to get an ample supply of these important nutrients without complex carbs.

REMEMBER

Portion control is an especially important part of meal planning to remember. As we discuss in Chapters 4 and 10, plan meals so that one-fourth of your plate is lean protein, one-fourth to one-third of your plate is whole grains, and the remainder of the plate is vegetables.

REMEMBER

We focus on whole grains because they have more fiber, B-vitamins, and other nutrients than refined grains do. Here are a few points to keep in mind when it comes to whole grains:

>> Look for products labeled *100 percent whole grain.*

>> Grains are naturally low in fat and salt, so avoid a lot of butter and cream sauces and the addition of table salt.

>> If you don't eat many whole grains currently, add them to your diet gradually to avoid gas and bloating. After all, you don't want to scare away your dinner guests.

Ancient grains such as quinoa, farro, and whole-wheat couscous create a great nutritional base for half the side dish recipes we share in this chapter.

The other half shows you how to incorporate more vegetables into your meal planning. Whether plucked from your own garden, picked up from a farmers' market, or purchased at your local supermarket, vegetables with such humble beginnings can turn into a scrumptious side by adding some aromatic flavor combinations. They can also help you eat the rainbow by adding a variety of colors to your plate. A rainbow of colors gives you important nutrients needed to promote heart health (see more in Chapter 5). As an added bonus, vegetables may even have some anti-aging qualities! How awesome is that?

REMEMBER

When you have hypertension, adding more potassium, magnesium, and calcium to your diet is important. Dark green, leafy vegetables, such as kale and Swiss chard, are especially rich in potassium, magnesium, beta-carotene, vitamin C, folate, and fiber — a perfect fit for the DASH plan. If you haven't tried many dark green, leafy vegetables before, check out the recipes for Moroccan-Style Farro with Kale and Crunchy Brussels Sprouts Slaw in this chapter.

Crunchy Brussels Sprouts Slaw

PREP TIME: 20 MIN | **YIELD: 4 SERVINGS**

INGREDIENTS

¼ cup extra-virgin olive oil

2 tablespoons sherry vinegar

2 teaspoons Dijon mustard

Freshly ground pepper to taste

1 pound Brussels sprouts, washed and dried

½ cup chopped pecans, toasted

½ cup dried cherries

¼ cup crumbled blue cheese

DIRECTIONS

1 In a small bowl, whisk together the oil, vinegar, mustard, and pepper. Set aside.

2 Remove the stems and slice the Brussels sprouts so they have the appearance of a slaw. (You can also shred the Brussels sprouts in the food processor by pulsing once or twice. This results is a bit more refined product.) Place them in a large bowl and add the pecans and cherries. Drizzle in the dressing and toss until the ingredients are coated.

3 Garnish with the crumbled blue cheese.

PER SERVING: *Calories 328 (From Fat 229); Fat 25g (Saturated 4g); Cholesterol 6mg; Sodium 176mg; Carbohydrate 24g (Dietary Fiber 6g); Protein 7g.*

TIP: Look for Brussels sprouts that have bright green leaves that are tightly packed without any yellowing or discoloration. Small ones are usually sweeter and more tender than large ones. They actually grow on a stalk, and if you can find them sold that way, they'll be the freshest tasting!

NOTE: Brussels sprouts are nutritional powerhouses and contain lots of fiber, potassium, and antioxidants.

VARY IT! You can substitute dried mixed berries or cranberries in place of the cherries and use any variety of nut (such as almonds or pistachios).

TIP: For another quick side-dish idea, cut the sprouts in half, add 1 tablespoon of olive oil, and add to an air fryer preheated to 375 degrees, arranging into a single layer. Air-fry for 15 minutes, shaking the basket (or rotating the pan if a larger unit) halfway through the cooking. The result is tender on the inside and crispy on the outside.

Cauliflower "Steak" Diablo

PREP TIME: 10 MIN	COOK TIME: 25 MIN	YIELD: 4 SERVINGS

INGREDIENTS

1 cauliflower head, washed

1 tablespoon extra-virgin olive oil

¼ cup low-sodium arrabbiata spaghetti sauce

¼ cup freshly grated Parmesan cheese

4 slices provolone cheese

Fresh basil leaves, chiffonade

DIRECTIONS

1 Preheat the oven to 450 degrees. Trim the cauliflower of leaves and cut the stem at the base. With the stem and core intact, and slice the cauliflower into four 1-inch "steaks."

2 Place the cauliflower "steaks" on a baking sheet covered with parchment paper or a silicone baking mat. Using a pastry brush, lightly brush both sides of the cauliflower with olive oil.

3 Roast until the cauliflower starts to brown, about 8 minutes.

4 Use a spatula to flip the cauliflower, and then evenly divide the sauce over the top. Sprinkle with Parmesan and provolone and roast for another 8 to 10 minutes. Check midway through baking, and bake just until the cheese is bubbly.

5 Garnish with the fresh basil.

PER SERVING: *Calories 172 (From Fat 90); Fat 10g (Saturated 6g); Cholesterol 25mg; Sodium 370mg; Carbohydrate 10g (Dietary Fiber 4g); Protein 13g.*

TIP: Reserve any cauliflower florets that break off to toss in a salad. If you can't find low-sodium arrabbiata sauce, just use a marinara or regular pizza sauce. (You can still kick it up a notch with some red pepper flakes!)

NOTE: Cauliflower is a cruciferous vegetable that also comes in the shades of orange, purple, and green. The flavor is the same, and they're equally high in nutrients and fiber.

VARY IT! Add cooked lean ground beef or a small amount of cooked Italian sausage. Add some black or Kalamata olives or any leftover vegetable. The sausage or olives will increase the sodium, though, so watch your food pairings!

Moroccan-Style Farro with Kale

PREP TIME: 10 MIN	COOK TIME: 40 MIN	YIELD: 4 SERVINGS

INGREDIENTS

1 cup farro

2½ cups water

¼ teaspoon ground allspice

2 tablespoons extra-virgin olive oil

5 cloves garlic, sliced

1 tablespoon finely chopped ginger root

1 bunch kale, trimmed and chopped (about 4 cups)

¼ cup golden raisins

1 tablespoon apple cider vinegar

1 tablespoon honey

½ teaspoon ground cumin

½ teaspoon cinnamon

½ cup Marcona almonds

DIRECTIONS

1 Place the farro, water, and allspice in a large saucepan. Bring to a boil, cover, reduce heat to medium-low, and simmer for 30 minutes, or until the farro is tender.

2 In a medium skillet, heat the olive oil and add the garlic and ginger. Sauté until the garlic is lightly browned. Add the kale and continue to cook until the kale is tender, about 5 minutes. Add the raisins and stir gently.

3 Transfer the kale mixture into the cooked farro and stir gently. Add the vinegar, honey, cumin, and cinnamon. Add the almonds just before serving.

PER SERVING: *Calories 422 (From Fat 153); Fat 17g (Saturated 2g); Cholesterol 0mg; Sodium 63mg; Carbohydrate 57g (Dietary Fiber 7g); Protein 14g.*

NOTE: Farro, a member of the wheat family, is a traditional Mediterranean grain that's high in fiber and is a good source of iron and protein. It has a nutty flavor and a chewy texture, and it makes a wonderful substitute for rice. It's easy to prepare and something different to impress guests. Pearled farro has the hull removed, which shortens the cooking time. Be sure to follow the cooking instructions on the package, as they may be different from what's listed in the recipe.

TIP: You can purchase kale already chopped, which makes it easy to include the wonderful green in side dishes, morning smoothies, and tossed salads.

TIP: Marcona almonds are Spanish almonds that are sweet and tender. If you can't find them, you can substitute blanched slivered almonds.

Roasted Veggie Pouches

PREP TIME: 5 MIN	COOK TIME: 20 MIN	YIELD: 4 SERVINGS

INGREDIENTS

½ teaspoon garlic powder

½ teaspoon dried rosemary, crushed

½ teaspoon dried oregano

½ teaspoon dried parsley

¼ teaspoon black pepper

12 baby carrots, cut in half

20 snow peas

2 small zucchini, thickly sliced

2 small yellow squash, thickly sliced

½ small red onion, sliced

2 tablespoons extra-virgin olive oil

DIRECTIONS

1 Preheat the oven to 400 degrees. Place four 12-x-18-inch sheets of heavy-duty aluminum foil on a work surface.

2 In a small bowl, combine the garlic powder, rosemary, oregano, and parsley. Set aside.

3 Divide the carrots, snow peas, zucchini, squash, and onion equally between the four pieces of foil. Drizzle with oil and toss the vegetables so they're lightly covered with oil. Sprinkle the seasoning over the top.

4 Fold the foil over the vegetables to make 4 rectangular pouches. Fold the short sides over several times to make a seal. Fold over and crimp the final edge to make a sealed pouch. Place the pouches on a baking sheet and roast in the preheated oven for 18 to 20 minutes.

5 When ready to serve, open the pouches carefully to release the steam. Serve in the foil or transfer to a dinner plate.

PER SERVING: *Calories 90 (From Fat 62); Fat 7g (Saturated 1g); Cholesterol 0mg; Sodium 26mg; Carbohydrate 7g (Dietary Fiber 2g); Protein 1g.*

TIP: To make this into a main dish, add 4 ounces of fish or chicken tenders to each pouch and increase the time in the oven to 20 to 25 minutes. Veggie pouches can also be grilled for the same amount of time. You can also do one big pouch for a family-size serving!

NOTE: Use any veggies and as many veggies that are in season and that your family enjoys! Keeping the size of the vegetable slices even will ensure even cooking.

VARY IT! There are so many ways to season these packets! Try Italian seasoning or other dried herb blends, but check the label for sodium. Fresh herbs are always great and are a better choice than high-sodium blends. If you choose to use fresh herbs instead of dry, triple the amount of the herb. For example, 1 teaspoon dried is equivalent to 1 tablespoon fresh.

Southwest Corn with Chipotle Peppers

PREP TIME: 10 MIN	COOK TIME: 10 MIN	YIELD: 4 SERVINGS

INGREDIENTS

1 tablespoon canola oil

3 medium shallots, peeled and chopped

1 tablespoon canned chipotle peppers in adobo sauce, finely chopped

2 cups corn kernels from 3 to 4 ears of grilled corn or thawed from frozen

2 tablespoons chopped fresh thyme

Fresh ground pepper to taste

Thyme sprigs for garnish (optional)

DIRECTIONS

1 Heat the canola oil in a medium skillet. Add the shallots and sauté until tender (about 2 minutes). Add the chipotle peppers and stir for 3 more minutes.

2 Add the corn to the skillet. Add the thyme and cook, stirring frequently, until the flavors are combined (about 5 minutes).

3 Add fresh ground pepper to taste.

4 Garnish with thyme sprigs (if desired) and serve at once.

PER SERVING: *Calories 113 (From Fat 36); Fat 4g (Saturated 0g); Cholesterol 0mg; Sodium 21mg; Carbohydrate 19g (Dietary Fiber 2g); Protein 3g; Potassium 212mg.*

NOTE: This recipe tastes even better with corn you've grilled rather than thawed or boiled. If you have the will and the way, place the corn cobs directly on the grill and cook for 15 minutes, turning every 5 minutes until the corn is done. Cut the corn from the cob using a sharp knife or mandolin. You can also find frozen grilled corn at specialty grocery stores.

TIP: Chipotles are also known as smoked jalapeños and have a deep, smoky, fiery flavor. These are packed in adobo sauce, which consists of tomatoes, vinegar, onions, and herbs and contains sodium. Remember to begin by adding just a little; you can always add more depending on the heat tolerance threshold of your palate.

VARY IT! Add a 14.5-ounce can of thoroughly rinsed black beans for added flavor, protein, and variety. Serve warm or at room temperature as a dip with unsalted, baked tortilla chips.

Bok Choy Stir-Fry

PREP TIME: 5 MIN	COOK TIME: 5 MIN	YIELD: 4 SERVINGS

INGREDIENTS

1 tablespoon peanut oil

2 tablespoons minced ginger root

2 large garlic cloves, minced

1 red bell pepper, cut lengthwise into thin strips (see Figure 20-1)

2 stalks celery, sliced diagonally

2 large green onions, thinly sliced on a sharp diagonal

1 head bok choy, thinly sliced, green leaf tops only

½ teaspoon sesame oil

Toasted sesame seeds (optional)

DIRECTIONS

1 Heat an electric wok or a heavy wok skillet over high heat. Add the oil and swirl to coat the bottom and sides of the wok. Add the ginger and garlic and sauté 20 seconds.

2 Add the bell pepper and celery and sauté until crisp-tender, about 2 minutes.

3 Add the green onions and bok choy and sauté until just wilted, about 2 minutes. Drizzle in the sesame oil.

4 Sprinkle with toasted sesame seeds (if desired) and serve immediately.

PER SERVING: *Calories 78 (From Fat 45); Fat 5g (Saturated 1g); Cholesterol 0mg; Sodium 155mg; Carbohydrate 8g (Dietary Fiber 3g); Protein 4g; Potassium 672mg.*

NOTE: If you can find it, baby bok choy looks like its big brother, but its stems and leaves are more uniform with a fresh, sweet flavor. Some say it's not as "cabbagey"!

TIP: The trick to perfect stir-frying is to cook using small amounts of food or in batches. It's best not to overcrowd the wok with too many ingredients at once.

How to Core and Seed a Pepper

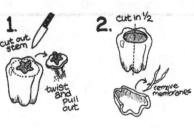

FIGURE 20-1:
How to core and seed a pepper.

Illustration by Elizabeth Kurtzman

Roasted Broccolini with Toasted Sesame Seeds

PREP TIME: 5 MIN	COOK TIME: 5 MIN	YIELD: 4 SERVINGS

INGREDIENTS

1 pound broccolini, rinsed in cold water and toweled dry

Nonstick cooking spray

1 tablespoon sesame oil

Freshly ground pepper to taste

1 teaspoon toasted sesame seeds

Pinch of red pepper flakes (optional)

DIRECTIONS

1 Preheat your oven to 400 degrees. Line a large baking pan with a silicone baking mat or parchment paper.

2 Place the broccolini on the baking pan, spray with nonstick cooking spray, and drizzle with sesame oil. Toss until evenly coated.

3 Place the pan in the preheated oven and roast for 4 to 5 minutes, just until the broccolini florets begin to turn golden in color. Remove them from the oven and toss with sesame seeds and red pepper flakes (if desired).

PER SERVING: *Calories 73 (From Fat 36); Fat 4g (Saturated 0.5g); Cholesterol 0mg; Sodium 38mg; Carbohydrate 7g (Dietary Fiber 3g); Protein 3g.*

NOTE: Broccolini is a cross breed of broccoli and Chinese broccoli. It has a dark green color and long, slender stalks. Some say it's sweeter and more tender than broccoli and requires a shorter cooking time. Trim the ends if they tend to be a bit woody. Otherwise, it's completely edible, from stem to floret!

TIP: Broccolini is one of the most nutritious cruciferous vegetables — a true powerhouse of vitamins, minerals, and the carotenoids beta carotene and lutein.

VARY IT! Omit the sesame oil and sesame seeds. Use only the cooking spray and sprinkle with a small amount of Gruyère or Parmigiano-Reggiano cheese, or dust lightly with cayenne, garlic powder, and paprika.

Chapter **21**

Meatless Main Dishes

This chapter is all about helping you take a plant-forward approach to your meals. We're not saying you need to give up meat entirely. Rather, we want to encourage you to cook up meatless main dishes at least once a week so that you include protein alternatives, like beans, legumes, tofu, edamame, quinoa, eggs, seeds, Greek yogurt, green peas, cottage cheese, nuts, and nut butters in place of meat — and you take positive steps toward meeting your DASH goals in the process. Keep in mind that you can use some of these dishes any time alongside smaller portions of meat to help you modify your carnivorous side.

The basis for plant-forward eating is foods that come from the soil. Foods of animal origin, if included at all, are considered a condiment or side dish rather than a focal point on the plate. There's a whole world of plant food out there that's just waiting to educate your palate. We're here to help you dive into it.

The Magic of Plant Food

When you add more plant foods to your diet, the health benefits are plenty. You reduce your intake of animal products, which translates to a reduction in saturated fat and cholesterol. At the same time, foods of plant origin contain so many properties that protect against disease. The extra fiber, potassium, magnesium, important antioxidants, beta-carotene, vitamins C and E, and most likely a reduction in sodium fit perfectly with the DASH plan. Weight loss and lower blood pressure are an automatic byproduct of your healthier choices!

Not too excited about the idea of meatless mains? We're willing to bet some of your favorite ethnic dishes are actually meatless: Mexican bean burritos, Greek spinach pie, and Italian spaghetti with marinara sauce, just to name a few. These are good choices, but you can improve them by adding even more veggies and beans, using corn tortillas, whole-wheat pasta, and healthier oils like extra-virgin olive oil. For example, in our Louisiana Red Beans and Rice (see the recipe later in this chapter), in place of high-fat sausage we add flavor using a variety of onions, garlic, and seasonings, and of course we use brown rice in place of the processed white rice. Lentils are a wonderful addition to your meal planning. They take less time to cook than beans and provide 12 grams of protein. When combined with a whole grain (as in our Braised Mediterranean Lentils with Quinoa recipe), they provide the same quality protein as meat!

Meatless dishes can be satisfying and full of flavor by including foods like beans, portobello mushrooms, and tofu, and by incorporating wonderful seasonings and aromatic vegetables like garlic and onion. Tofu is a versatile soy byproduct that takes on the flavor of whatever it's cooked with. It's high in protein, cholesterol-free, and low in calories, making it a nutrition treasure. It comes in silken and regular varieties and in soft, medium, firm, and extra-firm textures, allowing you to adapt a recipe to a type of tofu. Firm and extra-firm tofu work well in the Stir-Fry Tofu with Mushrooms in Sichuan Sauce recipe in this chapter.

TIP

Swapping out meat for the ingredients that give meatless main dishes their bulk can have the unexpected bonus of putting money back in your pocket. For example, buying a couple pounds of beans is significantly cheaper than buying a couple pounds of ground beef or turkey.

The road to a healthy blood pressure is paved in better food choices. It's not always about "giving up"; instead, it's about adding a variety of better choices. Try some of the savvy swaps listed in Table 21-1 to increase fiber and bump up your antioxidant intake to a new level with recipes from this very chapter.

TABLE 21-1   Food Swaps for Better Heart Health

If You're Craving This	Try This Instead
A greasy cheeseburger slider with sautéed onions	Black Bean 'n' Slaw Slider
Lasagne	Lasagna Spaghetti Squash Bowls
A cheesy stuffed enchilada casserole	Butternut Squash Enchiladas with Avocado Cream
A serving of beans and white rice with ham hocks and salt pork	Louisiana Red Beans and Rice

Louisiana Red Beans and Rice

PREP TIME: 10 MIN PLUS SOAKING TIME	COOK TIME: 2 HR	YIELD: 10 SERVINGS

INGREDIENTS

1 pound dry red beans, washed and drained

1 large onion, chopped

4 green onions, chopped

1 small green pepper, chopped

1 clove garlic, minced

1¼ teaspoons cayenne pepper

1¼ teaspoons black pepper

¼ teaspoon thyme

1 teaspoon celery flakes

¼ teaspoon oregano

1 tablespoon Worcestershire sauce

2 to 5 drops hot pepper sauce

6 ounces no-salt-added tomato paste

5 cups cooked brown rice

DIRECTIONS

1 Place the beans in cold water in a 4-quart pot and soak overnight.

2 Drain and rinse the beans and place them back in the pot. Add water to 1 inch above the beans. Add the remaining ingredients except the brown rice, bring to a boil, lower the heat, and simmer for 1 hour, covered. Stir several times during cooking.

3 Cook uncovered for an additional hour, continuing to stir to prevent the beans from sticking to the bottom of the pot.

4 Serve over steaming brown rice.

PER SERVING: *Calories 48 (From Fat 0); Fat 0g (Saturated 0g); Cholesterol 0mg; Sodium 120mg; Carbohydrate 10g (Dietary Fiber 3g); Protein 3g; Potassium 175mg.*

NOTE: Red beans and rice is a Louisiana creole classic typically made with sausage, smoked meat, or pork bones; we left those out to reduce the sodium content and keep it simple. This recipe makes an easy and yummy meal.

VARY IT! Make this recipe even easier by tossing the ingredients into a slow cooker and cooking the mixture on low for 7 hours. If you can be a little more flexible on your sodium count for this meal, substitute two 15-ounce cans of pinto beans, well rinsed and drained, in place of the dried beans.

Black Bean 'n' Slaw Sliders

PREP TIME: 20 MIN	COOK TIME: 6–8 MIN	YIELD: 6 SERVINGS

INGREDIENTS

2¼ cups bagged coleslaw mix with carrots

2 teaspoons lime juice

1 teaspoon canola oil

½ teaspoon honey

½ tablespoon chipotle peppers, minced

One 15-ounce can low-sodium black beans, rinsed well and drained

1 egg white, beaten

½ cup minced red onion

¼ cup whole-wheat panko bread crumbs

1 large garlic clove, minced

1 teaspoon cumin

½ teaspoon coriander

½ teaspoon chili powder

3 tablespoons fresh cilantro, chopped

6 whole-wheat slider buns

DIRECTIONS

1 Combine the coleslaw mix with the lime juice, canola oil, honey, and chipotle peppers and refrigerate for 30 minutes to let the flavors blend.

2 Mash the beans with a fork and mix together with the egg white, onion, bread crumbs, garlic, cumin, coriander, chili powder, and cilantro. Shape the bean mixture into six small patties. Set aside on a well-oiled, flat grill basket.

3 Preheat the grill and cook the patties until heated through, about 3 to 4 minutes on each side.

4 Serve on whole-wheat buns with the slaw.

PER SERVING: *Calories 212 (From Fat 27); Fat 3g (Saturated 0g); Cholesterol 4mg; Sodium 451mg; Carbohydrate 42g (Dietary Fiber 10g); Protein 10g; Potassium 321mg.*

NOTE: If you prefer, you can broil the burgers for 3 to 4 minutes on each side rather than grilling them.

TIP: You can eliminate the egg white in this recipe by simply moistening your hands with water or oil to shape the burgers. Handle the burgers with care when turning them on the grill.

VARY IT! In place of the coleslaw mixture, peel and shred jicama and red onion for a nice variety of flavors.

Braised Mediterranean Lentils with Quinoa

PREP TIME: 15 MIN	COOK TIME: 55 MIN	YIELD: 12 SERVINGS

INGREDIENTS

2 tablespoons extra-virgin olive oil

1 medium sweet onion, finely chopped

1 fennel bulb, thinly sliced

5 large cloves garlic, minced

1 teaspoon dried thyme

1 teaspoon dried basil

One 28-ounce can no-added-salt fire-roasted diced tomatoes

One 14.5-ounce can low-sodium vegetable broth

1½ cups green lentils

2 tablespoons tomato paste

2 cups tricolor quinoa, cooked according to package directions

1 cup cherry tomatoes, cut in half

4 ounces feta cheese, crumbled

DIRECTIONS

1 In a large deep skillet, heat the oil over medium heat. Add the onions and fennel, and sauté until the vegetables are soft and caramelized, about 10 minutes. Add the garlic, thyme, and basil and stir until fragrant.

2 Add the tomatoes, vegetable broth, lentils, and tomato paste, and bring the mixture to a boil over high heat. Reduce the heat to low, cover, and simmer for 45 to 50 minutes, or until the lentils are tender. Add up to 1 cup of water if the mixture gets too thick.

3 Serve the lentils over the quinoa. Garnish with cherry tomatoes and crumbled feta.

PER SERVING: *Calories 215 (From Fat 58); Fat 6g (Saturated 2g); Cholesterol 8mg; Sodium 140mg; Carbohydrate 31g (Dietary Fiber 6g); Protein 9g.*

TIP: Cook quinoa according to package or by using 2 cups quinoa and 3 cups water or low-sodium broth. Save any leftover quinoa for the Quick and Easy Shrimp Ancient Grain Bowl in Chapter 19. Cooked lentils can be frozen for about 3 months and refrigerated up to a week; cooked quinoa can be frozen for 8 to 12 months and refrigerated up to a week. Packaged lentils and quinoa will keep up to a year when stored in a dry, cool, and dark location.

TIP: To process the fennel, first trim off the stems and wash the bulb thoroughly under cool running water. Save the fronds for salads and the stems for making stock. Cut the bulb in half lengthwise, peel off the wilted outer layers, and cut out the core. Slice the fennel crosswise into thin slices or shave it on a mandolin.

TIP: Many stores carry grain pouches that can be microwaved for 90 seconds. Be sure to check the sodium content. Cooked from scratch, grains have zero sodium. To add more flavor, cook them with low-sodium vegetable broth instead of water.

VARY IT! Instead of quinoa, serve the lentils in a bowl of roasted spaghetti squash.

Lasagna Spaghetti Squash Bowls

PREP TIME: 15 MIN	COOK TIME: 1 HR	YIELD: 2 SERVINGS

INGREDIENTS

1 medium spaghetti squash, about 1½ to 2 pounds

1 tablespoon extra-virgin olive oil, divided

Freshly ground black pepper to taste

½ cup chopped onion

3 garlic cloves, chopped

1 cup store-bought low-sodium marinara sauce

½ cup part-skim ricotta cheese

1 teaspoon dried basil

One 6-ounce jar marinated artichoke hearts, drained and chopped

½ cup fresh mozzarella cheese, cut into small pieces

Fresh basil, for garnish

DIRECTIONS

1 Preheat the oven to 425 degrees. Line a baking sheet with aluminum foil.

2 Cut the spaghetti squash in half lengthwise through the stem. Scrape out the seeds and discard. Pour the oil into a small bowl and brush ½ tablespoon of the olive oil over the cut side of the squash with a pastry brush (reserve the remainder for Step 3). Lightly sprinkle with pepper. Place the squash, cut side up, on the foil-lined baking sheet and bake for 45 to 60 minutes. The squash is done when the flesh is tender and easily pulls away from the shell.

3 While the squash is baking, heat a large skillet over medium-high heat and sauté the onion and garlic in the remaining ½ tablespoon oil until the onion is soft. Reduce the heat and add the marinara sauce and simmer until the sauce is thickened, about 8 to 10 minutes.

4 In a small bowl, combine the ricotta cheese with the dried basil.

5 When the squash is completely cooked, use a fork to loosen the spaghetti-like strands from the shell, using the shell as a bowl.

6 Evenly divide the marinated artichoke hearts between each squash half. Top with the ricotta mixture, dividing evenly between each half. Spoon the marinara sauce evenly over each half. Then sprinkle ¼ cup mozzarella cheese over the top of each squash bowl.

7 Return the squash to the oven for 3 to 5 minute and heat until the cheese is melted.

8 Garnish with fresh basil and serve.

PER SERVING: *Calories 504 (From Fat 248); Fat 28g (Saturated 9g); Cholesterol 39mg; Sodium 211mg; Carbohydrate 46g (Dietary Fiber 4g); Protein 21g.*

TIP: Spaghetti squash can be tough to cut through. To make it easier, pierce the squash a few times with a sharp knife; then place it in the microwave for 3 to 5 minutes until the flesh is easier to cut through.

Stir-Fry Tofu with Mushrooms in Sichuan Sauce

PREP TIME: 10 MIN	COOK TIME: 15 MIN	YIELD: 4 SERVINGS

INGREDIENTS

12 ounces extra-firm tofu, drained and cut into cubes (see Figure 21-1)

1 tablespoon cornstarch

2 tablespoons low-sodium ketchup

2 teaspoons rice vinegar

1 teaspoon sugar

2 teaspoons reduced-sodium soy sauce

1 teaspoon sesame oil

1 tablespoon chili paste

2 tablespoons peanut oil

4 ounces button mushrooms, cut in half

2 cloves garlic, minced

2 green onions, sliced

4 ounces bean sprouts

4 ounces shredded carrots

DIRECTIONS

1 Drain the tofu well, using paper towels to soak up the extra liquid. Lightly dust with cornstarch.

2 In a small bowl, combine the sauce ingredients: ketchup, rice vinegar, sugar, soy sauce, sesame oil, and chili paste. Set aside.

3 Heat an electric wok or stir-fry pan over high heat. Add 1 tablespoon peanut oil and stir-fry the mushrooms until golden, about 2 to 3 minutes; then add the garlic and green onions for a few seconds. Add the bean sprouts and carrots and toss quickly in the hot oil until crisp-tender.

4 Remove the vegetables from the wok and set aside. Add the remaining tablespoon of peanut oil and the tofu, and stir-fry until the tofu begins to brown, about 2 to 3 minutes.

5 Add the stir-fry sauce and cook until bubbly, about a minute. Return the vegetables to the wok and toss all ingredients until completely covered with the sauce and heated through.

PER SERVING: *Calories 175 (From Fat 90); Fat 10g (Saturated 2g); Cholesterol 0mg; Sodium 352mg; Carbohydrate 14g (Dietary Fiber 2g); Protein 9g; Potassium 429mg.*

TIP: Tofu browns more easily when you remove the excess liquid.

VARY IT! Use your favorite veggies in this stir-fry and clean out the vegetable bin in the fridge.

PRESSING TOFU

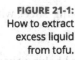

FIGURE 21-1: How to extract excess liquid from tofu.

1. TO REMOVE THE EXCESS LIQUID FROM THE COMPRESSED TOFU, WRAP THE CAKE IN A CLEAN KITCHEN TOWEL.

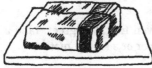

2. USE A PLATE TO PLACE ON TOP OF IT TO WEIGH IT DOWN. LET IT DRAIN FOR 10 TO 20 MINUTES (DEPENDING ON THE DESIRED FIRMNESS).

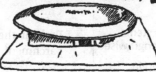

3. UN-WRAP AND PAT IT DRY. SLICE ACCORDING TO DIRECTIONS.

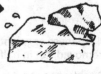

Illustration by Elizabeth Kurtzman

Easy Eggplant Parm

PREP TIME: 5 MIN	COOK TIME: 25 MIN	YIELD: 4 SERVINGS

INGREDIENTS

4 Japanese eggplants, stems removed, cut in half lengthwise

2 tablespoons extra-virgin olive oil

1 cup store-bought low-sodium marinara sauce, plus extra for serving

1 cup shredded part-skim mozzarella cheese

½ cup panko breadcrumbs

¼ cup finely grated Parmesan cheese

DIRECTIONS

1 Preheat the oven to 425 degrees. Line a baking sheet with parchment paper or a silicon mat.

2 Place the eggplant skin-side down on the lined baking sheet. Using a pastry brush, brush the eggplant on both sides with olive oil. Bake for 15 minutes, or until tender.

3 Lightly coat the eggplant with equal amounts of the marinara sauce and sprinkle each half evenly with mozzarella cheese.

4 In a bowl, combine the breadcrumbs and the parmesan cheese; divide evenly to coat the top of each eggplant half.

5 Return to the oven and bake another 10 to 12 minutes or until the cheese is bubbly and the breadcrumb mixture just starts to brown.

6 Serve with additional sauce if desired.

PER SERVING: Calories 347 (From Fat 140); Fat 16g (Saturated 6g); Cholesterol 22mg; Sodium 369mg; Carbohydrate 39g (Dietary Fiber 14g); Protein 16g.

TIP: Japanese eggplants are thinner and longer and have a more delicate flavor than globe eggplant. You can substitute 2 small globe eggplants, but cut into ½-inch slices and follow the remaining instructions.

TIP: Look for low-sodium marinara, which is a blend of imported Italian tomatoes, onions, garlic, basil, and olive oil. Be sure to compare labels to find the one lowest in sodium. Another option is to substitute a no-salt-added tomato puree and add your own salt-free Italian herb blend.

NOTE: Traditional eggplant parm is typically pan fried or deep fried and much higher in fat. Many recipes suggest salting eggplant to remove the bitterness. It's not necessary, though, and if you use the Japanese eggplant it's generally less bitter.

VARY IT! For more intense cheese flavor use a shredded Italian-style blend of mozzarella, Parmesan, and provolone. The sharper the cheese, the less you have to use to get great flavor!

Butternut Squash Enchiladas with Avocado Cream

PREP TIME: 20 MIN	COOK TIME: 55 MIN	YIELD: 6 SERVINGS

INGREDIENTS

2 small butternut squash, peeled and cut into small cubes (about 3 to 4 cups)

Freshly ground pepper to taste

½ teaspoon cumin

½ teaspoon chili powder

Nonstick cooking spray

½ small onion, chopped

2 garlic cloves, minced

1 tablespoon olive oil

½ cup frozen corn, thawed

Twelve 6-inch-diameter corn tortillas

2 cups low-fat shredded Mexi-blend cheese

One 16-ounce jar salsa verde

1 ripe avocado

8 ounces low-fat sour cream

¼ cup finely chopped cilantro

DIRECTIONS

1 Preheat the oven to 425 degrees. Spritz the squash with non-stick cooking spray and then toss the squash with the pepper, cumin, and chili powder. Place on a lined baking sheet and roast for 30 minutes, tossing once during the cooking process. When roasting is complete, reduce the oven temperature to 350 degrees.

2 Sauté the onion and garlic with the olive oil in a large skillet until tender, about 3 minutes. Add the squash and corn to the onion mixture. Set aside.

3 To soften the tortillas, wrap them in a paper towel and place in the microwave on high for 30 seconds to 1 minute. Divide the squash mixture evenly among the tortillas, placing the veggies in the center of the tortillas.

4 Top each with a tablespoon of cheese, roll them up, and arrange them side by side in a 9-x-13-inch glass baking dish. Pour the salsa verde over the enchiladas and sprinkle the remaining shredded cheese on top. Bake until the cheese is bubbly, about 20 minutes.

5 While the enchiladas are baking, mash the avocado until smooth and creamy. Blend in the sour cream and 2 table-spoons cilantro.

6 To serve, top the enchiladas with the avocado cream and the remaining fresh cilantro.

PER SERVING: *Calories 542 (From Fat 126); Fat 14g (Saturated 4g); Cholesterol 32mg; Sodium 300mg; Carbohydrate 84g (Dietary Fiber 10g); Protein 20g; Potassium 578mg.*

VARY IT! If you prefer, you can swap the corn tortillas for whole-wheat fat-free tortillas.

Creamy Polenta with Gingered Kale

PREP TIME: 10–12 MIN	COOK TIME: 35–40 MIN	YIELD: 6 SERVINGS

INGREDIENTS

3 tablespoons olive oil

1 tablespoon peeled and finely chopped fresh ginger

6 cloves garlic, sliced

4–5 cups chopped kale

⅓ cup raisins

½ teaspoon cumin

½ teaspoon cinnamon

1 tablespoon honey

1 tablespoon apple cider vinegar

½ cup sliced almonds

4 cups water

½ teaspoon salt

1 cup yellow cornmeal

2 tablespoons butter

DIRECTIONS

1 In a large skillet, heat the oil over medium–low heat. Add the ginger and garlic and sauté until light brown and fragrant, about 1 to 2 minutes. Add the chopped kale and cook slowly on low heat until the kale is tender, about 10 minutes.

2 Add the raisins, spices, honey, vinegar, and almonds and mix until well combined. Set aside for the flavors to blend or keep on very low heat until you cook the polenta.

3 Bring the water to a boil in a large saucepan and add the salt. Pour the cornmeal into the water in a steady stream and whisk continuously until it thickens slightly, about 5 minutes. Reduce the heat to low.

4 Cover the polenta and cook for another 20 to 25 minutes, watching it closely. Stir the polenta by scraping the sides and bottom of the pan every 10 minutes to smooth out any lumps that may form. Cover and continue to cook until the polenta is creamy. Remove from heat and stir in the butter. Spoon the polenta into soup bowls and top with the gingered kale.

PER SERVING: *Calories 308 (From Fat 135); Fat 15g (Saturated 4g); Cholesterol 10mg; Sodium 222mg; Carbohydrate 39g (Dietary Fiber 3g); Protein 6g.*

NOTE: Polenta solidifies when cooled. Leftovers can be sliced and grilled or sautéed. To make it creamy again, add milk, water, or broth and stir well.

TIP: Coarse-ground cornmeal works best. Avoid instant and quick-cooking products.

VARY IT! After the polenta begins to thicken, stir in your favorite low-fat cheese along with the butter. Top with the kale and a poached egg.

Chapter **22**

One-Pot and Sheet-Pan Meals

This chapter gets you dusting off your slow cooker and simmering up some big flavors and nutrition-conscious meals. It also introduces you to foil-pouch cooking. Both techniques are easy to prepare with minimal cleanup — talk about a winner!

Keeping It Simple with One-Dish Wonders

One way to get dinner on the table without breaking a sweat is to make a one-dish meal. Every ingredient goes into one pan or oven dish. Getting a meal into a slow cooker, sauté pan, or the oven usually takes only about 10 to 15 minutes of prep time. A one-dish meal is easy to cook, and the cleanup is easy, too. We feature several one-dish recipes in this chapter, but you don't have to limit yourself to them. You can create your own one-dish meals with a little imagination and whatever ingredients you have on hand.

TIP

When planning your own unique one-dish meals, follow this simple guideline: Include a protein, vegetables, and a grain (rice, whole-wheat tortillas, or whole-wheat pasta are best). Here are some ideas:

>> **Whole-wheat pasta with veggies and protein:** Pasta itself only takes 8 to 10 minutes to cook, and whole-wheat pastas pack added flavor, texture, and even fun shapes to your meal. You can add leftover diced chicken and vegetables right to the pot or quickly sauté some spinach and mushrooms to toss with the cooked pasta.

>> **Jambalaya:** Add your own healthy spin to this Louisiana tradition by using low-fat chicken sausage and adding more tomatoes and peppers to the rice.

>> **Stir-fries:** What do you get when you mix a nonstick pan with sliced chicken or lean beef and 2 cups of sliced vegetables? Dinner! Use about 2 teaspoons of oil in the pan, cook the meat first, and then add the vegetables. Serve over a cup of whole-grain rice.

Wrapping Up Dinner Fast with Foil

Using a foil pouch is a great way to cook a meal, whether you purchase foil bags or make aluminum-foil pouches yourself at home (see Figure 22-1). Meats and poultry stay moist, and vegetables cook quickly using this method. This easy cooking technique is a great way to get the children involved because they can help assemble the pouches. Here's how to create and cook a foil-pouch meal:

1. **Using either heavy-duty foil or double-layered standard foil, cut a 12- to 15-inch square of foil for each pouch.**

    Basically, the pouches should be big enough to allow air space to surround the food.

2. **Spray the foil with cooking spray to keep food from sticking to it.**

3. **Place meat on the center of the foil square, followed by high-moisture vegetables such as tomatoes and onions to keep the meat moist.**

4. **Taking opposite ends, fold up each side so the edges meet at the top, then fold the top over two or three times until it almost meets the food, and finally fold in each open side until the pouch is well sealed.**

    Always seal the foil by folding the ends together so no steam will escape.

REMEMBER

5. **Place your pouches on a grill plate and cook them for 15 minutes or place them on a baking sheet and cook them in a 375-degree oven for 20 to 25 minutes.**

Meat generally is cooked to a safe temperature after 20 to 25 minutes, seafood 8 to 10 minutes, and vegetables 5 to 8 minutes. Vegetables such as carrots and potatoes take a longer time to cook, 20 to 30 minutes unless you cut them into smaller pieces.

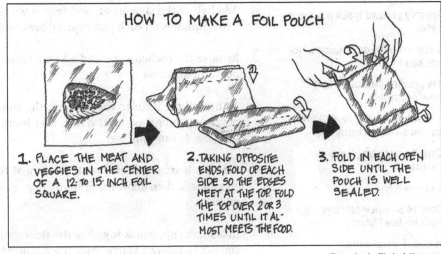

HOW TO MAKE A FOIL POUCH

1. PLACE THE MEAT AND VEGGIES IN THE CENTER OF A 12 to 15 INCH FOIL SQUARE.

2. TAKING OPPOSITE ENDS, FOLD UP EACH SIDE SO THE EDGES MEET AT THE TOP. FOLD THE TOP OVER 2 OR 3 TIMES UNTIL IT ALMOST MEETS THE FOOD.

3. FOLD IN EACH OPEN SIDE UNTIL THE POUCH IS WELL SEALED.

Illustration by Elizabeth Kurtzman

FIGURE 22-1:
It's easy to create a foil pouch for cooking.

Bold and Beefy Instant Pot Stew

PREP TIME: 20 MIN	COOK TIME: 50 MIN	YIELD: 6 SERVINGS

INGREDIENTS

1 tablespoon extra-virgin olive oil

1 pound lean beef stew meat

Freshly ground black pepper to taste

1 cup sun-dried tomatoes, not packed in oil

1½ pounds (about 10 to 12) new potatoes

1 medium onion, peeled and cut into 1-inch chunks

One 8-ounce bag baby cut carrots

1 cup water

One 14.5-ounce can low-sodium beef broth

½ cup dry red wine

1 to 2 tablespoons salt-free Italian herb mixture (a blend of oregano, thyme, garlic powder, and rosemary)

2 tablespoons flour or cornstarch

¼ cup cold water

Chopped parsley, for garnish

Crusty bread (optional)

DIRECTIONS

1 Turn the Instant Pot to Sauté, and then select More. Wait for the pot to heat up; then add the oil.

2 Add half of the stew meat, and season with pepper. Cook for 3 to 4 minutes on each side or until browned.

3 Remove the cooked meat and add the remaining meat to the pot until browned.

4 Return all the meat to the pot with the sun-dried tomatoes, potatoes, onions, carrots, water, beef broth, wine, and herb mixture; stir to combine.

5 Seal the Instant Pot and set it to Manual High Pressure for 30 minutes; then allow the pressure to release naturally for 10 minutes.

6 In a small cup, whisk together the flour and cold water until smooth to create a slurry. Pour the mixture back into the pot, and turn the pot back to Sauté. Simmer for 5 minutes or until the stew has thickened.

7 Serve in soup bowls, garnished with parsley and crusty bread, if desired.

PER SERVING: *Calories 413 (From Fat 64); Fat 7g (Saturated 2g); Cholesterol 50mg; Sodium 282mg; Carbohydrate 61g (Dietary Fiber 8g); Protein 25g.*

TIP: If you don't have an Instant Pot, combine all the ingredients except for the flour or cornstarch and ¼ cup water to a slow cooker, cover and cook on low for 8 to 9 hours, or until the beef and vegetables are tender. Stir the flour into ¼ cup water and mix until smooth. Add ½ cup of stew broth to the flour mixture. Gradually stir the mixture into the hot stew. Cover and adjust the temperature to high heat and continue cooking for about 10 minutes, or until slightly thickened.

TIP: Store leftovers in the refrigerator for 4 days or freeze up to 3 months.

Hearty Southwest Slow-Cooker Soup

PREP TIME: 15 MIN	COOK TIME: 6 HR	YIELD: 8 SERVINGS

INGREDIENTS

3 tablespoons canola oil

1 medium onion, chopped

1 small red bell pepper, chopped

3 large cloves garlic, minced

One 16-ounce jar of your favorite salsa (we like chipotle-flavored)

1 quart low-sodium chicken stock

Three 6-ounce chicken breasts, each cut into 6 pieces

1 cup frozen or fresh corn

One 16-ounce can low-sodium black beans, rinsed and drained

1 tablespoon chili powder

1 teaspoon cumin

½ teaspoon oregano

1 cup shredded low-fat Mexi-cheese

Fresh cilantro, chopped

DIRECTIONS

1 Heat the oil in a small skillet over medium heat. Add the onions, red bell peppers, and garlic. Sauté until the vegetables are soft and fragrant, about 8 minutes.

2 In the slow cooker, add the salsa, chicken stock, chicken breast pieces, corn, beans, chili powder, cumin, oregano, and the onion mixture.

3 Cook on low for 6 hours. Remove the chicken breasts and chop them into smaller, bite-sized pieces. Serve garnished with 2 tablespoons shredded cheese and fresh cilantro.

PER SERVING: *Calories 285 (From Fat 90); Fat 10g (Saturated 2g); Cholesterol 60mg; Sodium 452mg; Carbohydrate 19g (Dietary Fiber 5g); Protein 29g.*

NOTE: You can feed an army with this fail-proof pot of soup. Have a leftover ingredient that's not listed? Throw it in the mix.

TIP: This recipe is great for leftover vegetables and chicken. Use leftover rotisserie chicken, rinsed and without the skin, in place of the raw chicken.

TIP: Use a slow cooker liner for even easier cleanup.

Caribbean Chicken Foil Pouches

PREP TIME: 10 MIN | COOK TIME: 20 MIN | YIELD: 2 SERVINGS

INGREDIENTS

Two 4-ounce boneless, skinless chicken breast halves

1 cup diced pineapple, canned or fresh

½ small red onion, sliced

6 multicolored sweet bell peppers, sliced into rings

½ cup low-sodium barbecue sauce

DIRECTIONS

1 Preheat a gas grill to high. Place two 12-x-15-inch sheets of heavy-duty aluminum foil, shiny side down, on a work station.

2 Place one chicken breast half in the center of each piece of foil.

3 In a medium bowl, combine the pineapple, onion, peppers, and barbecue sauce. Divide the mixture between the two pieces of chicken.

4 Bring the opposite edges of the foil together. Double-fold the foil at the top. Crimp the edges of the pouch on the sides in a tight seal to allow the steam to cook the chicken and vegetables while preserving the juices.

5 Place the pouches on the preheated grill, close the grill cover, and cook for 12 to 15 minutes. When done, open each pouch slightly to allow the steam to escape.

PER SERVING: *Calories 248 (From Fat 23); Fat 3g (Saturated 1g); Cholesterol 54mg; Sodium 185mg; Carbohydrate 37g (Dietary Fiber 3g); Protein 19g.*

TIP: Choose small chicken breasts or use chicken tenders for a portion-controlled substitute. One serving is 2 or 3 chicken tenders. Double the foil if you don't have heavy-duty foil to prevent any leakage.

NOTE: You can also bake the foil pouches for 18 to 20 minutes in an oven preheated to 425 degrees. For a more accurate method of ensuring doneness, use an instant-read thermometer to register 165 degrees.

TIP: Foil pouches can be prepped ahead of time and stored in the refrigerator until it's time to grill. They're a hit for dinner, at a campout, or for a quick snack. Eating them out of the foil makes for easy cleanup!

VARY IT! Top the chicken with basil pesto, cherry tomatoes, and fresh mozzarella for an Italian flavor. Or add bell pepper and onion slices, black beans, and salsa for a Mexican flair. Or try snap peas, carrot strips, and succulent shrimp with sesame ginger dressing. Involve the whole family and get creative!

Sheet-Pan Lemon-Herb Barramundi with Asparagus

PREP TIME: 10 MIN	COOK TIME: 15 MIN	YIELD: 4 SERVINGS

INGREDIENTS

2 tablespoons extra-virgin olive oil

1 tablespoon butter

2 lemons, zested

3 tablespoons lemon juice

2 garlic cloves, minced

½ teaspoon cayenne pepper

1 teaspoon dried thyme

Four 4-ounce Barramundi fillets, thawed

1 bunch asparagus, washed and trimmed

Freshly ground pepper to taste

DIRECTIONS

1 Preheat the oven to 425 degrees. Line a sheet pan with parchment paper or a silicon baking mat.

2 In a small saucepan, combine the oil, butter, lemon zest, lemon juice, garlic, cayenne pepper, and thyme; simmer until the flavors blend, about 2 minutes. Let cool slightly.

3 Place the fish and asparagus spears on the lined baking sheet. Season lightly with pepper.

4 Drizzle the lemon butter sauce over the fish and vegetables. Bake for 10 to 15 minutes or until the fish flakes easily with a fork and the flesh is opaque. Serve with lemon slices and drizzle any remaining sauce over the fish, if desired.

PER SERVING: Calories 233 (From Fat 111); Fat 12g (Saturated 3g); Cholesterol 61mg; Sodium 90mg; Carbohydrate 5g (Dietary Fiber 2g); Protein 26g.

NOTE: Barramundi is a highly sustainable farm-raised fish with pinkish-white flesh, a wonderfully mild flavor, buttery texture, and a meaty bite. It is renowned for its versatility and is high in omega-3 fatty acids. Good substitutes for barramundi are red snapper, grouper, or halibut.

TIP: Be careful not to overcook! To make sure the fish is done, use an instant-read thermometer. The internal temperature should be less than 145 degrees. When you remove it from the heat source, the flesh continues to cook. (This is called *carryover heat*.) Remove it before the center is at the desired doneness.

VARY IT! Instead of roasting, you can easily pan sauté the fish over medium-high heat or broil for 5 to 6 minutes and serve with a citrus salsa, using cut-up oranges, cilantro, lime juice, minced garlic, and red onion.

Chapter **23**

Sweet Endings

RECIPES IN THIS CHAPTER

- ↻ **Wine-Poached Pears**
- ↻ **Strawberries with Peppered Balsamic Drizzle**
- ↻ **Vanilla Chia Seed Pudding with Toppings**
- ↻ **Mango Banana Soft Serve**

Many people are accustomed to having a sweet treat sometime during the day, and often it's a dessert at the end of a meal. A meal plan that offers more variety will make it easier to include the key DASH nutrients. The DASH diet allows two to five servings of fats and sweets, depending on a person's calorie requirements. Fruits and vegetables are the foundation of the DASH diet because of the nutritional contributions. Saving your fruit serving (or some form of it) for your treat may provide you the motivation to stick with your plan.

TIP

Eating with the seasons provides the best and most flavorful choices. Find out what's in season where you live, and opt for those fruits and vegetables. You'll get variety throughout the year as what's in season changes.

The recipes in this chapter use a minimum amount of sweeteners and an interesting use of fruit.

Wine-Poached Pears

| PREP TIME: 5 MIN | COOK TIME: 35 MIN | YIELD: 4 SERVINGS |

INGREDIENTS

2 cups dry red wine (such as Cabernet, Pinot Noir, or Merlot)

5 tablespoons sugar

½ cup orange juice

1 to 2 tablespoons orange zest

1 cinnamon stick

2 whole cloves

4 firm, ripe pears, free of blemishes, peeled, stems intact

Vanilla Greek yogurt (optional)

Toasted almond slices (optional)

Fresh mint (optional)

DIRECTIONS

1 In a 4-quart saucepan, combine the wine, sugar, orange juice, orange zest, cinnamon stick, and cloves. Stir until the sugar dissolves.

2 Add the pears and bring the liquid to a boil. Cover and simmer 15 to 20 minutes, turning every 5 minutes until the pears are tender and uniform in color.

3 Transfer the pears to a dish and allow them to cool. Remove the cinnamon and cloves from the liquid and continue to simmer the liquid until it's thickened and reduced by half, about 15 to 20 more minutes.

4 When ready to serve, either warm or at room temperature, drizzle the pears with a few tablespoons of the warm syrup. Garnish with a dollop of Greek yogurt, almond slices, and fresh mint, if desired.

PER SERVING: *Calories 278 (From Fat 2); Fat 0g (Saturated 0g); Cholesterol 0mg; Sodium 7mg; Carbohydrate 50g (Dietary Fiber 6g); Protein 1g.*

TIP: Bosc pears are ideal because they keep their shape when cooked. Use ripe pears — the harder ones won't soften up even with cooking. Pears are ripe when they yield to pressure but are still firm.

VARY IT! Add ½ teaspoon ground cardamom with the wine mixture for an extra warm, elegant finish. Any leftover pears are great chopped in a crisp salad with blue cheese, toasted walnuts, and vinaigrette made with the sauce blended with extra-virgin olive oil.

Strawberries with Peppered Balsamic Drizzle

PREP TIME: 1 HR 5 MIN	COOK TIME:	YIELD: 4 SERVINGS

INGREDIENTS

2 cups fresh strawberries, washed and cut in half

1 tablespoon balsamic vinegar

1 tablespoon brown sugar

Pinch freshly and finely ground black pepper

4 ounces vanilla Greek yogurt

Fresh mint, for garnish

DIRECTIONS

1 In a bowl, combine the strawberries, balsamic vinegar, sugar, and pepper. Gently stir to be sure the berries are coated. Cover and set aside at room temperature for 1 hour; then refrigerate until ready to serve.

2 Divide the strawberries evenly into 4 bowls and top with a dollop of yogurt. Garnish with a sprig of fresh mint, and serve.

PER SERVING: *Calories 65 (From Fat 2); Fat 0g (Saturated 0g); Cholesterol 0mg; Sodium 15mg; Carbohydrate 0g (Dietary Fiber 2g); Protein 3g.*

TIP: The recipe will require less sugar if you use more expensive vinegar. Aged Italian balsamic is a great choice. You can also use store-bought balsamic glaze.

VARY IT! Try flavored balsamic vinegars like lemon or chocolate! You can substitute ice cream in place of the yogurt. If you're in a really decadent mood, serve the strawberries and ice cream over grilled pound cake or angel food cake. You can also use the strawberries as a topping for waffles or a filling for crêpes. Of course, these would be special treats, outside of your normal DASH routine.

SUGAR: ALL GOOD, ALL BAD, OR SOMEWHERE IN BETWEEN?

Many misconceptions surround sugar. Natural sugars, such as fructose (found in fruit) and lactose (found in milk), have redeeming value because they also provide nutrients and antioxidants to keep you healthy. Added sugars, which are used in foods and beverages during processing and production, provide empty calories and have few nutrients. One of the key recommendations of the 2015–2020 Dietary Guidelines for Americans is to reduce the intake of calories from added sugars. A DASH meal is not heavy on fats or refined carbohydrates. Foods such as white pasta, white rice, bagels, sweetened cereals, and pretzels may not be the best choice — they provide calories without significant vitamins, minerals, or protein and are considered to have low nutrient density. But fruits, vegetables, low-fat dairy, nuts, beans, and lean meats are great choices.

Vanilla Chia Seed Pudding with Toppings

PREP TIME: 5 MIN PLUS 4 HR FOR REFRIGERATING	YIELD: 10 SERVINGS

INGREDIENTS

1 cup vanilla Greek yogurt

2 cups reduced-fat 2 percent milk

½ cup chia seeds

1½ tablespoons maple syrup

½ teaspoon vanilla extract

Pinch salt

DIRECTIONS

1 In a large bowl, whisk together the yogurt, milk, chia seeds, maple syrup, vanilla, and salt until blended.

2 Cover and refrigerate 3 to 4 hours or overnight. When ready to serve, whisk again if needed, to smooth out any clumps that may have formed.

3 Spoon into dessert cups and top with your favorite toppings (see the Tip below).

PER SERVING: *Calories 92 (From Fat 32); Fat 4g (Saturated 1g); Cholesterol 4mg; Sodium 49mg; Carbohydrate 10g (Dietary Fiber 3g); Protein 5g.*

TIP: Use whatever toppings you love most. Some ideas include fresh or thawed berries, fresh or thawed peaches mixed with peach preserves and pinch of cardamom, sliced bananas and strawberries with chocolate syrup, low-sugar canned pie filling, a dollop of pumpkin pie filling, or caramel sauce with toasted walnuts.

TIP: Leftover pudding can be stored in an air-tight container in the refrigerator until ready to serve. It will last about 4 to 5 days in the refrigerator.

NOTE: Chia seeds are an easy way to get omega-3 fatty acids, which are important for heart health. A single 1-ounce serving of chia seeds contains 5 grams of omega-3s. When the chia seeds get wet, they turn into a kind of gel — this is soluble fiber, also good for a healthy digestive system.

VARY IT! If you're craving chocolate, add 3 tablespoons of cocoa powder to the original recipe and increase the maple syrup to 3 to 5 tablespoons.

Mango Banana Soft Serve

PREP TIME: 10 MIN PLUS 4 HR | YIELD: 6 SERVINGS

INGREDIENTS

1 large ripe banana

One 16-ounce package frozen mango chunks

1 to 2 tablespoons sugar

1½ tablespoons lime juice

1½ tablespoons canned light coconut milk

Mint leaves, for garnish

DIRECTIONS

1 Peel the banana, cut it in half, place in a resealable freezer bag, and freeze until solid, at least 4 hours.

2 In a large bowl, combine the mango and sugar and let stand for 5 minutes. (If you prefer a little more tang, skip the sugar.)

3 Place the mango, banana, lime juice, and coconut milk in a high-speed blender and pulse for 3 to 4 minutes using the tamper to scrape down the sides until the mixture is thick and smooth.

4 Spoon the soft serve into bowls, and serve immediately for a softer consistency or freeze until ready to serve. Garnish with mint leaves if desired.

PER SERVING: *Calories 85 (From Fat 8); Fat 1g (Saturated 1g); Cholesterol 0mg; Sodium 3mg; Carbohydrate 21g (Dietary Fiber 2g); Protein 1g.*

TIP: Already cut-up frozen fruit is the best trick for making a frozen treat. If you've got fresh fruit, freeze it on a large baking sheet; then make your own resealable bags after it has frozen.

NOTE: If you decide to freeze all or a portion of the recipe, pour it into an airtight container. When ready to serve, defrost at room temperature for about 10 minutes or in the microwave for 20 to 30 seconds to make it easier to scoop. You can store this soft serve in the freezer up to 2 weeks.

VARY IT! Substitute pineapple for the mango or any combination of fruit that you enjoy. Add sweetened or unsweetened shredded coconut for a taste of the tropics. Don't have unsweetened coconut milk? Add the same amount of Greek yogurt or skip it all together.

5
The Part of Tens

Keep your bank account and your blood pressure on the right track with our tips for eating the DASH way on a budget.

Find out several easy and delicious ways of adding flavor to your food without picking up the salt shaker.

Make your DASHing good habits a way of life with our list of positive lifestyle changes that curb hypertension.

Need to convert ounces to grams or cups to milliliters? You can find a helpful metric conversion appendix at the end of this part.

Chapter **24**

Ten Tips for Following DASH on a Budget

Eating healthy doesn't have to be expensive. This chapter shares ten simple tips to get you eating the DASH way without depleting your bank account.

Plan Meals and Snacks for the Week

Decide which recipes to make based on your pantry and freezer staples. Then prepare your grocery list by checking for store specials and coupons and making a list of all the items you intend to purchase.

TIP

Use your grocery store loyalty cards for extra rewards. Also, eat before you shop to keep from buying foods that aren't on your list.

Include Canned and Frozen Fruits and Vegetables

Canned vegetables are often higher in sodium, but they're economical and convenient. Rinsing them can lower total sodium content, or you can choose reduced-sodium varieties. Canned fruit is just as nutritious as fresh. Frozen fruits and vegetables are also convenient and budget-friendly.

WARNING

Avoid frozen packages with sauces, and read labels for added saturated fat and sodium. Avoid fruit that is canned in syrup; opt for fruit canned in its own juice instead.

Purchase in Bulk

Buy in bulk, especially when stores are having promotions. Foods such as meat, pasta, rice, and canned goods are easy to stockpile because they last a long time in the freezer or pantry. If they're on sale, buy as much as you can afford and store them until the next big sale.

TIP

Buy a side of beef or a family pack at the grocery store or meat market. When you get home, split it into two or four servings and freeze in resealable freezer bags. This way you'll have better quality meat that will last you a long time. You can also purchase whole-grain breads that are on sale and freeze some for later use. They'll keep for up to three months in the freezer.

TIP

Consider shopping at discount stores as well. Some stores offer deep discounts, and many have their own store brands. Most of the time you get an equal-quality product for so much less.

Select In-Season Produce and Store It Properly

Not only is in-season produce more readily available, but it also has a better flavor and is more budget-friendly. Buy some fruit that still needs time to ripen if you don't plan to use it right away. Be sure to store fruits and vegetables properly to avoid waste. Items such as grapes, berries, and cherries should be stored in the refrigerator, and washed when ready to eat.

TIP

If you have the space in your freezer, buy extra in-season produce and freeze some so you can have it on hand in the off-season months. Berries, for example, are super easy to freeze. Just rinse, let dry, then place into zippered freezer bags (these come in handy for a frozen sweet treat or for yogurt smoothies).

Buy Store Brands

Buying store brand items can save you quite a bit of cash without sacrificing important nutrients. When you compare different brands of canned vegetables or cottage cheese, for example, odds are the store brand is more economical for the same good quality.

Skip Convenience Foods

Convenience foods (think precut fruits and vegetables, sliced fresh chicken breast, premade kebobs) can really add up at the cash register. Some can also be very high in sodium (think frozen dinners and meals-in-a-box). Preparing items yourself inevitably saves money and is usually healthier. Sometimes the timesavings is worth it, but you're paying more for more prep.

Buy Food from Local Farmers

The best-quality produce comes from your local farmers because the food doesn't have to travel very far to get to your table. Find out about CSAs (Community Supported Agriculture) in your area, buy into a farmer's crop for the season, or hit up a nearby farmers' market.

Grow Your Own Vegetables and Herbs

Whether in a plot in your backyard, a pot on your patio, or in a community garden, you can grow fresh, flavorful, and inexpensive produce for your meals. Fresh herbs, tomatoes, spinach, salad greens, onions, and peppers are the easiest for the novice gardener to grow. You can even grow herbs in a pot on the kitchen counter.

Cook at Home

Eating out can be expensive. Save money by cooking meals at home. Prepare bigger batches of some food items (such as grain dishes or vegetable soups) and freeze some for later use in individual containers. Also, try incorporating leftovers into your meals. Cook a meal (or ingredients such as lentils or roasted vegetables) once and use it in a variety of ways for a few days.

Go Meatless Once a Week

Buying meat, poultry, and fish for every day of the week adds up. Try eating more plant-based protein (beans, peas, and lentils) with vegetables, as well as eggs and peanut butter. These low-cost items have a long shelf life and are available year-round. Because DASH includes small portions of lean meats overall, you can stretch a 4-ounce portion of lean beef, pork, or poultry to create servings for four people.

Chapter **25**

Ten Ways to Add Flavor without Salt

O ne of the fundamental goals of the DASH lifestyle is to reduce your dietary sodium. Any kind of salt (such as table salt, sea salt, kosher salt and *fleur de sel*) contributes flavor to foods and balances the effects of sour, bitter, and sweet, but it also contributes a lot of sodium. (Salt is made up of 60 percent sodium and 40 percent chloride.) The good news is you have numerous options for adding flavor to your foods *without* salt or with less of it. All you have to do is embrace *flavor-building* — the process of using multiple, complementary ingredients and techniques to create new flavors in a dish. Flavor-building just takes a bit of practice and is well worth the learning curve. It makes your food so pleasurable and so tantalizing that you don't feel the need to add salt to make your food palatable. Plus, learning to recognize and manipulate all the different components of flavor ultimately makes you a better cook. This chapter presents our top ten ways to build flavor without salt. Enjoy!

Sauté, Grill, Roast, and Oven-Crisp

Sautéing, grilling, and roasting are cooking methods that bring out the natural caramelizing properties in foods and really seal in the natural flavors and juices of meats and vegetables. Learning to do a quick sauté is a versatile skill to master in the kitchen. Sautéing simply involves using a sauté pan to cook foods at high temperatures for short periods, giving you a moist, tender-crisp result. When you sauté chicken, for instance, you brown the chicken on both sides in a small amount of vegetable oil, add some flavoring (perhaps garlic or shallots), and then add some liquid (wine or low-sodium chicken broth) to finish cooking. For an example of melt-in-your-mouth sautéed seafood, try the Seared Scallops with Pistachio Sauce in Chapter 19.

TIP

Grilling doesn't have to dry out your meats and veggies. Seasoning foods properly and then refrigerating them for one or more hours before grilling can create moisture and allow the foods to absorb more flavor. Grilling sears in flavor, creating a "crust" on the outside that keeps juices in. Grilling is generally a quick-cook method, so keeping an eye on the food, or using a meat thermometer, to avoid overcooking is key. For an example grilled meat, try the juicy and delicious Grilled Pork Tenderloin Medallions in Chapter 19.

Roasting is done in an open pan in the oven. It involves beginning at a higher temperature to promote exterior browning (caramelizing) and then reducing the temperature for the remainder of the cooking time. Long and slow roasting times for meats or vegetables promote tenderness and allow more flavors to develop. To keep meats moist when you roast them, add cooking liquid (such as water, low-sodium broth, stock, or tomato sauce), which allows the meat to create its own juice throughout the cooking process.

Oven crisping provides a similar texture as deep frying, without the excess fat. The Curry-Crusted Roasted Salmon in Chapter 19 is an example of the crisp texture you can get by using the oven-crisping method instead of deep-fat frying.

Add Herbs and Spices

Herbs and spices can add great flavor to your dishes. They're the backbone of many recipes, lending a cultural and regional flair to food, as well as antioxidants and visual appeal. Herbs are the leafy parts of plants; they provide a crisp, clean taste. Spices are the bark, roots, seeds, and flowers of tropical plants; they work well in longer cooking to provide rich flavor.

The trick to incorporating herbs and spices in your cooking is to use the ones you really love. For instance, if you're not fond of oregano, which may be an ingredient in a tomato sauce recipe, substitute another herb that you do enjoy, such as basil, parsley, or rosemary. You can purchase salt-free herb blends at the store or mix up your own blends with various jarred herbs you have in the pantry. Try mixing 3 tablespoons dried parsley, 1 tablespoon powdered sage, 2 tablespoons dried rosemary, and 1 tablespoon garlic powder in a small bowl. Use immediately or store in an airtight jar for a week.

TIP

To bring out the aroma of dried herbs, such as rosemary, thyme, and oregano, crush them between your fingers before adding them to a dish. If you're substituting dried herbs for fresh, remember that 1 teaspoon of dried herbs equals 1 tablespoon of fresh herbs. For an example of how adding fragrant herbs can channel a trip to the south of France, try the Herbes de Provence Lamb Chops in Chapter 19.

Squeeze in Some Citrus

A bit of lemon, lime, or orange zest can make the flavors of a dish come alive. Citrus juices can also add intense flavor when reduced or combined with other spices. Some delicious examples are fresh corn on the cob with lime chili butter rather than salt, and an orange juice reduction added to salad dressings and sauces. Grilling a lemon half adds a wonderfully sweet, tart sensation to grilled fish. For an example of a how a burst of citrus can liven up the flavor of a dish, try the Shrimp Avocado Ceviche in Chapter 18.

Toss in Onions, Peppers, Garlic, and More

Aromatic vegetables such as onions, garlic, scallions, shallots, leeks, and chives add a distinctive flavor and aroma whether sautéed, roasted, or raw. Use them to build flavors, adding the pungency of raw onion, the earthiness of roasted garlic, or natural sweetness with the browning and caramelization of sautéed onions and garlic.

TIP

A small amount of garlic (one clove) can enhance the flavor of a variety of foods, from meats like pork and beef to vegetables to salad dressing. Garlic also has heart-healthy benefits, providing those important phytochemicals and antioxidants. Start by adding a clove of crushed garlic to your favorite dish or infuse it into olive oil for cooking.

Or try using pepper. Sweet peppers (such as poblanos or mini sweet peppers) or hot peppers (such as jalapeño, chipotle, or Serrano peppers) can kick food up a notch. Whether sliced raw into salads or roasted and mixed into vegetable dishes or casseroles, they add more flavor to food along with potential antioxidant properties. For an example of how to boost flavor and kick up the heat using chilies, try the Southwest Corn with Chipotle Peppers in Chapter 20.

Use Fresh Ginger and Horseradish

Fresh ginger adds a flavor punch that can't be matched. Fresh ginger root is available in the produce section of your grocery store and is easy to use. Store it in a brown paper bag and it will keep in the vegetable bin of your refrigerator for about 4 to 6 weeks. You can store it longer in the freezer — simply pop it into a plastic zippered bag and freeze, and then take it out to grate and return it to the freezer. You can also use ginger to give oil a mild ginger flavor: Cut a small, coin-like piece of ginger (you don't have to peel it) and place it in hot oil. Cook it for a few minutes, taking care not to burn it, and then remove and discard the ginger. It gives a delicious Asian flair to sauces, stir fries, and noodle dishes.

Horseradish is an underused flavor agent. You can purchase it fresh or jarred. A little bit goes a long way, adding heat and punch to a sauce or stew. It also makes a great condiment — add it to mayonnaise or plain yogurt to make a sandwich spread. For an example of the flavor punch you get from horseradish, try the Open-Faced Roast Beef Sandwich with Horseradish Sauce in Chapter 18.

Cook with Oils and Flavored Oils

Add extra-virgin olive oil, avocado, or walnut oil to a garden-fresh salad mix or top off a stir-fry with a dash of sesame oil. You can infuse neutral oils (such as canola, safflower, and grape seed oils) with spices, citrus zest, hot peppers, and herbs to give them unique flavors as well. Use them alone to drizzle over food or to enhance flavor in the cooking process. These additions not only boost flavor but also give you another way to add heart-healthy fats to your diet. Try a drizzle of orange-zest-infused olive oil on salmon before grilling.

Pour in Vinegars, Wine, and Liqueur

Flavored vinegars can really wake up your taste buds without added salt. You can choose a wine vinegar (made from red wine, white wine, rosé wine, champagne, rice wine, or sherry), cider vinegar (made from apples), or balsamic vinegar (made from Trebbiano grapes and aged in barrels). You can flavor infused vinegars with roasted garlic, chili peppers, herbs, vegetables, or fruit. You can use wine and spirits as flavor builders, too. Use them in a sauce or as a flavoring. Delicious additions include sherry in a cream sauce, a splash of amaretto with cooked carrots, or brandy poured and flamed over a dessert. For an example of how vinegar can elevate a sweet treat from good to fantastic, try the Strawberries with Peppered Balsamic Drizzle in Chapter 23.

Puree and Chop Vegetables

Using vegetables to make a puree, coulis, or salsa is a great way to infuse flavor into a dish. These wonderful alternatives replace high-fat and high-salt sauces, and they add not only flavor but color and nutrition too! For a delicious vegetable coulis, blend a roasted red bell pepper with a small amount of homemade stock. Pureed vegetables can also thicken soups, stews, and sauces without the addition of fat. Salsas and relishes are generally chunky mixtures made from a variety of vegetables or fruits, with the addition of one or two intense flavors, such as chile peppers and cilantro. For an example of how to use a vegetable puree as a flavor enhancer and thickener, try the Velvety Vegetable Soup with Tarragon Cream in Chapter 18.

Make Rubs and Marinades

You can use a rub or marinade as a seasoning or a tenderizer. Dry or wet rubs can provide flavor profiles that vary from sweet and hot, like Jamaican jerk seasoning, to a full-bodied raw garlic rub. A *dry rub* is a combination of spices and herbs that are blended together and rubbed into meat. A *wet rub* is a combination of spices and herbs blended with liquid ingredients — usually oil — and rubbed over the meat's surface. You can adjust a homemade rub to have as much heat as you desire by adding more or less cayenne, freshly ground pepper, jalapeños, and other fragrant spices. *Marinades* are liquids that contain an acidic ingredient to tenderize tough meat or add flavor. Wine, citrus juice, and yogurt can serve as the base of a marinade, dressed up with herbs, spices, and even fruit. Be sure to read labels on any premade rubs and marinades you purchase and look for low-sodium, sodium-free, or salt free versions — they add flavor to food without sodium. For an example of how a dry rub with vinegar can take ho-hum chicken and transform it into a Caribbean favorite, try the Jamaican Jerk Chicken with Cha-Cha Salsa in Chapter 19.

Sprinkle on a Wee Bit of Cheese

Small amounts of sharp, pungent white cheeses, such as Romano, Parmesan, or Asiago, can really boost the flavor of a dish. Just 1 or 2 tablespoons of freshly grated cheese adds tons of flavor. Better yet, this flavor boost may help promote consumption of more veggies. For instance, a teaspoon of Parmesan may add an enticing punch to spinach, and a tablespoon of shredded mozzarella added to sautéed zucchini may tempt the most hesitant of vegetable eaters. For an example of how a little bit of cheese can go a long way toward improving the flavor of a dish, try the Braised Mediterranean Lentils with Quinoa in Chapter 21.

Chapter **26**

Ten Lifestyle Changes to Curb Hypertension

Hypertension can be serious when not treated properly, but for most people it's a very manageable condition. The best way to manage hypertension is by setting long-term goals rather than focusing on nonexistent quick fixes. In this chapter, we share the ten best lifestyle changes you can make to create optimal health and lower your blood pressure. Controlling hypertension doesn't happen overnight, but you can turn the corner by following our tips.

REMEMBER

Before you implement any major changes to your diet or exercise regimen, talk to your doctor first to make sure what you're planning is medically safe. Then check in with your doctor regularly to keep her abreast of your progress and challenges to ensure the best management of your hypertension.

Lose Weight and Keep It Off

Weight loss is often the number-one treatment for hypertension, and even a small drop in pounds helps. Being overweight strains your body and your heart, and losing weight will usually help to improve your blood pressure.

After you've lost the weight, the key is to keep it off. A healthy diet is not a one-and-done situation. To maintain that weight loss you worked so hard to achieve, you must maintain the lifestyle changes that got you there: eating the right amounts of the right foods (lean meats, vegetables, fruits, dairy, grains, less salt, and smaller portions of treats) and exercising 20 to 30 minutes per day. You'll be rewarded with the energy and vitality you crave.

TIP

Sticking to lifestyle changes often means continuously setting new goals to avoid a setback. A great tool to help you set diet and exercise goals — and stick to them — is *Calorie Counter Journal For Dummies*, by coauthor Rosanne and Meri Raffetto (Wiley).

Develop an Exercise Routine

Along with eating right, regular exercise keeps your weight under control, improves your cardiovascular health, and reduces your stress level, all of which help you curb hypertension in the long run. *Regular* is the magic word here. Scheduling a 20- to 30-minute walk five days a week is a great way to begin moving regularly. Do whatever you can at first, and then add minutes each week. After you're up to 30 to 45 minutes of walking, gradually increase your pace until you can walk a mile in 15 to 20 minutes.

TIP

Weight-bearing exercise is important too, especially as you age because muscle and bone loss occur at a more rapid rate. Adding workouts with weights or resistance bands two or three times a week to your aerobic activity is a great plan. Some forms of yoga can help, too.

Stick to DASH

Although one of the goals of DASH eating is to reduce sodium, saturated fat, and cholesterol in the diet, the DASH diet is more about what to *add* to your diet than what you should *limit*. Fruits and vegetables, for instance, are very important sources of potassium and magnesium (which help lower blood pressure), antioxidants (such as vitamins C and A), and fiber (which helps keep cholesterol in check). DASH also encourages you to include more monounsaturated fats and low-fat dairy products. Following the DASH dietary guidelines has been proven to lower hypertension. Enjoy the recipes in Part 4, which all incorporate aspects of the DASH plan, and check out Part 3 for even more information on what to eat and how to navigate restaurants and get-togethers so you can stay true to your DASH eating plan for the long haul.

Eat Less Salt

A high-salt diet has been shown to raise blood pressure in some people, so reducing your intake of high-sodium foods and the amount of salt you use in cooking is a good idea (daily goal: 1,500 to 2,300 milligrams). Because more than three-fourths of the salt in most peoples' diet comes from prepared foods, the first step is to read food labels and reduce your consumption of highly processed packaged foods. Eating out less often (and eating smaller portions) will also help, because restaurant foods tend to be highly salted. By cutting back in stages, you'll find that your cravings will gradually subside.

REMEMBER

Ingredient lists and product labels usually refer to salt in terms of sodium, a building block of salt, but may also include other forms of sodium such as monosodium glutamate (MSG), which is typically found in Asian foods and some processed products. Also, be aware that salt commonly hides in restaurant foods.

Add Good Fats to Your Diet

Hypertension is a risk factor for heart disease; so is high blood cholesterol. Consuming heart-healthy fats may help improve the balance of good and bad cholesterol in your blood stream. On the other hand, saturated fats from red meat and tropical oils may make it worse. Vegetable oils such as olive, canola, avocado, and peanut oils are your best bet because they're high in heart-smart monounsaturated fat. Other vegetable oils are higher in polyunsaturated fat, which isn't harmful but seems to have a neutral effect (see Chapter 5 for more details). Adding nuts, seeds, avocados, olives, and monounsaturated oils to your diet is a good idea, but keep in mind that good fats have just as many calories as the bad stuff. Try walnuts or plain roasted sunflower seeds in salads or mixed into vegetable dishes or in stir-fries. Nuts can also be a nutritious snack as long as you don't overindulge (about 15 to 20 nuts is sufficient).

Avoid Drinking Alcohol Excessively

Although one glass of red wine or other alcoholic beverage a day may be beneficial to your blood circulation and heart health, overindulging is not. If you're male, drinking more than two drinks a day can lead to heart damage, high blood pressure, and high triglycerides. For women, the threshold is over one drink daily; this level can also increase the risk for breast cancer. The U.S. Centers for Disease Control and Prevention defines *heavy drinking* as consuming 15 or more drinks per week for men and 8 or more drinks per week for women. One drink is equivalent to a 5-ounce glass of wine, a 12-ounce beer, or 1½ ounces of 80-proof liquor. So keep your alcohol intake moderate for heart health — and if you don't drink alcohol, there's no need to start. Make other heart-healthy lifestyle choices instead, such as adding more grapes and colorful fruits and vegetables to your diet and exercising regularly.

Don't Use Tobacco Products

Smoking causes coronary heart disease, contributes to stroke, and increases the risk of *peripheral vascular disease* (obstruction of the large arteries in the arms and legs, resulting in pain and possible tissue death which may lead to amputation). Chewing tobacco isn't much better because it raises blood pressure, harms the arteries, and increases the risk of a wide variety of cancers. Tobacco is also a factor in dementia. Basically, there's nothing good about it. If you use tobacco products, talk to your doctor. Although quitting isn't easy, there are products and programs that can help.

Stress Less

Stress has both direct and indirect effects on blood pressure. Work, family, health, and your personal life may affect your overall stress level, causing poor-quality sleep and unhealthy food choices, both of which can contribute to hypertension. Finding ways to manage stress helps you cope more effectively with day-to-day life and simply makes you feel better. You can reduce stress in a number of ways. One of the best strategies is to engage in regular exercise. For starters, put on your sneakers and take a walk. Yoga is another excellent stress reducer, and many people find that a meditation practice helps to calm the mind and body.

TIP

Even simple breathing exercises can help reduce stress. Try taking long, slow breaths: Inhale to a count of four; then exhale to a count of eight.

Enlist Your Family and Friends

Having the support of family and friends can keep you on track with your lifestyle changes, turning eating well and exercising regularly into a shared and social experience. Let your family know that by choosing a healthy way of life, you have made a commitment to your well-being both now and into the future. Emphasize that you need their help and positive support. If they decide to get onboard, that's fantastic; if not, don't let that discourage you. It may help to ask a friend to meet you for a walk or at the gym so you can maintain a regular exercise program, but don't make your plans subject to anyone else's obligations. Do it for yourself, and you'll find that it gets easier over time.

WARNING

If your workout buddy can't make it one day, don't use his absence as an excuse to slack off. You owe it to yourself to stick with your program, no matter who else comes along for the ride. After you get going, you'll feel great!

Follow Your Doctor's Orders

If you've been diagnosed with hypertension, be sure to follow your doctor's advice and keep regular appointments, including an annual physical exam. Take any prescribed medications as directed and keep track of your own blood pressure. If you have any concerns about the medication or treatment your doctor recommends, ask questions. Blood pressure medication is not a one-size-fits-all proposition. Thanks to the variety of medications available, your doctor can almost always find an option, or a combination, that works for you.

Metric Conversion Guide

Note: The recipes in this book weren't developed or tested using metric measurements. There may be some variation in quality when converting to metric units.

Common Abbreviations

Abbreviation(s)	What It Stands For
cm	Centimeter
C., c.	Cup
G, g	Gram
kg	Kilogram
L, l	Liter
lb.	Pound
mL, ml	Milliliter
oz.	Ounce
pt.	Pint
t., tsp.	Teaspoon
T., Tb., Tbsp.	Tablespoon

Volume

U.S. Units	Canadian Metric	Australian Metric
¼ teaspoon	1 milliliter	1 milliliter
½ teaspoon	2 milliliters	2 milliliters
1 teaspoon	5 milliliters	5 milliliters
1 tablespoon	15 milliliters	20 milliliters
¼ cup	50 milliliters	60 milliliters
⅓ cup	75 milliliters	80 milliliters
½ cup	125 milliliters	125 milliliters
⅔ cup	150 milliliters	170 milliliters
¾ cup	175 milliliters	190 milliliters
1 cup	250 milliliters	250 milliliters
1 quart	1 liter	1 liter
1½ quarts	1.5 liters	1.5 liters
2 quarts	2 liters	2 liters
2½ quarts	2.5 liters	2.5 liters
3 quarts	3 liters	3 liters
4 quarts (1 gallon)	4 liters	4 liters

Weight

U.S. Units	Canadian Metric	Australian Metric
1 ounce	30 grams	30 grams
2 ounces	55 grams	60 grams
3 ounces	85 grams	90 grams
4 ounces (¼ pound)	115 grams	125 grams
8 ounces (½ pound)	225 grams	225 grams
16 ounces (1 pound)	455 grams	500 grams (½ kilogram)

Length

Inches	Centimeters
0.5	1.5
1	2.5
2	5.0
3	7.5
4	10.0
5	12.5
6	15.0
7	17.5
8	20.5
9	23.0
10	25.5
11	28.0
12	30.5

Temperature (Degrees)

Fahrenheit	Celsius
32	0
212	100
250	120
275	140
300	150
325	160
350	180
375	190
400	200
425	220
450	230
475	240
500	260

Index

Numbers

A

B

E

Easy Eggplant Parm recipe, 304

eating slower, 237–238

echocardiogram, 82

eggs
  Confetti Hash with Poached Eggs recipe, 258
  Open-Faced Egg Sandwich recipe, 254
  stocking refrigerator with, 190

EKG (Electrocardiogram), 99

Electrocardiogram (EKG), 99

electrolytes, 135

elevated blood pressure, 80

endocrine organs, 135

endometrial cancer, 141

enriched, defined, 71

ephedra, causing hypertension, 84

essential hypertension, 90

ethnic restaurants, finding healthy food options at, 232–233

ethnicity, contributing to diabetes, 125

exercise
  aerobic, 14
  asanas, 241
  to clear out brain fog, 132
  enlisting exercise partners, 245
  hypertension and, 86, 334
  ideas for regular exercise, 241–243
  importance of, 14
  lowering stress with, 89
  Pilates, 14
  to promote sleep, 237
  recording routine, 53
  types of, 86
  for weight loss, 118

expiration dates, on food, 176

extra salt, 19

F

face, arms, speech, time (FAST) test, 105–106

Facts Up Front, 171

family
  putting on DASH diet, 10
  support from, 244–245, 337

family history
  contributing to diabetes, 125
  contributing to primary hypertension, 89

FAST (face, arms, speech, time) test, 105–106

fast food places, finding healthy options at, 231–232

fats, limiting, 12, 13

fiber
  importance of, 174, 176
  reducing cholesterol levels with, 34

fibromuscular dysplasia, 83

fish
  freezing, 222
  lean
    benefits of, 12
    choosing, 73
    grocery shopping for, 180–181
    servings of, 13
  Lemon Pepper Tuna and White Bean Salad recipe, 265
  Sesame-Infused Steamed Haddock recipe, 284

fitness trackers, 50

flavanols, 69

flavanones, 69

flavor-building
  with cheese, 331
  with citrus fruits, 329
  dry rub, 331
  with homemade sauces, 198–199
  horseradish, 330
  marinades, 331
  oils, 330
  plank-cooking, 202
  roasting, 327
  salt substitutes, 63
  spices, 197–199, 328–329
  with vegetables, 329, 331
  vinegars, 330
  without salt, 327–331

foil pouches, cooking with, 308–309

food bags, reusable, 195

food groups, combining, 252

food intake, recording, 53

food labels, 178

N

NASH (nonalcoholic steatohepatitis), 109

National Health and Nutrition Examination Survey (NHANES), 89

National Heart, Lung, and Blood Institute (NHLBI), recommended total fat from, 172

National Heart, Lung, and Blood Institute's Family Heart Study, 33

natural labeled foods, 178, 185

natural sugars, 319

nephrons, 135

NHANES (National Health and Nutrition Examination Survey), 89

NHLBI (National Heart, Lung, and Blood Institute), 172

no salt added claim, food packaging, 174

nonalcoholic steatohepatitis (NASH), 109

nonfat (skim) milk, calcium in, 65

nonfat (skim) yogurt, calcium in, 65

non-high-density lipoprotein (non-HDL) cholesterol, 34–36, 35, 97–98

non-meat protein, 180

nonsteroidal anti-inflammatories (NSAIDs), 83

normal blood pressure, 80

NSAIDs (nonsteroidal anti-inflammatories), 83

nut milk, 182

nutrient goals, 49

nutrient-dense, defined, 211

nutrition

  misleading nutrition claims, 175–176

  nutrition counseling, 19

  over medicine, 28–30

Nutrition Facts label

  calories and calories from fat, 171–172

  cholesterol, 173

  overview, 170–171

  protein, 175

  sodium, 173–174

  total carbohydrate, 174–175

  total fat, 172–173

nuts

  adding to current diet, 46–48

  Banana Nut Hot Oatmeal recipe, 256

  benefits of, 12, 13

  eating for cancer prevention, 142

  Fruit and Nut Chicken Salad Lettuce Wraps recipe, 266

  Seared Scallops with Pistachio Sauce recipe, 275

  serving sizes of, 74

  stocking pantry with, 188

O

obesity

  contributing to diabetes, 125

  health problems, 115–116

  hypertension and, 37, 85

  levels of, 107

  in relation to cancer, 41

  sleep apnea and, 109

obstacles, planning for, 54–55, 153

oil mister, to portion oil, 196

oils

  flavor-building with, 330

  limiting, 12, 13, 142

  olive oil, 189

omega-3 fatty acids, 36, 74, 176

omega-6 fatty acids, 72

Omni-Heart (Optimal Macronutrient Intake Trial to Prevent Heart Disease)

  diet testing, 27–28

  in relation to diabetes, 40

  studies on limiting oils, 12

1% milk, calcium in, 65

one-dish meals

  guidelines for, 307–308

  recipes for

    Bold and Beefy Instant Pot Stew, 310

    Caribbean Chicken Foil Pouches, 312

    Hearty Southwest Slow-Cooker Soup, 311

    overview, 307

    Sheet-Pan Lemon-Herb Barramundi with Asparagus, 313

  using foil pouches with, 308–309

100% stamp, Whole Grains Council, 174

one-pot meals, 225

About the Authors

Sarah Samaan, MD, FACC, FACP, FASE: A Vanderbilt-trained physician, Dr. Samaan has been practicing cardiology in the Dallas–Fort Worth metroplex since 1995. She is a physician partner at the Baylor Heart Hospital in Plano, Texas, where she has served as the co-director of the Women's Cardiovascular Institute and practices at Legacy Heart Center. Dr. Samaan is board certified in cardiology, echocardiography, and nuclear cardiology.

Dr. Samaan has been named as a "Texas Super Doctor" by *Texas Monthly* magazine since 2006.

Dr. Samaan's other books, including *Best Practices for a Healthy Heart: How to Stop Heart Disease Before or After It Starts* (The Experiment Publishing), focus on heart disease prevention for both men and women, with an emphasis on a heart-smart lifestyle. *The Smart Woman's Guide to Heart Health* (Brown Books) was awarded *ForeWord Magazine*'s Bronze award for Women's Issues.

A frequent speaker to patient and professional groups on lipid disorders and other cardiac-related topics such as nutrition, hypertension, and women and heart disease, Dr. Samaan has also served as a spokesperson for the American Heart Association. She is a member of the American Society of Nuclear Cardiology, American Society of Echocardiography, American College of Cardiology, and American College of Physicians.

Dr. Samaan received her Bachelor of Science degree from Texas A&M University and her Doctor of Medicine degree from Vanderbilt University in Nashville, Tennessee. She served her residency in internal medicine at the University of California in Irvine and completed her fellowship in cardiology at the University of New Mexico in Albuquerque.

Dr. Samaan practices yoga, runs, hikes, and rides horses. She enjoys training and competing in the equestrian sport of dressage.

Opinions presented are those of Dr. Samaan and not of HealthTexas Provider Network, Baylor Health Care System, or its controlled affiliates.

Rosanne Rust, MS, RDN, LDN: Rosanne Rust is a registered, licensed dietitian with more than 34 years of experience in the field of food and nutrition. Her work experience has included both inpatient and outpatient nutrition counseling across the life span, with emphasis in cardiovascular nutrition, weight control, and wellness. She currently works as a freelance writer, blogger, and nutrition communications advisor to the food industry and other health professionals. Her brand, Chew the Facts, aims to help consumers enjoy eating for better health.

Rosanne received her Bachelor of Science degree in Clinical Dietetics from Indiana University of Pennsylvania and her Master of Science degree in Nutrition from the University of Pittsburgh. She did her internship at Mercy Hospital of Pittsburgh. She is a member of the Academy of Nutrition and Dietetics and several professional practice groups, including Sports, Cardiovascular, and Wellness Nutrition; Nutrition Entrepreneurs; and Food and Culinary Nutrition.

Her previous titles in the *For Dummies* series include *Hypertension Cookbook For Dummies*, *Restaurant Calorie Counter For Dummies*, *Calorie Counter Journal For Dummies*, and *Glycemic Index Cookbook For Dummies* (all published by Wiley).

A wife and mother of three boys, Rosanne practices what she preaches, follows DASH guidelines, and enjoys regular exercise and the outdoors. She loves both the seaside and the mountains and, of course, good food and festive entertaining with family and friends.

Cindy Kleckner, RDN, LD, FAND: An award-winning nutrition and culinary expert, speaker, and author in the Dallas–Fort Worth area, Cindy helps clients improve diet and enjoy optimal health by combining the science of nutrition with the culinary arts. She is an adjunct professor who teaches nutrition at the Collin College Institute of Hospitality and Culinary Education.

A specialist in cardiovascular health, corporate wellness, weight management, sports, and culinary nutrition, Cindy received a Bachelor of Science degree from Indiana University of Pennsylvania and completed her dietetic internship at Texas Health Resources (formerly Presbyterian Hospital of Dallas).

She is a former president of the Dallas Academy of Nutrition and Dietetics and media spokesperson of the Texas Academy of Nutrition and Dietetics. Cindy is active in many professional specialty groups, including Food and Culinary Professionals; Nutrition Entrepreneurs; and Sports, Cardiovascular, and Wellness Nutrition. Cindy was recognized by the Academy of Nutrition and Dietetics as a Fellow for her professional accomplishments and commitment to the field of dietetics. She was recently inducted into the prestigious Les Dames d'Escoffier Dallas Chapter.

Additional accomplishments include coauthoring *What's Cooking at the Cooper Clinic* (It's Cooking, Inc.) and contributing nutrition chapters for Dr. Kenneth H. Cooper's books *Overcoming Hypertension*, *Preventing Osteoporosis*, and *The New Aerobics for Women* (all published by Bantam). She also coauthored *Hypertension Cookbook For Dummies* and developed recipes for *Gluten-Free Cooking For Dummies*, 2nd Edition (Wiley).

Cindy works individually with clients as a nutrition coach and in groups through her high-energy presentations, culinary demonstrations, and Kitchen Boot Camp program to educate, inspire, and entertain. Her passion is to translate the science of nutrition into practical solutions for busy people to help motivate positive behavioral change.

Cindy enjoys training and competing in tennis with the Tennis Competitors of Dallas and the U.S. Tennis Association. Her passions combine her love of family, travel, and cooking whole food from cultures around the world. Follow Cindy on her LinkedIn page at www.linkedin.com/in/cindy-kleckner-rdn-ld-fand-45a154a.

Dedication

We would like to dedicate this book to all our current and former patients, as well as all consumers seeking a healthier lifestyle and all those families who have lost someone to heart disease. May this book help you reduce your risk and create your happiest and healthiest life.

Authors' Acknowledgments

We would like to acknowledge our whole team that made this book possible.

Rosanne and Cindy would like to thank their agent, Matt Wagner at Fresh Books, Inc., and Wiley Senior Acquisitions Editor Tracy Boggier, for bringing this project to us. Matt's support, guidance, and attention to detail are very much appreciated. Sarah would also like to thank her agent, Linda Konner, for her wisdom and steadfast support.

Of course, our team of editors helped us create an excellent book. We'd like to thank our awesome project editor, Elizabeth Kuball; and technical editor recipe tester, and nutrition analyst, Rachel Nix.

Sarah would like to thank Gary Cooper for encouraging her to dream a little bigger, and for his love and tolerance. She is grateful beyond words to her mother, Dr. Jean Moffatt Samaan, who forged her own extraordinary life despite the constraints of her time. And she is indebted to her patients, who inspire and challenge her every day.

Rosanne would like to thank her husband David, for his love and unending support. She also is so grateful to her sons, Matthew, Max, and Marcus, for tolerating her distractions in her home office and her writing through the years. She's proud that they have become such independent, responsible young adults. Each of them will always hold a very special place in her heart.

Cindy would like to thank her family, the people who make life worth living. Her deepest love and appreciation go to her husband of 40 years for his support and encouragement and for always making her laugh. She's so grateful for her sweet granddaughter Maya, and her wonderful sons (and awesome taste testers), Brian and Neil, who outgrew her lap but never her love and cooking.

Publisher's Acknowledgments

Senior Acquisitions Editor: Tracy Boggier

Project Editor: Elizabeth Kuball

Copy Editor: Elizabeth Kuball

Technical Editor: Rachel Nix

Nutrition Analyst: Rachel Nix

Recipe Tester: Rachel Nix

Proofreader: Debbye Butler

Production Editor: Mohammed Zafar Ali

Cover Photos: © Cristina Pedrazzini/ Science Photo Library/Getty Images

Take dummies with you everywhere you go!

Whether you are excited about e-books, want more from the web, must have your mobile apps, or are swept up in social media, dummies makes everything easier.

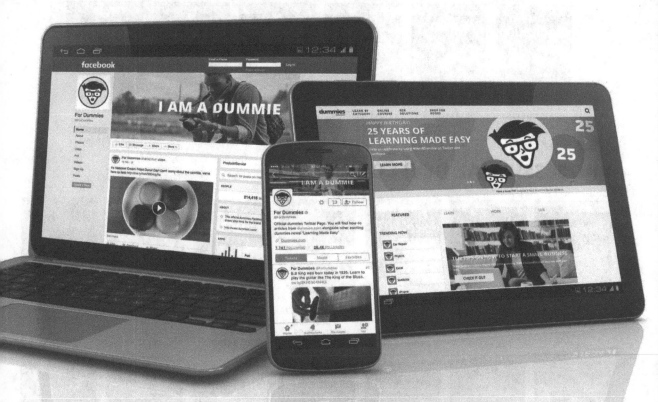

Find us online!

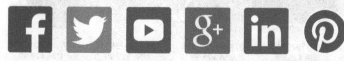

dummies.com

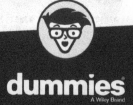

dummies
A Wiley Brand

PERSONAL ENRICHMENT

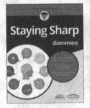 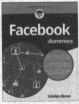 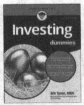 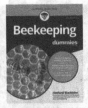 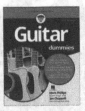 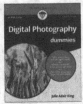

Staying Sharp
9781119187790
USA $26.00
CAN $31.99
UK £19.99

Facebook
9781119179030
USA $21.99
CAN $25.99
UK £16.99

Guitar
9781119293354
USA $24.99
CAN $29.99
UK £17.99

Investing
9781119293347
USA $22.99
CAN $27.99
UK £16.99

Beekeeping
9781119310068
USA $22.99
CAN $27.99
UK £16.99

Digital Photography
9781119235606
USA $24.99
CAN $29.99
UK £17.99

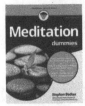 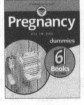 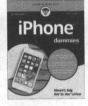 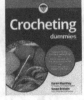 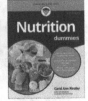

Meditation
9781119251163
USA $24.99
CAN $29.99
UK £17.99

Pregnancy
9781119235491
USA $26.99
CAN $31.99
UK £19.99

Samsung Galaxy S7
9781119279952
USA $24.99
CAN $29.99
UK £17.99

iPhone
9781119283133
USA $24.99
CAN $29.99
UK £17.99

Crocheting
9781119287117
USA $24.99
CAN $29.99
UK £16.99

Nutrition
9781119130246
USA $22.99
CAN $27.99
UK £16.99

PROFESSIONAL DEVELOPMENT

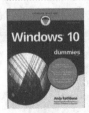 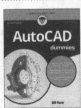 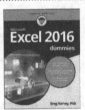 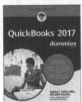 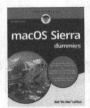 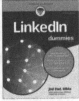

Windows 10
9781119311041
USA $24.99
CAN $29.99
UK £17.99

AutoCAD
9781119255796
USA $39.99
CAN $47.99
UK £27.99

Excel 2016
9781119293439
USA $26.99
CAN $31.99
UK £19.99

QuickBooks 2017
9781119281467
USA $26.99
CAN $31.99
UK £19.99

macOS Sierra
9781119280651
USA $29.99
CAN $35.99
UK £21.99

LinkedIn
9781119251132
USA $24.99
CAN $29.99
UK £17.99

Windows 10
9781119310563
USA $34.00
CAN $41.99
UK £24.99

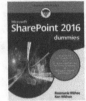 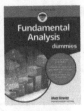 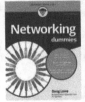   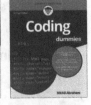

SharePoint 2016
9781119181705
USA $29.99
CAN $35.99
UK £21.99

Fundamental Analysis
9781119263593
USA $26.99
CAN $31.99
UK £19.99

Networking
9781119257769
USA $29.99
CAN $35.99
UK £21.99

Office 2016
9781119293477
USA $26.99
CAN $31.99
UK £19.99

Office 365
9781119265313
USA $24.99
CAN $29.99
UK £17.99

Salesforce.com
9781119239314
USA $29.99
CAN $35.99
UK £21.99

Coding
9781119293323
USA $29.99
CAN $35.99
UK £21.99

dummies.com

dummies
A Wiley Brand